PLANTS FIRST

A PHYSICIAN'S GUIDE TO WELLNESS THROUGH A PLANT-FORWARD DIET

DR. KATIE TAKAYASU

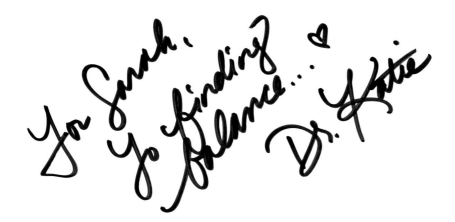

VICTORY BELT PUBLISHING

LAS VEGAS

Cover and recipe photos by Julia D'Agostino

Photo shoot kitchen team: Sydney Sheehan, Maggie Wehri, Lisa Clarke, Cathrin Bowtell, Ashling Keenan, and Jun Takayasu

Cover design by Kat Lannom

Interior design by Charisse Reyes

Illustrations by Eli San Juan and Allan Santos

Printed in Canada

TC 0121

CONTENTS

PREFACE:
HOW TO BE WELL

Wellness is more than a state of being.
It's a state of action.

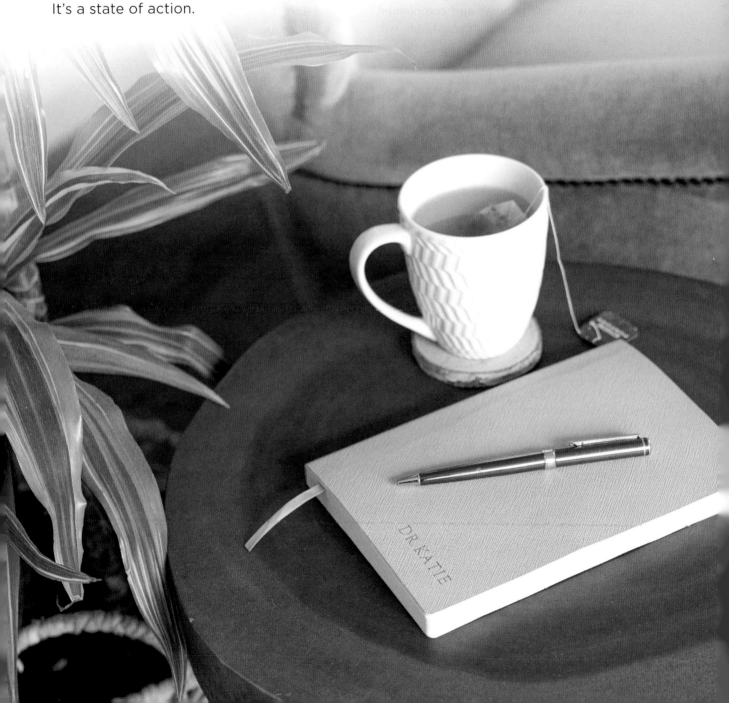

I wrote this book for anyone who wants to do a better job of taking care of themselves.

Whether you come to the table well versed in plant-rich nutrition or you are just starting your journey away from packaged foods and sugar, this book will arm you with the knowledge you need to make better decisions. And it's making better choices on a daily basis that will lead you to a state of wellness.

I have more than ten years of experience guiding patients and clients through complex health challenges with the goal of finding authentic wellness. I bridge the gap between traditional Western medicine and complementary health practices in an approachable way, helping others recognize their own innate wisdom for finding balance in mind, body, and spirit. And then I help them set the stage for true healing by incorporating plant-rich nutrition and gentle lifestyle shifts into their daily routines.

Our bodies want to be well, and with literally every move we make, our bodies are trying to return to a state of wellness. If we pay attention, we recognize the search for balance is a constant flow from feeling well to not-so-well.

For example, if you have a few drinks on Saturday night, your body does its best to detoxify that alcohol, leaving you with a headache and nausea, telling you it needs time to rid itself of those harmful metabolites.

If you eat too much sugar and processed foods, your body responds to that load of glucose by ramping up its release of insulin, often doing such a good job that it overcompensates, leaving you feeling lethargic, like a limp spaghetti noodle on the floor.

If you overexert yourself with high-intensity interval training, your body gets overly achy while it removes lactic acid buildup from your muscles, leaving you feeling fatigued while your adrenaline and stress hormones recover your heart rate back to baseline.

If you stay up too late working on a project and shortchange your sleep, your body requests an extra dose of caffeine the next morning despite its increase in cortisol to get you out of bed, all in an attempt to override the buildup of adenosine in your brain that invariably happens sooner than you'd want.

And if you stop paying attention to your Spiritual Self because you're so busy fighting the fires of your everyday life, your mind just keeps bouncing from task to task, trying to find something to hold on to, making focus and concentration virtually impossible.

Your body is just trying to find balance.

I have grounded my medical career and personal life on the truth that if we give ourselves the circumstances to succeed, our bodies reward us with feeling well. It's all in the name of finding the right balance.

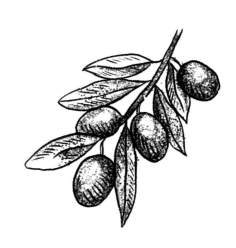

HOW TO USE THIS BOOK

While I know it's tempting to skip straight to the recipes, I recommend reading the book from the beginning, as my goal is to distill my years of medical training and knowledge into an approachable package that will arm you with an understanding of how personal experience, science, and habits come together to create wellness.

I begin with why you should trust me with your health. My introduction is your window into my start on the farmlands of northwest Ohio eating beef and corn. I give you a front seat to the theater of my issues with managing my weight throughout childhood and young adulthood, the unmasking of chronic anxiety in medical school and residency, my journey from infertility to becoming a mama, and how I manage chronic pain. I want you to know that I seek wellness from the purest of places. Finding my own balance is what has allowed me to find healing.

Then we move on to the nitty-gritty of science, pared down for you in a form that is easy to understand even if you've never cracked open a biology textbook. My book is chock-full of scientifically backed information that sets the stage for why we should choose a plant forward lifestyle; namely, it comes down to decreasing inflammation.

Inappropriate inflammation is the root of all evil in the body. Chapter 1 discusses how inflammation is a necessary part of our immune system's response to foreign invaders; we need it to survive. You'll understand that inflammation becomes a problem when the immune system goes overboard and produces excessive amounts of irritating hormones and chemicals, all in an attempt to make us well again. This over-the-top inflammatory activity damages cells, tissues, and organs and manifests as feeling sick, tired, or just plain unwell. I dig deep into how inflammation presents itself, especially when it comes to conditions like cardiovascular disease, metabolic disease, and cancer, which are overwhelming our healthcare system and impacting the lives of those we care about. I use medical evidence to show you why, when comparing all of the various diets and eating plans that exist, our single best strategy is to choose more plants.

After discussing why we do better with a plant-rich, nutrient-dense diet, I explain how to put that lifestyle into practice. I guide you to recognizing your own *Wellness Intuition* and hormonal balance, your individualized way of approaching which foods and life rhythms feel good in your body, and how to find the right balance of fiber, fat, and protein to help you feel your best.

Then, in Chapter 6, I anchor our macronutrient conversation in *Dr. Katie's Anti-Inflammatory Diet,* my approach to getting the nutrients we need on a daily basis. I walk you through the nuts and bolts of what you need to know about vegetables, fruit, whole grains, plant-forward proteins, healthy fats, and much more. I also talk about the all-important 80/20 rule, which means that you don't have to be "perfect" and eat only vegetables. What's important is finding a balance in your diet and doing a good job *most of the time.* I get that not everyone likes or feels good eating every food, so we'll chat about how to navigate food sensitivities and aversions if you just can't wrap your mind around something like kimchi. After you read Chapter 6, you'll view your daily choices in a new way, and I hope you'll be inspired to make even better decisions at the grocery store and in your kitchen.

Then we move on to chapters about ensuring adequate hydration, managing and recognizing satiety, and getting the proper vitamins and minerals on a plant-rich diet, as well as finding balance with the important pillars of gentle physical exercise, adequate rest, and attending to your Spiritual Self.

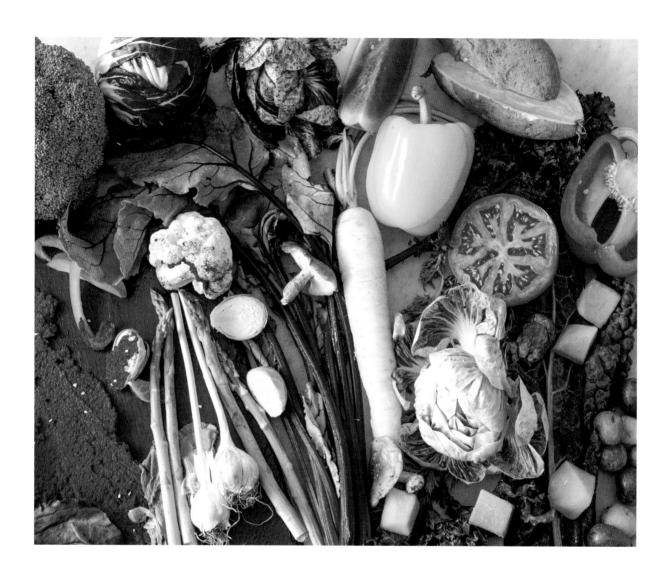

"What's *important* is **finding a balance** in your diet and **doing a good job** most of the time."

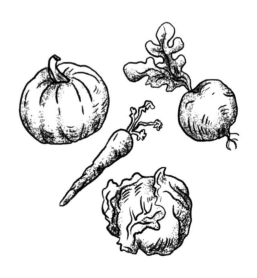

This brings us into the space of *Dr. Katie's Life Kitchen,* my approach to taking all this information and making it practical. I lead you through topics like why we need to home-cook our meals in the name of ingredient control, how to save time in the kitchen, how to prioritize food choices like organic produce and wild-caught fish, and how to troubleshoot issues like bloating and gas when you increase your consumption of plant-forward proteins, and then move into essential ingredients and tools that should make their way into your kitchen.

Following that are my recipes: gorgeous combinations of flavors, colors, textures, and nutrients that I think a plant-forward eater will enjoy making and eating. They were all designed with deep attention to the balance of fiber, protein, and fat so that you will get up from your dining table feeling satiated and energized instead of wanting to curl up for a nap.

Finally, I walk you through the *Dr. Katie Detox,* my approach to reminding yourself how to eat, sleep, and flow through your day for optimal health. I give you the key components to the tried and tested *Dr. Katie Detox Intensive,* a quick, get-down-to-business approach to detoxing using the power of plants that I developed with my business partner, Integrative Health Coach Courtney Evans. You'll discover that you can reset your body quickly and efficiently by reconnecting to eating for nourishment and satiety while rebalancing your daily habits. Best of all, you don't need anything other than the recipes in this book to make it happen.

STANDING THE TEST OF TIME

A lot of controversy exists in the research world when it comes to what to eat. Health information is constantly changing. A few of the ideas in this book may become dated as our medical knowledge grows, but most of it will stand the test of time because it's what we've known to be true through centuries of living passed down through the generations who've come before us. Eating broccoli is not going to go out of style. Take heart in knowing that most of the information in the book will remain accurate, but if you read this book many years from 2021, know that some nuances may have shifted as we've become smarter.

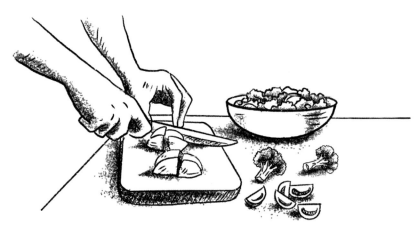

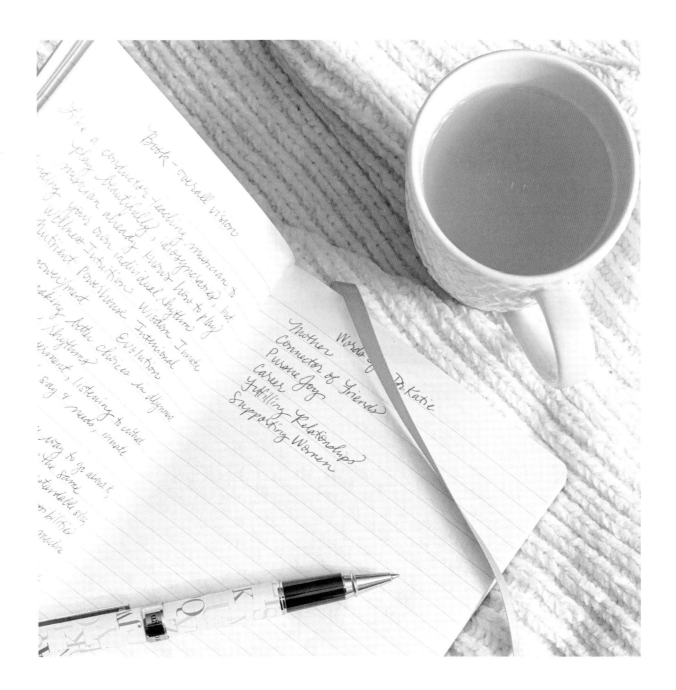

FINAL THOUGHTS

I sincerely believe in the inner wisdom and *Wellness Intuition* we all hold in our physical, mental, emotional, and spiritual bodies. Trust that you inherently know how to live your life. I want you to reconnect to what feels good in your authentic life because the downstream effects in your health will truly revolutionize the way you feel.

I am confident in my ability to guide you toward that place of self-healing.

Let's do this.

INTRODUCTION

A personal journey of finding balance and helping others find their balance: from being an uncomfortable girl to anxious doctor to desiring mother to chronic pain manager—with grace and humor along the way.

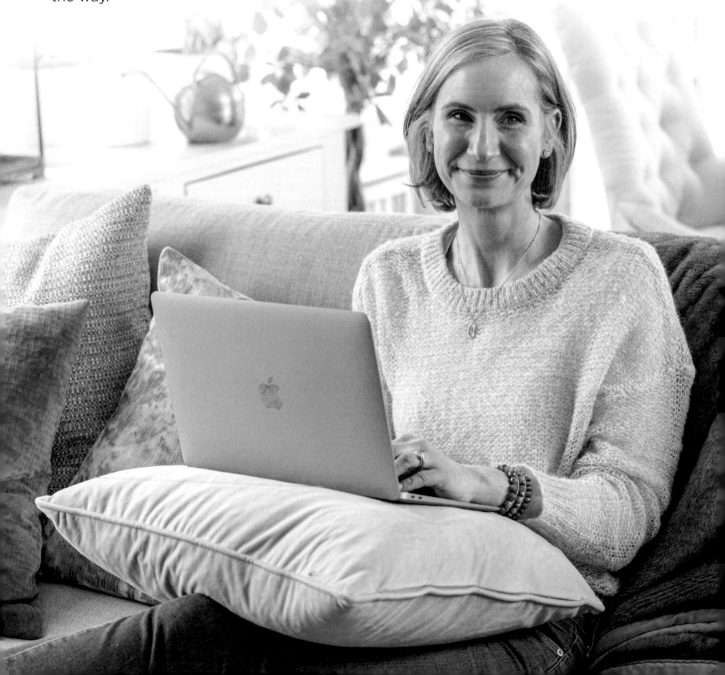

I haven't always been a healthy eater or lived a well-balanced lifestyle.

My journey to living a more well-balanced life came to fruition out of personal struggle. I imagine you have struggled, too—maybe with weight and body shame, mood balance, growing your family, or managing chronic pain.

This book is written for those of you who want to shift your lifestyle because you recognize what you're doing now is not serving you.

Let me take you on a journey of becoming Dr. Katie so you can understand why I believe so wholeheartedly that our food choices and balanced lifestyles matter.

BEING AN UNCOMFORTABLE GIRL

My story starts on the farmlands of northwest Ohio, in a small rural town. My childhood home was picturesque—a big brick house full of kids and music, a vibrant vegetable garden and McIntosh apple trees in the backyard, surrounded by fields of corn that created a sense of safety, and country roads with no lines where we waved to everyone who drove past because we probably knew them.

From childhood until medical school, I was quite chubby, nearing obesity at points as my weight fluctuated. In fact, I weighed more at my high school graduation than I did when pregnant with my twin boys.

My chubbiness was accompanied by feeling uncomfortable in my body. Despite being smart and well liked and known regionally as an accomplished pianist, I felt unhappy with myself. For many years, I carried an enormous heaviness of shame about my body, and it severely affected my self-esteem. I can so easily go back to being that girl who felt Less Than because she was self-conscious, embarrassed, and ashamed about her weight. Unfortunately, my insecurities fueled cruel comments and actions toward my peers and family members as a way to divert the negative feelings inside me, which made close friend relationships difficult.

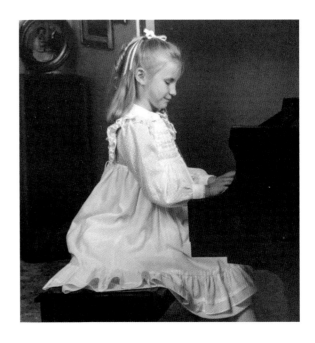

My mom cooked most of our meals following what I now consider to be a slightly healthier Standard American Diet. Supper was the most balanced meal because it included a vegetable or two with a starch—sometimes pasta or rice but mostly corn or potatoes—with the star of the show being the animal protein. There were days, however, when I didn't eat any vegetables and filled up on breakfast cereal, boxed macaroni and cheese, and frozen pizza. My favorite school lunch was a breaded pork tenderloin sandwich with creamed rice, canned peaches, and low-fat chocolate milk. And let's not forget about the evil but delightful SnackWell's Vanilla Creme Sandwich Cookies that lived in our pantry. I could put away an entire box of those treats too easily.

Looking back, I realize it wasn't my fault I had issues with my weight and overeating because I was eating foods that were *designed to make me fail.* The more I ate those tasty packaged cookies and other processed foods, the more my brain wanted and the more my body told me to eat. It was like crack to a cocaine addict. I now recognize that I was a prisoner in the brain's dopamine-fueled reward circuit combined with the hormonal effects of "store-this-as-fat" insulin and "I'm-not-full-yet" ghrelin secretion. Processed foods are a recipe for disaster.

I thought I needed willpower to be thinner. *I'll just eat one Oatmeal Creme Pie. I'll just have a small bowl of Special K or Raisin Bran. I'll just eat a handful of M&Ms.* Now I know that one is never enough because processed foods are designed to find the brain's Bliss Point, creating a hormonal cascade that sends us reeling back to the package to stuff our faces.

From age eight until my mid-twenties, there was never a time I wasn't on a diet. I knew the calorie count and grams of fat in most packaged foods and Taco Bell and McDonald's menu items. I constantly thought about what I had just eaten or would eat at my next meal. Getting my driver's license was both a blessing and a curse because then I had free access to drive-thru binges on french fries, McFlurries, and chili cheese burritos—accompanied by diet soda, of course.

Sometimes my diets were successful, like the summer when I turned sixteen and stopped eating fruit and sweets but continued to eat multiple slices of bread with butter each day along with a cup of milk at every meal and eggs or chicken three times a day. Calorie restriction does work in the short term, but it's not sustainable. As soon as I started eating fruit and sweets again, I not only suffered from diarrhea but gained 50 pounds over the course of two years until I hit my peak weight as a senior in high school. Instead of being proud of my academic and musical accomplishments, I was constantly fixated on how fat I looked. I cringe when I think about the intrinsic shame I felt as a valedictorian delivering the graduation welcome address to a gymnasium full of people who I feared were judging my failure to remain thin.

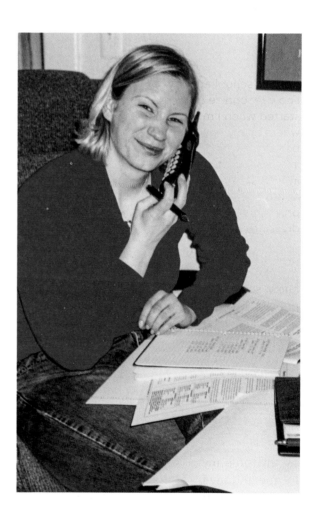

I went on to develop slightly better habits at the University of Michigan. I have funny memories of a good friend calling me "Four Food Groups Girl" in the cafeteria, with two of the food groups being dairy and animal protein, which I ate at most meals. I remember asking my boyfriend (now devoted husband) Jun, "Where's the protein?" when he made me a dinner of spaghetti with red sauce at his apartment. But the question at that time was never "Where are the vegetables?"

Despite my yo-yo challenge with weight in college, I did begin to recognize the power of regular physical movement. My freshman residence hall was next to the rec center, and I made it a habit to run laps around the indoor track several times a week while I listened to the local pop station on my armband radio. I knew my concentration was better and my period cramps more tolerable when I exercised regularly. I also took my first yoga class in college from a flexible, introverted hairy guy who wore tiny shorts, but at the time I failed to understand that yoga could be more than just boring choreographed stretching.

TIRED, WIRED & SAD

Medical school at Wright State University in Ohio was tough. I went through what I now recognize as full-on anxiety and depression. My anxiety and depression started when I moved to a new condo where I was lonely and a new school where all my new classmates seemed to know everything I didn't know. I quickly began drowning in a sea of overwhelmingly complex science while a fire hose of information pummeled me all day long. I stopped sleeping well for the first time in my life. Everything I ate tasted and smelled like the formaldehyde from the anatomy lab. One night I made a salad for dinner (topped, of course, with salty processed pink deli turkey, shredded low-fat cheese, and bottled low-fat Italian dressing) and threw it away after a few bites because I just couldn't eat.

Not eating had never been my normal. I knew something was wrong. I quickly lost 10 pounds. My grandmother told me I looked thinner at Thanksgiving—the hallmark compliment to a chubby girl; Grandma hasn't seen me in a few months and thinks I look thin!

Thankfully, over time, I adjusted to the demands of medical school and developed some amazing friendships that sustain me to this day. My anxiety and depression were soothed by Sunday night "Family Dinners" where Jun, by this time my husband, would make dinner for me and my friends after a long weekend of studying, and then we would all watch *Grey's Anatomy* together. I recognize now that finding community with friends and family is a critical piece of anchoring the Spiritual Self. Jun has always been—and continues to be—my rock.

I also believe that psychotherapy helped me to stabilize my moods. To this day, I always tell patients, "The best money spent is on therapy." There's nothing like talking to someone who is objective and paid to listen. I started weekly therapy sessions with the Chief Resident in Psychiatry at Wright State during my first year of medical school. Using the power of cognitive behavioral therapy, he helped me to recognize patterns in my thoughts and actions that I started to shift. I still use those tools today.

As I neared graduation with my MD and MBA, I had to choose a medical specialty. I considered a variety of specialties, and I was—of course—swayed by work schedules and income potential and considerations for "lifestyle." I ultimately chose family medicine because it just felt like home to me. My dad is a family doctor, and the model of taking care of the whole patient—physically, mentally, and spiritually—was how I wanted to be present with patients.

The transition from the relative ease of my last year of medical school and graduate work to residency in New York City was rocky. Jun and I wanted a change of pace from our suburban lifestyle, so we sold most of our belongings and moved to the Big Apple with a few suitcases and dreams of exciting city life. I started residency in urban family medicine at Columbia University/New York Presbyterian while Jun was still working in Ohio and commuting back and forth on weekends. A brand-new job as a brand-new doctor in a brand-new city without a sense of grounding from my rock made for many long days and nights.

There's no way to say this delicately: residency was brutal. Our work hours seemed never-ending, and everything felt like an emergency. On my first day of my intern pediatrics rotation, I arrived to find out that I was on call that night. No one had bothered to tell me. I had to find some ill-fitting scrubs to wear and deal with the fact that I wouldn't be brushing my teeth for thirty hours. I carried a walkie-talkie phone on my hip to communicate with nurses, and it never stopped ringing. There was no time to eat, no time to rest or sleep, no time to pee. I remember finding a private bathroom to do my business and stopping mid-stream to answer the phone, praying the nurse didn't realize the echo of my voice was from the bathroom tile. That evening on the floor, a tiny human aspirated while eating and died. Imagine the level of adrenaline and cortisol in my body as I did micro chest compressions with my thumbs and

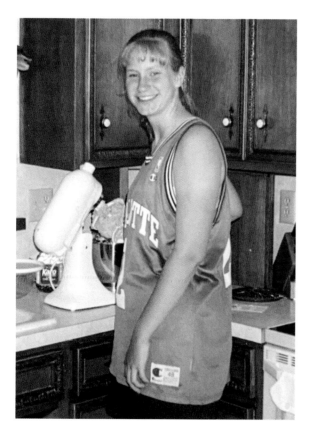

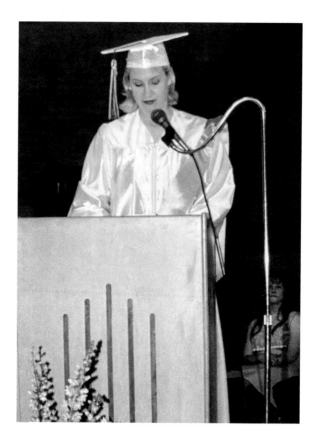

beseeched God to bring the baby back. Deaths are always sad no matter how old the patient, but I will never forget the gut-wrenching wails of the mother who lost her only child a few short months after welcoming him into the world.

My self-care during residency was nonexistent. I was not eating well, moving enough, sleeping enough, or attending to my Spiritual Self. My only sense of safety was being in my one-bedroom Upper West Side apartment with my husband on the couch watching TV and eating pizza with a big glass of wine. Working thirteen days straight with only one day in between to catch a breath is no way to live.

Jogging became an efficient way to exercise and see the city, but after injuring my knee while training for a half marathon, I found that I could no longer run without pain. That injury basically ended my workout regimen of jogging around the reservoir in Central Park. (By the way, if your body hurts, please listen to it. Our bodies have an innate wisdom that is all too easy to ignore when it's inconvenient—even I do it.)

I searched for exercise alternatives, and for a while I was happy enough to walk on a treadmill while reading *US Weekly*. Then my husband signed us up for a fancy gym membership and got me into a 6 p.m. trial yoga class. At the time

I was super irritated about the class because I was working nights and had left the hospital only a few hours earlier. But that evening, in my sleep-deprived state, shortly before reporting for duty again at 8 p.m., I truly found yoga. I had done yoga in college with the introverted hairy dude, but this experience was different. My now-beloved teacher Mindy helped me figure out how to slow my busy mind by focusing on my breath and movement. For the first time, I found my movements graceful and my body beautiful. Each class was a connection to a deeper sense of Self. My Real Self. The Self I had almost lost.

Around that same time, I stopped eating the free hospital food because I recognized it just made me feel more tired. I stopped eating from the trays of gooey lasagna and salty chicken lo mein served at educational conferences. I stopped buying flavored yogurt in the cafeteria and snacking on my favorite comfort of orange soda and pizza-flavored Combos. I started taking more care of my nutrition by packing my meals, sometimes taking an entire day of food with me. It was not convenient to walk around in search of a refrigerator at every medical site I went to, and sometimes my meals were lukewarm when I ate them. I'm frankly surprised I didn't get a food-borne illness. The big plates of delicious processed carbs my friends were eating started to look less appetizing to me because I noticed how lethargic I felt both mentally and physically after eating them. I noticed that more real food in my diet not only helped my energy level but also eased my chronic constipation.

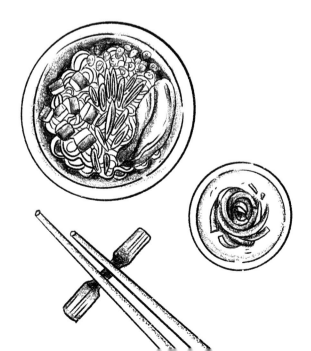

"I started *taking more care of my nutrition* by **packing my meals,** sometimes taking an **entire day of food** with me."

NO FRUIT OF THE WOMB

After I became a Chief Resident, my husband and I decided it was time to think about a family. I'd been on birth control for over ten years, and when I stopped taking the pill, I never really resumed a normal menstrual cycle. You don't need to be a doctor to figure out that having no period is not conducive to getting pregnant the good old-fashioned way. Oh, how I wanted to jump in the sack and make a baby like everyone else I knew.

My primary care doctor at the time was ambivalent about my concern for not having a period, and the way she dismissed my worries made me feel unheard and unimportant. I asked around for recommendations of another physician and found Dr. Jeremy, my favorite family doctor of all time. I started tearing up as I told him my worries. Upon hearing my story, he gently said, "It must feel so hard to not have your body work the way it's supposed to."

Being present with someone's feelings, letting them know they are heard and understood, is often the most important gift we can give those we care about. His acknowledgment was just what I needed to begin grieving the loss of normal.

I knew I needed help from a specialist, so I found an infertility doctor whom my husband and I called Guacamole because he had the personality of an avocado. He was terse and scientific and procedure-oriented with no bedside manner. Guacamole recommended IVF because my ovarian reserve was "severely compromised." This curt statement shocked me at first but ultimately just made me deeply sad. After all my years of schooling to become a doctor–the hardest thing I'd ever done–while responsibly taking the pill to prevent unwanted pregnancy, it was revealed that my little ovaries had almost no eggs. I felt a void in my heart that overwhelmed every moment and took away most of the pleasure from my already diminished life as a medical resident.

Dr. Jeremy recommended acupuncture to me, and that's when literally everything in my life started to shift. Every weekly check-in with my acupuncturist, Kelly, was a ray of hope that my body was not broken. During one session, I was moved to tears–not the little tears that gently roll down your cheeks, but the kind of big, ugly sobbing that comes from your soul hitting rock bottom. Earlier that week I had gone to yoga, and Mindy's theme had been the Goethe quote "At the moment of commitment, the Universe conspires to assist you." As I calmed myself down by meditating on that quote, a parade came down the street outside. The rumble of the drums, the music blasting from a speaker, and the cheering and clapping from the spectators stirred my Spirit to recognize that the Universe could conspire to assist me.

"At the **moment of commitment,** the *Universe* conspires to assist you."

Being on the acupuncture table that day ultimately led me to pursue Integrative Medicine. I came to realize that my journey to eat real, nutrient-dense food, find joyful daily movement, and regain my connection to my Spiritual Self were the backbones of Integrative Medicine. I landed an Integrative Medicine fellowship at Stamford Health shortly after a successful fertility treatment of ovulation induction and intrauterine insemination (IUI).

I felt so well during my pregnancy with my twin boys. Sure, I was large and in charge and uncomfortable. I peed on myself if I laughed too hard. I couldn't empty the dishwasher because the pelvic pressure and weight of the pregnancy were so intense when I bent over. I had absurd amounts of swelling in my legs that prevented every shoe from fitting and necessitated the wearing of thick and uncomfortable support stockings from the moment I got up in the morning. But I felt a deep sense of my physical body doing God's work. I felt a connectedness with and an appreciation for my body I had never experienced before, especially during yoga as I navigated around my amazing belly. Ultimately, I vaginally delivered my healthy little boys at full term guided by an amazing team of doctors, many of whom were my coworkers from prior residency rotations.

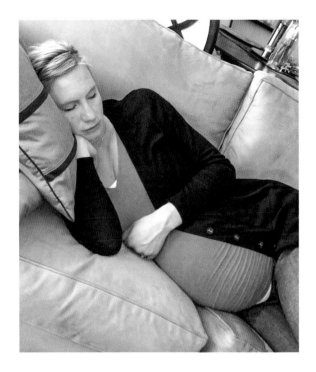

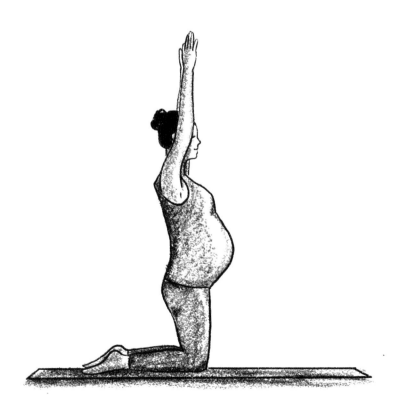

LIVING WITH CHRONIC PAIN

Shortly after the boys' birth, I bent down one day to pick one of them up from the crib and felt a sharp, excruciating pain in the right side of my low back. The pain was so severe it took my breath away, and I almost dropped my baby. It went away a moment later, so I dismissed the pain and went on with my day.

A few days later, however, I was pushing our twin stroller across the street and a taxi turned the corner without seeing us. I sprinted out of the way and again had a sudden searing pain in my low back. I knew something was wrong.

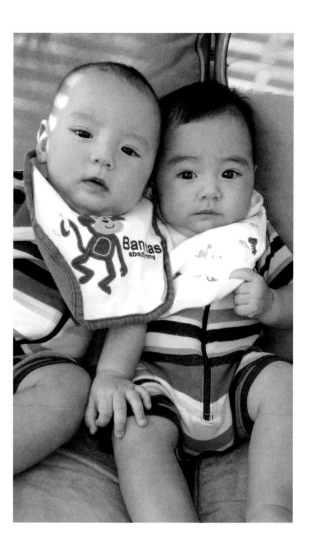

Ultimately, I was diagnosed with ligament instability in my low back and pelvis due to the relaxing effects of pregnancy hormones on my overly flexible joints. I had always thought that being flexible was a gift, but as with most things in life—sweets, alcohol, caffeine, even sleep—too much of a good thing is not a good thing. I was prescribed some strengthening exercises, a steroid injection, and a back brace and told to rest and use ice. The immediate inflammation died down, but the instability was still lurking under the surface.

Two years later, I did the amazing Cliff Walk in Newport, Rhode Island, a feast for the senses with the roaring Atlantic Ocean sea spray on one side and gorgeous historic mansions on the other. While climbing, I slipped on a mossy rock, but my muscles were not strong enough to stabilize me. I fell hard and could barely move without awful pain. Getting back to the car was almost impossible. I subsequently recovered but had several more episodes of sudden severe pain after menial events like tripping over a rug and taking a two-mile jog.

I saw several medical specialists, including one who said I was missing entire supporting ligaments in the right side of my pelvis, which caused me to rely too much on my hamstring muscles for support. The ligaments had likely torn during pregnancy and delivery and couldn't be repaired without a hysterectomy and major surgery. I was a walking disaster.

These days, I usually wake up feeling fine, but certain run-of-the-mill activities like running, sitting, driving, and too much forward folding in yoga cause me pain. I have workarounds, like a standing desk at work and an understanding husband who does most of our family driving, but daily pain interrupts everything and puts a damper on joy. While others can sit in a standard chair, I need a cushion to create padding for my chronically inflamed hamstring and quadratus femoris muscles. While others can take a casual jog, I notice pain the moment I stop running that leaves me unable to sit comfortably for days. I dutifully stretch, foam roll, and strength train my butt and leg muscles to support me and do my best to focus on being strong and what I *can* do, not what I can't.

Over time, I have grown to understand how to manage chronic pain. My focus has shifted away from identifying with my pain; now, I recognize that pain is something that happens *to*

HELPING OT
WITH INT

My passion for helping
making positive life
changes didn't c
part of a deca
space for ch

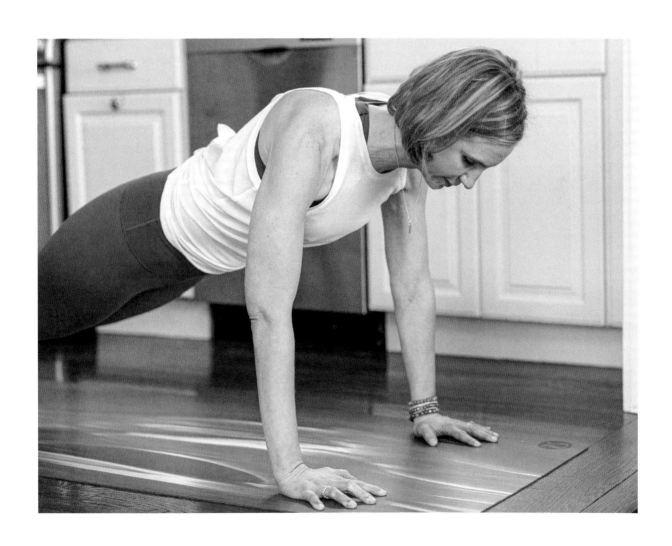

...g others find balance is rooted in my own experience of
...style choices to create an environment for harmony. Those
...me about overnight. My quest to finding balance took the better
...e and happened in tiny increments as I intentionally created the
...ange.

...althy habits have a delicate way of
...king. My slow shifts sometimes felt incon-
...quential. At first, I was simply eating more
vegetables instead of processed food, or taking a walk instead of watching TV, or mindfully
staying present during yoga instead of making
to-do lists in my head. But I wasn't just *doing*
those things. Those healthy shifts were actually
changing *me* because I had created the space
for positive *internal* change.

I often tell patients that I don't have a silver bullet to cure them of their ailments—but
what I do have are Integrative Medicine strategies that, when taken all together, amount to
big change on the inside. I use this philosophy
in my medical practice, where I combine traditional Western medicine with evidence-based
complementary modalities to help patients heal
naturally with acupuncture, mind-body medicine, botanical medicine, nutrition, and lifestyle
optimization.

Over the past several years, I've become a
champion of plant-forward eating and women's
health. I help patients find holistic approaches
to issues including perimenopause, infertility, pregnancy-related conditions, and pain
management for a variety of conditions from
migraine headaches to irritable bowel syndrome to pelvic pain. I help patients discover
their own practical strategies for prioritizing healthy habits. I consider myself more of a
coach than a doctor because I guide patients
to recognize their own sense of wholeness in
the mind, body, and spirit. When we take care
of our whole selves, we can take care of others
more authentically.

I feel like an angel who gets her wings
every time a patient says to me, "I started eating more vegetables, and I notice that I just feel
better." The light in their eyes as they recognize
their intrinsic power to make incredible shifts
is what fuels me through my work as a doctor.

I hope you eat more vegetables, too. Let
me show you how to make gentle shifts in your
life in the spirit of wholeness, with grace and
humor along the way.

Love,

Dr. Katie

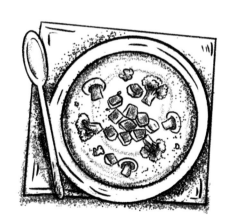

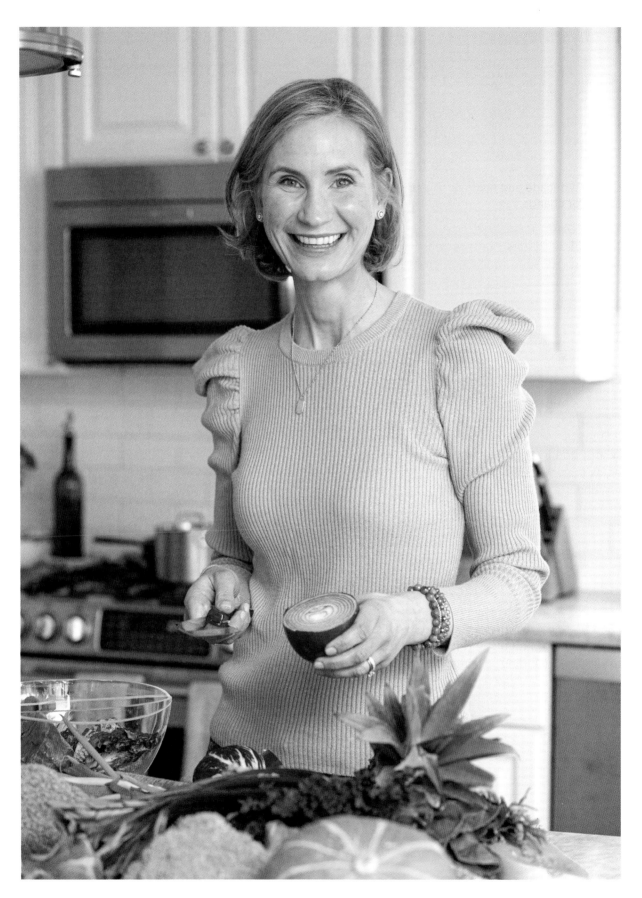

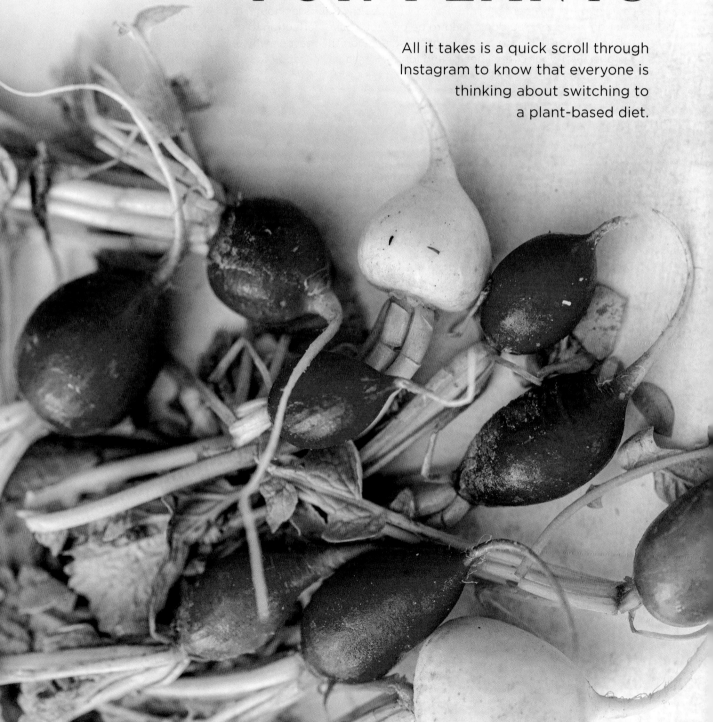

CHAPTER 1

THE CASE FOR PLANTS

All it takes is a quick scroll through Instagram to know that everyone is thinking about switching to a plant-based diet.

We are bombarded with information about why it might be a better idea to eat plants, from Netflix documentaries on vegan athletes to tweets shaming the meat industry to podcasts about centenarians living in Blue Zones. We get emails from our favorite bloggers with Meatless Monday dinner menu ideas. We see flashy Instagram stories on snatching a table at a trendy plant-forward restaurant in Greenwich Village after queuing for three hours in anticipation of a tender maple and miso-glazed leek amuse-bouche.

But *thinking* about being more plant-forward and *doing it* are two separate things. They are connected by knowing not only the *why* but also the *how* to get it done.

This book is the why *and* the how.

As a physician and devotee of delicious food, I have distilled the important take-homes from science and created *Dr. Katie's Life Kitchen,* where I keenly follow the 80/20 rule, recognizing that 80 percent compliance with healthy habits is enough to make a huge impact on wellness. You don't need to be perfect. Leave perfection to the Instagrammers!

This chapter gets into the nitty-gritty science on the reasons why eating more plants is beneficial for your overall health and longevity. You'll be happy to know that eating plants is better for the environment and your wallet, too. Stick with me and learn why a plant-rich diet is the way to go.

WHY YOU NEED THIS BOOK

I'm a practical person who loves food and happens to be a doctor, and my perspective is all about balance.

Balance does not mean everything in life gets the same weight. It means we figure out what's most important, prioritize those pearls, and then allow everything else to flow around them.

Most of us know we can do a better job of taking care of ourselves. The problem is that everyday life gets in the way. How is one supposed to eat perfectly balanced meals while chauffeuring kids around, or managing the complex care of an elderly parent, or working a full-time job only to realize there's another full-time job waiting at home?

You need this book for precisely this reason: most of us know generally which actions would help us eat better, sleep more soundly, minimize stress, lose weight, and prevent disease, but we get stuck.

When polled, up to 84 percent of women feel some dissatisfaction with their bodies and lifestyle habits.[1] We know when we don't feel well, but we become paralyzed with the massive amount of information out there. We don't know if we should listen to the online fitness instructor telling us to do more high-intensity interval training and decrease our carbohydrate intake

---

[1] C. D. Runfola, A. Von Holle, S. E. Trace, et al., "Body dissatisfaction in women across the lifespan: results of the UNC-SELF and Gender and Body Image (GABI) studies," *European Eating Disorders Review* 21, no. 1 (2013): 52–9.

in favor of more protein. We get weighed down with worry about the hidden dangers of lectins in store-bought beans and feel pressured to buy the fat-burning, metabolism-boosting supplements a neighbor swears by. The amount of information available is almost paralyzing. You need a way to get unstuck.

This is your lucky day.

I wrote this book precisely with you in mind.

My journey to helping others find balance in their nutrition started with my own realization that I felt better when I ate more plants, and I've used my doctor brain to sort through the evidence and combined it with my need for lifestyle ease in the quest for sustainability. After all, what good is change if it only lasts the two days you create space to have breakfast while sitting down?

INTEGRATIVE MEDICINE & THE CARE OF YOUR MIND, BODY & SPIRIT

The framework I'll use starts with understanding the philosophy of Integrative Medicine.

Traditional Western medicine stems from a time when fighting disease was paramount. One hundred years ago, the top causes of death were infections like tuberculosis, influenza, pneumonia, and infectious diarrhea.[2] These infections are still around today, but the advent of better public health systems, vaccines, and medications like antibiotics have changed the landscape of traditional care to turn these prior killers into more like big inconveniences. For most of us, if we get the flu, we might need to take a few days off work or school chained to the bed or couch while we take Tamiflu. And yes, we feel horrible with body aches, malaise, fever, and cough, and a few of us may need support in a hospital setting, but overall death rates have dropped considerably since data started to be recorded last century, and certainly since we've started wearing masks.[3]

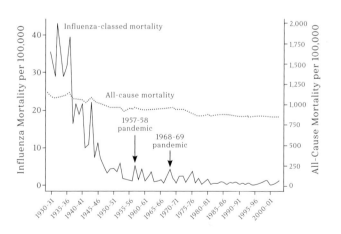

[2] R. A. Hahn, M. Chang, R. G. Parrish, et al., "Trends in mortality among females in the United States, 1900–2010: progress and challenges," *Preventing Chronic Disease* 15 (2018): 170284.

[3] P. Doshi, "Trends in recorded influenza mortality: United States, 1900–2004," *American Journal of Public Health* 98, no. 5 (2008): 939–45.

In the 1940s, the average seasonal rate was 10.2 deaths per 100,000 people from influenza, which decreased to 0.56 per 100,000 by the 1990s. This deserves a big round of applause!

So if we aren't dying of pneumonia and influenza and are living longer lives, what's taking us out? Now our top causes of death—heart disease, stroke, cancer, diabetes, and chronic respiratory disease such as emphysema—are largely driven by poor lifestyle choices.[4]

DEATH RATES THROUGH THE 20TH CENTURY, UNITED STATES, 1900 TO 1998

Total mortality rates by cause of death, measured as the number of deaths per 100,000 population. Death rates are given as all-age rates (not age-standardized). Data for specific causes of death may be missing or intermittent where it enters or falls out of the top 10 reported causes of deaths in any year.

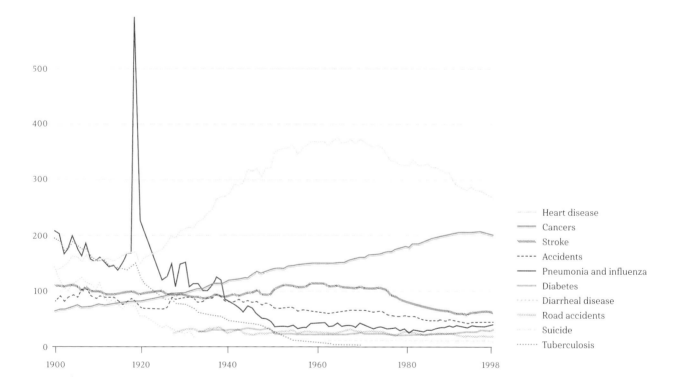

We can see from the graph that rates of death from infectious disease dropped off by the mid-twentieth century. And check out the fact that heart disease and stroke, which peaked earlier last century, begin to drop as the millennium approached. Hooray for medical advances in detecting and treating acute heart attacks and stroke!

But look closely to see the steady increase in deaths due to cancer and the fact that heart attack and stroke are still major causes of mortality. What's the common denominator there? Many, including me, argue that it's inflammation caused by poor lifestyle choices.

---

[4] B. Bastian, V. B. Tejada, E. Arias, et al., "Mortality trends in the United States, 1900–2018," *National Center for Health Statistics*, 2020.

The cost of our habits is far greater than the $1.99 soda at the gas station or the packaged cheese crackers at the supermarket. We are nearing a point of unsustainability in spending on healthcare that is crippling our national budget.

Integrative Medicine takes a closer look at the lifestyle choices that become the root cause of disease. I love this graphic of a tree where above ground we see conditions like diabetes, hormonal imbalance, and autoimmune disease. Below the surface, however, lurk the real reasons for the disease conditions that plague our healthcare system.

- High blood pressure
- Anxiety
- Depression
- Thyroid issues
- Hormone imbalances

- Cancer
- Allergies
- Autoimmune disease
- Diabetes
- Chronic fatigue

- Inflammation
- Stress
- Poor diet
- Toxins
- Lack of sleep
- Poor relationships

- Poor digestion
- Genetics
- Trauma
- Toxic thoughts
- Lack of exercise

Consider how inflammation, lack of exercise, poor dietary choices, excessive alcohol use, tobacco smoking, and lack of community and social interaction could be changed for the better. Doctors call these *modifiable risk factors* because they aren't necessarily a part of our genetic destiny. I like to say you can't choose your parents (or their genes), but you can choose how to live each day.

To address these modifiable risk factors, Integrative Medicine focuses on the biopsychosocial model, which recognizes that a patient's choices are a weaving of biological, psychological, and social factors. The fabric of your being is not just your genes or what's happening in your physical body; it's also rooted in what's happening in your mental and emotional spaces, all taken in the context of your environment.

Take, for example, my lovely patient Sabrina. She's a jovial thirty-year-old who came to me as a referral from her primary care doctor for help with managing headaches and weight loss, which at face value seems simple. But during our first conversation and over the subsequent months of seeing her once weekly for acupuncture, I've grown to understand how her life has been knitted together. Unfortunately, she has a history of trauma from childhood that has been subsequently reinforced by several romantic relationships fettered with emotional abuse and alcoholism. She chronically clenches her jaw because she's so stressed, and when her world is spinning out of control, she leans on highly processed sweets, which have led to an increase in fasting insulin and blood sugar. Little by little, we're working toward making her diet more plant-rich, taking into account the challenge of living with her mom, who prepares most of their food. Along with her psychotherapist and craniosacral therapist, we're slowly addressing her total mind-body-spirit connection. This will be an ongoing journey for Sabrina, but I am excited that she's embracing new tools to overcome her chronic health challenges.

Although I am a doctor, I consider myself more like a health coach for my patients because our doctor-patient relationship is less directive and more collaborative. One of my friends jokes that I am "like an MD on steroids" because after I finished the normal track of medical school and residency, I spent several extra years in an Integrative Medicine fellowship learning the complementary medicine tools that exist on the other side of the aisle.

One of the reasons I receive so many referrals from other doctors in the community is because my knowledge is rooted in the cold, hard science of medicine finessed by knowledge of preventive medicine, behavioral change, and ways to treat disease without pharmaceuticals or expensive procedures. I see patients like Sabrina every day, and addressing her health takes a multifactorial approach. Traditional doctors know that medication and surgery are not the only ways to treat disease, but most physicians are never taught how to think outside the disease management system. In fact, most medical students receive only a fraction of the training they need to understand and promote health. The average medical student gets about twenty-three hours of nutritional training, but the range goes from two to seventy hours based on surveys.[5] I distinctly remember four hours—one half day—of formal education on nutrition in my medical school, and at the time it felt kind of "fluffy" compared to the rigors of biochemistry we were learning. It's not your doctor's fault that they don't know how to coach your cholesterol problem using lifestyle tools. They were only taught to manage heart disease using drugs like atorvastatin

and procedures like stents and catheterization. Integrative Medicine is the link from disease management to health promotion.

The backbone of Integrative Medicine is lifestyle, which I divide into four simple categories: eating, moving, sleeping, and paying attention to our spiritual needs.

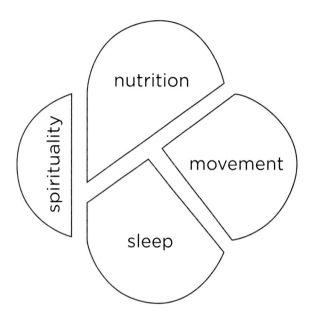

The three necessary things we do on a daily basis are eat, move, and sleep, and the fourth category denotes mindfulness of spiritual needs. I think about lifestyle—how we take care of our physical, emotional, mental, and spiritual selves—as the fertile ground in which the "seeds" of medications, surgeries, herbs, supplements, acupuncture, physical therapy, and psychotherapy are sown. Imagine trying to plant a flower in a barren field where the soil has been stripped of nutrients and lacks support from sunshine and water. Obviously, that flower wouldn't thrive. Your lifestyle choices regarding food, exercise, sleep, and spirituality can fertilize your soil and help your health and well-being flourish.

---

[5] K. M. Adams, K. C. Lindell, M. Kohlmeier, and S. H. Zeisel, "Status of nutrition education in medical schools," *American Journal of Clinical Nutrition* 83, no. 4 (2006): 941S–44S.

So the question becomes whether you need an Integrative Medicine doctor. The short answer is probably yes. Most of us need a personal guide to embark on a path of lifestyle change, but that guide could come in many forms. My shift toward a healthier lifestyle in residency was guided by a forward-thinking primary care physician in combination with my acupuncturist and yoga teacher, but eventually I wanted more and more knowledge, which ultimately led me to fellowship training. Today I learn from those three guides plus a health coach, psychotherapist, and physical therapist. Giving you the tools you need to take care of your physical, mental, emotional, and spiritual self can take a village. But your first step could be working with an Integrative Medicine doctor in combination with this book.

UNDERSTANDING THE RESEARCH ON DIETS

A lot of controversy exists in the research world when it comes to knowing what to eat. That's why you're reading this book, right? Before I dive into which types of foods to eat and why, it's important for me to explain a little about food research.

Research is the basis for practicing evidence-based medicine. Evidence-based medicine simply entails using the information scientists have gathered to inform medical treatment decisions, ultimately helping medical professionals to streamline care. Evidence-based medicine is why we recommend statins to those who've had prior heart attacks to prevent further damage and why we want your blood pressure to stay below 120/80. The research tells us that these metrics work.

Unfortunately, research on nutrition isn't so clear-cut. Much of the existing research on diet and longevity is confusing and doesn't point us directly toward a single way of healthy eating. It's virtually impossible to sift through the research and find the exact right answer so you know what to buy at the grocery store and serve for dinner.

There are multiple reasons for the confusion. One is that it's difficult to do studies on diet and longevity because they entail forward-looking prospective research. In this type of research, you're waiting for something to happen. Humans aren't lab rats that can be contained in a controlled environment. Imagine trying to gather tens of thousands of participants who are all somewhat similar, eating a relatively similar diet, and then following them for ten, twenty, or thirty years, waiting for them to have a heart attack or stroke or develop cancer, all the while asking them to report their habits to you. Some may drop out of the study or change their phone numbers and be impossible to reach. Or what if they start out in the "I eat meat" cohort of the study and suddenly change to a vegan diet after a close family member has a health scare? How does a researcher deal with all of these variables?

A second reason it's difficult to do research on diet is that it's expensive. Most research is funded by big pharmaceutical companies who are interested to see if their new blockbuster drugs in the pipeline are going to be the next Prozac or Viagra. This narrows the research available for the public to use when making decisions about our health. We also need to consider the effects of the animal industry on research that's done and information that's shared with consumers. Ever wonder why dairy is considered a separate food group and given its own spot on the updated MyPlate guidelines established by the United States Department of Agriculture? It's because the dairy industry has a strong influence over the people who make these recommendations, which creates bias. The same influence exists between organizations like the American Heart Association and their sponsors, which include companies like General Mills, Kellogg's, Kraft Heinz, Nestlé, and PepsiCo along with a whole host of fast-food chains. Unfortunately, there's not much money in proving a plant-forward diet is the way to go because the farmers who grow kale don't have deep pockets to fund kale research or hire lobbyists to advocate for their greens.

A third reason it's difficult to do research on diet is that it's hard to control for external factors that inherently raise a person's risk for mortality or morbidity. For example, it would be virtually impossible to conduct a large study looking at the effects of a plant-forward diet and control for all of the factors that might influence someone's risk of death, including family history and environmental hazards like groundwater safety and exposure, or understand exactly what someone's exercise habits are. To make research even more convoluted, participants are notoriously bad at recall when it comes to reporting what they eat, so the collected data may not be accurate.

Researchers certainly find ways to work around these problems, and well-done research attempts to minimize confounding variables. But it's not a perfect system.

So what do we do to navigate the uncharted waters of choosing what foods to eat? Very simply, we use the best information available across many platforms along with a healthy dose of common sense to piece together what is most likely the ideal way to fill a plate. And guess what? That's exactly what I've done for you in this book. So let's hop to it!

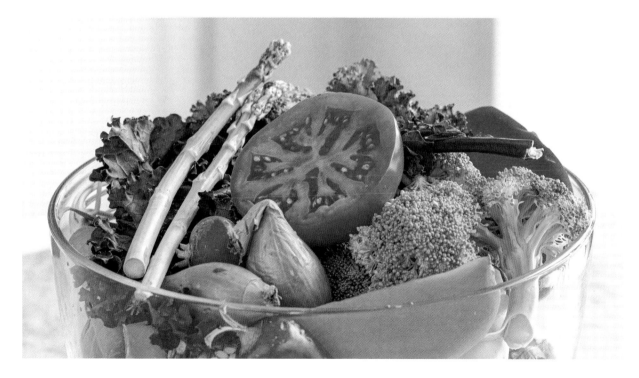

WHAT IT MEANS TO PUT PLANTS FIRST

Before I head into the science, let me start by defining what I consider to be the ideal diet. It's no secret that plant-rich foods are at the forefront. This section is just a primer on which foods are encouraged in a plant-forward diet. In Chapter 6, I get into the nitty-gritty.

Beyond the issues with research laid out on the previous pages, it's confusing to know what to eat because so many different diets exist. One of your friends is following a Paleo diet, and he stopped eating beans and lentils. Another friend wanted to lose weight, so she's doing a ketogenic diet and swore off whole grains like brown rice in favor of more steak. Your mother-in-law has heart disease and is terrified of plaque buildup in her arteries, so she's ditched all of the extra fat in her diet and barely uses any olive oil. You're left wondering what's wrong with beans, lentils, brown rice, and olive oil.

The answer: nothing is wrong with those foods. In fact, I'm going to show you that foods like beans, lentils, brown rice, and olive oil are *good* for you. The reasons all of those diets work is because of what they commonly take out: highly processed, inflammatory foods that don't serve your body.

Unfortunately, most people reverse the success they have following an elimination diet because they can't manage to eliminate those foods forever. That's why your friend following keto looked lean while she was sticking to the plan but easily gained weight as soon as she resumed eating pizza. It's virtually impossible to follow a restrictive diet for the rest of your life. It's just too limiting.

One of the best pieces of advice I've ever heard about figuring out what to eat is to look at the areas where all of the different diets out there overlap. In simpler words, look for commonalities rather than exclusions. Doing so saves you from deciphering what to eliminate from your diet and focuses you on what to prioritize. Let's take a look at the overlap:

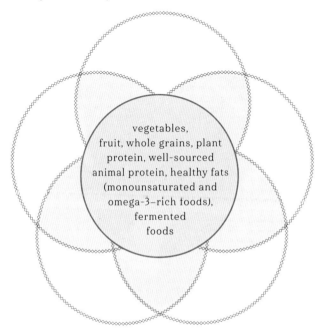

vegetables, fruit, whole grains, plant protein, well-sourced animal protein, healthy fats (monounsaturated and omega-3–rich foods), fermented foods

Look at all that you can enjoy! Zeroing in on the shared area of this diagram helps us understand that if we focus most of our attention on good stuff, we inherently eat less of the not-so-good stuff.

These commonalities lead us toward adopting a *plant-forward* lifestyle. A plant-forward diet emphasizes plants of all types alongside smaller amounts of animal foods like dairy, eggs, and meat. I recommend that about 80 percent of every meal should be plant-based foods, like vegetables, fruit, whole grains, legumes, nuts, and seeds. The other 20 percent can be high-quality animal products, with special emphasis on omega-3-rich wild fish (like salmon) and grass-fed, pasture-raised, organic dairy, eggs, poultry, and red meat.

Do you see how this reflects the 80/20 rule of life? The 80/20 rule states that what we do 80 percent of the time is what matters most. We don't need to fret about the remaining 20 percent. If it's your child's birthday and you want a slice of your favorite chocolate cake, then have a slice of cake after you've had a plant-rich meal. If you're jonesing for feta cheese on your salad, go for it if it's organic and not from artificial hormone-laden, factory-milked cows. The trick is to find balance with these less desirable foods. And that's where inflammation comes in.

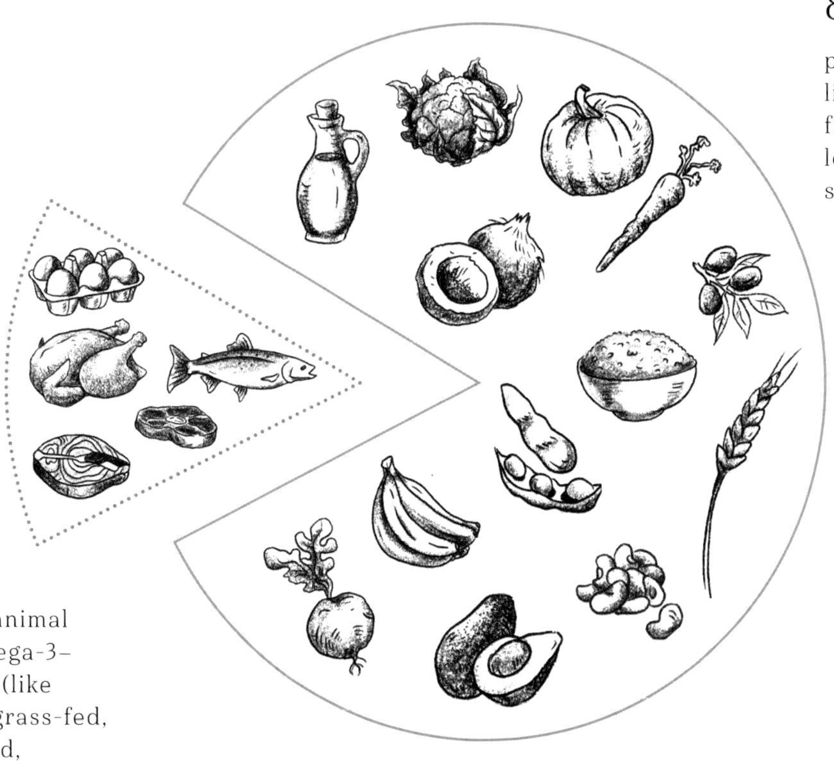

80%

plant-based foods, like vegetables, fruit, whole grains, legumes, nuts, and seeds

20%

high-quality animal products, omega-3–rich wild fish (like salmon) and grass-fed, pasture-raised, organic dairy, eggs, poultry, and red meat

INFLAMMATION: YOUR BEST FRIEND & WORST ENEMY

The most important reason to eat a plant-forward diet is that it's the best strategy for combating inflammation. Dialing down inflammation is the key to a long and healthy life.

If we drill down to the root cause of most diseases and health conditions, many experts agree that inflammation is the culprit.[6] Inflammation is the body's defense mechanism—the default pathway when the body senses danger lurking.

Not all inflammation is bad. In fact, we need short-term inflammation to survive and recover. Inflammation is how the immune system ramps up to combat an infection like a seasonal cold, or damage to the skin from a sunburn, or damage to a ligament following an ankle sprain. Inflammation is how the body begins the healing process.

We often experience inflammation in our bodies physically as swelling, redness, pain, or heat. A great example of this necessary short-term inflammatory process is the immediate impact of a bee sting. Within minutes of a little stinger irritating your skin, your body sends in a powerful cascade of help that causes swelling, itchiness, pain, and redness; the area sometimes even feels hot to the touch. You might want to put ice on your skin to help with the swelling and pain or take an antihistamine to combat the itchiness. The area might feel sore for a few days, but eventually the inflammation would resolve, and your skin would look normal again.

But what happens when inflammation continues? What if you were stung by a bee and several weeks later, the area was still red, swollen, and painful? You would be concerned, right?

Short-term, or *acute*, inflammation is usually helpful to the body's recovery, but long-term, or *chronic*, inflammation is a different story. What's tough about long-term inflammation is that it's not always visible, so we may not know it's there.

Chronic inflammation sticks around longer than it's supposed to, sometimes lasting months, years, or even a lifetime and is fueled by poor lifestyle choices. It is different from short-term inflammation because the body senses more and more danger, so it continues to ramp up its response with more and more helpers. Except most times these helpers just create more problems. The release of inflammatory cells like cytokines and other enzymes leads to tissue damage from free radical production and irregular repair in the body that compounds over time as the body attempts repeatedly to recover from the initial insult. In short, chronic inflammation weakens the body.

One example of chronic inflammation is osteoarthritis. What may start out as an innocent—maybe even imperceptible—knee injury

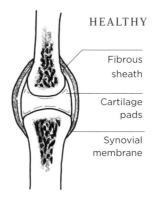

HEALTHY

Fibrous sheath

Cartilage pads

Synovial membrane

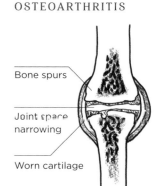

OSTEOARTHRITIS

Bone spurs

Joint space narrowing

Worn cartilage

---

[6] R. Pahwa, A. Goyal, P. Bansal, and I. Jialal, "Chronic inflammation," StatPearls [Internet], https://www.ncbi.nlm.nih.gov/books/NBK493173/, last updated November 20, 2020.

when playing tennis at age twenty-five may develop into chronic pain over the course of many years as the body destroys its healthy joint tissue and forms new irregular bone.

Modern medicine has direct ways of decreasing chronic inflammation. For knee osteoarthritis, a person could take nonsteroidal anti-inflammatory drugs like naproxen or ibuprofen or get steroid injections. Many of my patients manage osteoarthritis for years with an anti-inflammatory arsenal of a plant-forward diet, daily turmeric supplements, weekly acupuncture, and diligent physical therapy exercises along with occasional steroid injections from their friendly orthopedic surgeon. But sometimes the body's long-term inflammation cascade is just too powerful. In osteoarthritis, inflammation can erode the joint, making it too painful to walk or live a high-quality life, and ultimately necessitates joint replacement surgery.

This kind of chronic inflammation exists all over the body, and the problem is that most times we don't see or feel the effects.

The inflammatory changes that we see in a knee joint affected by osteoarthritis are the same basic changes found in the clogged blood vessels of heart disease, or the destruction of nerve cells in diabetic neuropathy, or the growth of a new tumor in cancer.[7] It all comes down to too much inflammation. The problem is we don't see this festering inflammation until the body reaches a tipping point that necessitates our attention.

Inflammation often goes unnoticed until we start to have an uneasy feeling of chest tightness when mowing the lawn, or notice our toes feel numb in our shoes, making us clumsy, or realize we've lost weight and felt profoundly fatigued and then find a lump in our breast. Those types of signs tell us something is seriously wrong and usually cause us to see a doctor.

Before the tipping point is reached, however, there are subtle signs of inflammation that we often ignore. We chalk up chronic bloating and stool irregularities to irritable bowel syndrome. We ignore the five pounds we put on during the holiday season thinking we'll get back to our regular weight in January when we hit the workout routine again and ditch the pumpkin pie. We ignore the morning puffiness in our faces and broken nonrestorative sleep after drinking too much wine at the school fundraiser. We ignore the pimply rash we get on our upper arms and energy slump every time we eat a delicious bagel at work on Fridays because we think we deserve a treat after a long week of intense meetings.

But these subtle signs are tiny cries for help. Our bodies gently call our attention to change, but we're often too busy or stressed or ambivalent to listen. When we don't pay attention, inflammation lurks under the surface and builds until the tiny cries for help become too loud to ignore. Then we're in real trouble.

The good news with inflammation is that it's almost never too late to intervene. We can always work on anti-inflammatory improvements to our health habits. And it starts with eating more plants.

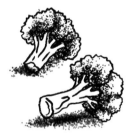

[7] S. Yagihashi, H. Mizukami, and K. Sugimoto, "Mechanism of diabetic neuropathy: where are we now and where to go?" *Journal of Diabetes Investigation* 2, no. 1 (2011): 18–32; A. Lopez-Candales, P. M. Hernández Burgos, D. F. Hernandez-Suarez, and D. Harris, "Linking chronic inflammation with cardiovascular disease: from normal aging to the metabolic syndrome," *Journal of Nature and Science* 3, no. 4 (2017): e341; L. Coussens and Z. Werb, "Inflammation and cancer," *Nature* 420, no. 6917 (2002): 860–7.

INFLAMMATION & LONGEVITY

An anti-inflammatory lifestyle is not only the key to a long life, but also the key to a high-quality life.

When I think about a high-quality existence, my mind immediately goes to my ninety-one-year-old grandma Margie who still lives on the family farm, drives a cute SUV, and mows her own lawn with a John Deere tractor. She's a social butterfly, and as friends have moved to nursing homes or passed away, she's found many new pals who are ten to fifteen years younger. She loves her daily exercise program on the local PBS station and eats hearty oatmeal every day for breakfast along with one cup of coffee. She's the chief cheerleader of the "Basketball Grandmas" at high school sporting events and the designated driver to polka dancing parties. She is the epitome of living a long, full life.

We come into this world with only one way out. Most of us don't like to think about death. I'm not morbid, either, but looking under the hood at the top causes of death and disability in the United States helps us understand why it's important to decrease inflammation.

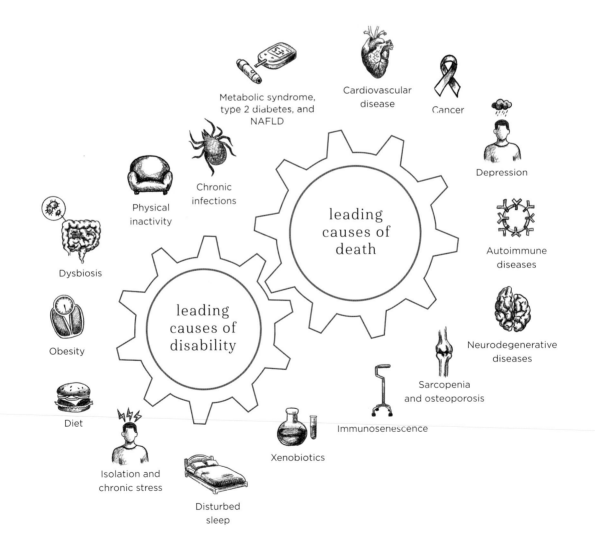

These were the leading causes of death in the United States in 2019 according to the Centers for Disease Control:[8]

Heart disease	659,041
Cancer	599,601
Accidents (unintentional injuries)	173,040
Chronic lower respiratory diseases	156,979
Stroke (cerebrovascular diseases)	150,005
Alzheimer's disease	121,499
Diabetes	87,647
Chronic kidney disease	51,565
Influenza and pneumonia	49,783
Intentional self-harm (suicide)	47,511

And these were the leading causes of disability in the United States in 2005 according to the Centers for Disease Control:[9]

Arthritis or rheumatism	8,552,000
Back or spine problems	7,589,000
Heart trouble	2,988,000
Lung or respiratory problem	2,224,000
Mental or emotional problem	2,203,000
Diabetes	2,012,000
Deafness or hearing problem	1,908,000
Stiffness or deformity of limbs/extremities	1,627,000
Blindness or vision problem	1,460,000
Stroke	1,076,000

I think we should care as much (or more) about disability as we do about death. Why? Because most of us will develop a disorder in our lifetimes that we'll have to live with for many years, affecting our quality of life. The data here show there's a good chance we could live many years with a chronic condition that makes life really hard.

As a doctor—and as a human on this wild ride called life—I don't just care about when I leave this planet. I care about how I spend my time and the quality of my life. I want to be shopping for my groceries and making lunch for my grandchildren when they come to visit like my Grandma Margie does. The key to a long, healthy life is decreasing inflammation. And how do you decrease inflammation? It comes down to eating a healthy diet, engaging in regular physical activity, getting proper sleep, avoiding environmental toxins, and decreasing psychological stressors.[10] In other words, our daily rhythms are our best weapons against long-term inflammation.

Each time you put something in your mouth, you're making a choice about inflammation or anti-inflammation. Food is, ultimately, calories and energy, but it's also *information* to our bodies. I'll talk more in future chapters about what specific choices to make, but the most crucial piece of nutrition to understand is that a real food, one that exists in Nature, is generally anti-inflammatory. Thankfully, we get to influence our bodies several times a day with each meal or snack. We don't need to feel compelled to be perfect because it's the overall balance of macronutrients, vitamins, minerals, and calories over time that's important. And that word *balance* is crucial to choosing the right foods.

---

[8] Centers for Disease Control, National Center for Health Statistics, "Leading causes of death," https://www.cdc.gov/nchs/fastats/leading-causes-of-death.htm, last updated March 1, 2021.

[9] Centers for Disease Control, "Prevalence and most common causes of disability among adults—United States, 2005," *MMWR Weekly* 58, no. 16 (2009): 421–6, https://www.cdc.gov/mmwr/preview/mmwrhtml/mm5816a2.htm#tab2.

[10] D. Furman, J. Campisi, E. Verdin, et al., "Chronic inflammation in the etiology of disease across the life span," *Nature Medicine* 25 (2019): 1822–32.

Balancing inflammation in the body is emerging in medical research as the underlying key to longevity and higher-quality living. We used to think that inflammation was linked to only a few select disorders. One of the most important medical discoveries over the past decade has connected the immune system and inflammatory processes to a wide variety of mental and physical health problems that dominate worldwide causes of death and disability.[11] In fact, chronic inflammation is recognized as the most significant cause of death in the world because it is linked to heart disease, stroke, cancer, diabetes, chronic kidney disease, nonalcoholic fatty liver disease, autoimmune disease, and neurodegenerative conditions.[12]

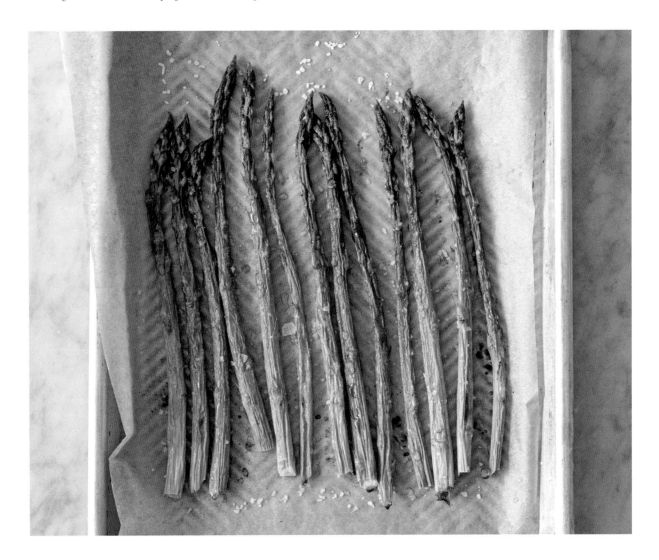

---

[11] D. Furman, et al., "Expression of specific inflammasome gene modules stratifies older individuals into two extreme clinical and immunological states," *Nature Medicine* 23 (2017): 174–84; M. G. Netea, F. Balkwill, M. Chonchol, et al., "A guiding map for inflammation," *Nature Immunology* 18, no. 8 (2017): 826–31; G. M. Slavich, "Understanding inflammation, its regulation, and relevance for health: a top scientific and public priority," *Brain, Behavior, and Immunity* 45 (2015): 13–14; J. M. Bennett, G. Reeves, G. E. Billman, and J. P. Sturmberg, "Inflammation–nature's way to efficiently respond to all types of challenges: implications for understanding and managing 'the epidemic' of chronic diseases," *Frontiers in Medicine* 5 (2018): 316.

[12] GBD 2017 Causes of Death Collaborators, "Global, regional, and national age-sex-specific mortality for 282 causes of death in 195 countries and territories, 1980–2017: a systematic analysis for the Global Burden of Disease Study 2017," *The Lancet* 392 (2018): 1736–88.

It's easy to see how finding a lifestyle that decreases inflammation would be beneficial to living a long, high-quality life. How we feed our bodies is at the root of decreasing inflammation. The typical American diet is high in refined grains, alcohol, and ultra-processed foods, which crowd out vegetables, fruits, and other fiber-rich foods we need to keep our immune systems happy and inflammatory markers low.

There's robust evidence to connect ultra-processed diets and mortality. Using health surveys and causes of mortality, the National Center for Health Statistics in the United States has shown that dietary trans-fatty acids, low dietary omega-3 fatty acids, and high dietary salt are some of the food-based risk factors associated with the highest mortality rates among American adults.[13] Where do we get all that trans-fat and salt? And why is our healthy omega-3 consumption so low? It's because we're eating ultra-processed food that isn't *real food.*

Similarly, a recent study reported in the *Journal of the American Medical Association (JAMA)* of about 44,000 French adults followed for seven years found that just a 10 percent increase in ultra-processed food consumption was associated with a 14 percent greater risk of all-cause mortality.[14] This type of information kinda makes you want to put down that can of prepared cream of broccoli soup and make your own, doesn't it?

Consumption of ultra-processed foods changes the way the immune system responds, leading to downstream total-body inflammation. Let's get super specific and talk about macrophages, one type of our white blood cell immune fighters. Macrophages go around eating pathogens like bacteria to prevent us from getting sick. (Remember the movie *Jaws*?

I think about that scary shark every time I think of macrophages.) Macrophages protect us by engulfing rogue pathogens and digesting them with acid to take them out of commission. These important cells are the first line of defense in our immune surveillance when it comes to preventing common illnesses. Thank your macrophages the next time your kid has strep throat and you somehow avoid getting sick, too.

Interestingly, research shows that an ultra-processed, high-salt diet skews maturing macrophages toward pro-inflammatory cell types.[15] Why is this important? Macrophages being steered toward inflammation has a downstream effect on other white blood cells that help with immune surveillance, raising our risk for common illnesses that an otherwise functional immune system might fend off.

Adding more fuel to the fire, research shows that an ultra-processed, high-salt diet also changes our microbiome mix. Our microbiome is the environment of good little bacteria called probiotics that live in our intestines and help us digest our food. High-salt diets disturb one of our most prolific types of bacteria, called *Lactobacillus*. Those little *Lactobacillus* bacteria want to eat fiber from asparagus and onions, not salty potato chips! It's important to note that our gut not only digests food but is also a significant part of our immune system and barrier protection from the external world. (Your gut is another part of your body to thank the next time you eat something that doesn't *quite* taste right but you magically don't develop food poisoning.) *Lactobacillus* is critical because it regulates those same inflammatory T_H-17 cells by keeping the intestinal barrier strong, thus reducing total-body, systemic inflammation.[16]

---

[13] G. Danaei, E. L. Ding, D. Mozaffarian, et al., "The preventable causes of death in the United States: comparative risk assessment of dietary, lifestyle, and metabolic risk factors," *PLoS Medicine* 6, no. 4 (2009): e1000058.

[14] L. Schnabel, E. Kesse-Guyot, B. Allès, et al., "Association between ultraprocessed food consumption and risk of mortality among middle-aged adults in France," *JAMA Internal Medicine* 179, no. 4 (2019): 490–8.

[15] D. N. Muller, N. Wilck, S. Haase, et al., "Sodium in the microenvironment regulates immune responses and tissue homeostasis," *Nature Reviews Immunology* 19 (2019): 243–54.

[16] See note 15 above.

Yikes! Who wants total-body inflammation and an increased risk of death from eating processed foods? Those zucchini in the refrigerator drawer are looking more appealing now, aren't they?

I bet you're already on the train of limiting processed food in your diet. After all, you're reading this book and thinking about increasing your plant consumption. The more serious question regarding longevity is which types of food to include once you decide to eat a diet that focuses on more wholesome, natural foods. Steak is a real food. So are chicken, eggs, and milk. So why do I advocate eating less of those foods if they are natural?

It comes back to finding balance. As a doctor, when I try to make sense of all of the research that exists, even I can get lost in the weeds. But taking the 10,000-foot view with my Integrative perspective, I hang my hat on prioritizing the foods known to be anti-inflammatory in the right combination to satisfy the body's needs for protein, fiber, fat, vitamins, and minerals along with the evidence we have for decreasing specific causes of death and disability.

INFLAMMATION, CARDIOVASCULAR DISEASE & OBESITY

Let's move on to the number one killer and leading cause of disability among Americans: cardiovascular disease. Guess what, my friend? Plants are your secret weapon against this huge problem and its underlying inflammation.

In the medical world, we consider issues like carotid artery disease, stroke, diabetes, and peripheral vascular disease (which includes conditions like abdominal aortic aneurysms) to be cardiovascular disease equivalents. This means if you have diabetes, your doctor is thinking about your care as if you'd already had a heart attack. These kinds of medical-thinking shortcuts help us assess a patient's future risk of complications and provide more efficient care.

Let's face it: it's hard to talk about preventing heart attacks, strokes, and diabetes without addressing the underlying element of obesity.

We have an obesity epidemic in the United States. Since the middle of last century, the waistlines of Americans have steadily grown as more processed foods have found their way into our diets and we engage in less physical activity than generations past. Being obese raises the likelihood of developing high blood pressure, and persistent hypertension is one of the major risk factors for strokes, heart attacks, heart failure, arterial aneurysms, and chronic kidney failure.[17]

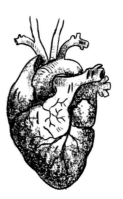

[17] L. Akil and H. A. Ahmad, "Relationships between obesity and cardiovascular diseases in four southern states and Colorado," *Journal of Health Care for the Poor and Underserved* 22, Suppl 4 (2011): 61–72.

BMI IS NOT THE WHOLE STORY

I don't want to fat-shame those who are not at their ideal weight. I have had many patients who didn't meet the criteria for a "normal weight"—typically earmarked by a body mass index (BMI) between 18.5 and 25—who were really fit and had healthy habits. Almost everyone in the medical field has dismissed the idea of BMI as outdated and not reflective of true health, but it gives us some benchmarks for weight management so that we can direct our goal-setting with patients.

BMI is not that helpful when it comes to addressing ideal weight because it doesn't take into account constitution, meaning the idiosyncrasies of a person's genetic tendency to be one way or another. It's not my fault that I tend to gain weight around my hips and thighs, giving me a pear shape, in the same way it's not your fault that you tend to gain it around the middle in more of an apple shape. We're stuck with the genes we have, but it's important to recognize that wearing jeans that are bigger around the waist to accommodate a lot of abdominal fat is not a good strategy when it comes to managing your future risk of heart attacks, stroke, or diabetes.

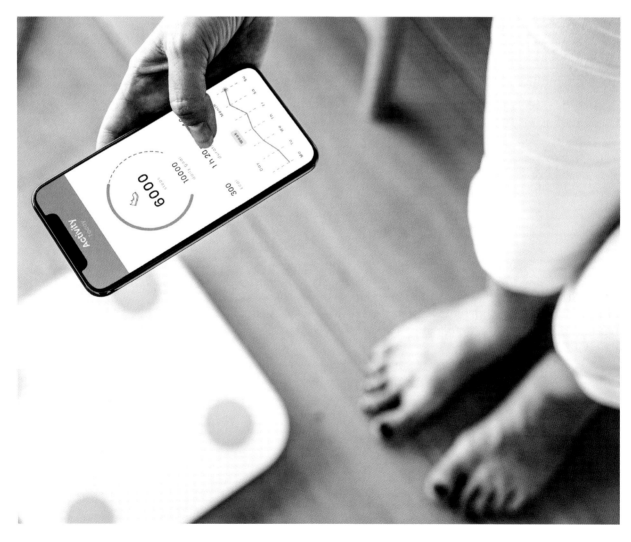

BODY FAT & LEAN BODY MASS

Body fat percentage might be a better assessment for obesity than BMI. We know that once body fat creeps north of about 25 percent for a man or 32 percent for a woman, it's in tough territory when it comes to weight management.

But the last time you were at your doctor's office, did they measure your body fat? No, they didn't. Why? Because that's not the way doctors are trained to think about weight. And while you may come across personal trainers, health coaches, and other smart allied health professionals who use this kind of data, few doctors have access to a device that properly measures body fat.

Once you know your body fat, you can easily calculate your lean body mass. Simply subtract the amount of body fat (in pounds) from your total body weight.

Lean body mass matters a lot because it ultimately drives the rate at which you burn calories, otherwise known as metabolism. The higher the ratio of lean body mass to total body mass, the more efficient your metabolism. I can't tell you how many patients come into my office complaining about how little they can eat before they start to gain weight, even if they are of a "normal" BMI. Unfortunately, BMI doesn't come close to helping us understand our ability to burn the calories we take in.

Lean body mass maintenance and metabolism are key to achieving and sustaining a healthy weight over the course of time, and maintaining a healthy weight is a big factor in the prevention of inflammation and, ultimately, heart attacks, strokes, and type 2 diabetes. Unfortunately, our lean body mass decreases as we age. We lose between 2 and 8 percent of our lean body mass every decade after the age of thirty if we aren't actively trying to build or maintain it.[18]

METABOLISM & THE HORMONES CORTISOL & INSULIN

Body composition changes are especially evident when we go through midlife. For aging men, a less robust metabolism is largely influenced by lower levels of the hormone testosterone in midlife, since testosterone is an important promoter of lean muscle mass. (That's why some bodybuilders take extra testosterone; it builds muscle mass.) For women, there's also a lessening of testosterone, but the majority of the decline in metabolism comes from the relatively lower amount of circulating sex hormones like estrogen and progesterone during perimenopause and after menopause, when menstrual periods stop altogether, which affects both metabolism and the risk factors of metabolic disease. Interestingly, the menopause-related decrease in metabolism happens whether a woman goes through natural menopause, surgically has her ovaries removed (going through what is called "surgical menopause"), or loses ovarian function due to another cause, like chemotherapy.

---

[18] D. Paddon-Jones and B. B. Rasmussen, "Dietary protein recommendations and the prevention of sarcopenia," *Current Opinions in Clinical Nutrition & Metabolic Care* 12, no. 1 (2009): 86–90.

Metabolic syndrome is the name given to the combination of high insulin levels and insulin resistance, high cholesterol and triglycerides, and high blood pressure accompanied by weight gain around the waist. Metabolic syndrome is often a precursor to developing more serious cardiovascular issues like heart attacks, strokes, and type 2 diabetes.

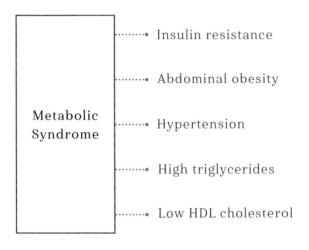

Metabolic Syndrome	Insulin resistance
	Abdominal obesity
	Hypertension
	High triglycerides
	Low HDL cholesterol

Understanding the midlife metabolism shift and the accompanying risk factors is a little bit like understanding which came first in the chicken-or-egg phenomenon. It's tough to know whether it's the decrease in lean body mass that takes the first hit, leading to a decrease in metabolism, or whether the metabolism decrease happens first, leading to a downward shift in lean body mass and a corresponding uptick in body fat. Regardless, if someone continues to eat their normal number of calories in midlife, they will gain weight, raise their risk of developing metabolic syndrome, and ultimately increase their risk of death and disability from cardiovascular-related disease.

It's not just perimenopause and midlife that change body composition and metabolism. Other hormonal shifts lead to changes in body mass, too. We go through so many hormonal transitions in our lives. Some of them involve our sex hormones, such as during puberty when estrogen and testosterone soar and all hell seems to break loose in our bodies. Contrast that to breastfeeding, when ovarian hormones are relatively low but the brain hormone prolactin is high, which allows women to nurse our babies. We experience a major hormonal change during super stressful times when cortisol production from the adrenal glands ramps up to help us rise to the occasion of fighting or fleeing from our stressors.

With all of the ups and downs, it's not hard to see why some women say their bodies are never the same after having kids or why many of us packed on the "quaran-ten" of a ten-pound weight gain during a pandemic.

Let's take a side step here and look a little more closely at the hormone cortisol and its friend insulin in the context of blood sugar and weight gain.

Any time blood sugar increases—whether you eat a Snickers bar or increase cortisol production by working late into the night on a big presentation for work—your body releases insulin from the pancreas to keep blood sugar normal. Insulin is the hormone that tells your body to store calories as fat, ultimately leading to weight gain.

Forward-thinking doctors also regard insulin as an inflammatory marker when it's elevated in a fasting state. But understand that insulin is necessary for life. Those with type 1 diabetes who cannot make their own insulin get very ill very quickly if they don't have insulin. Type 2 diabetes—the type associated with obesity and metabolic syndrome—is different from type 1. While type 2 is also a problem with blood sugar, the underlying reason is not that the body doesn't *make* insulin, but more that the body's insulin *stops working*. When we constantly challenge our bodies with increases in sugar—either from processed food or from stress—our bodies continue to pump out insulin, except the cells eventually stop listening to the signal. That's when insulin resistance develops and weight gain compounds, which are precursors to type 2 diabetes.

I use all this information to show you that talking with patients about weight is not easy for doctors because so many factors are at play. That's why so many physicians either don't do it well or don't do it at all. I can't tell you how many patients walk into my office baffled about what to eat. The only advice they receive after hearing their cholesterol is high is to "eat less cholesterol, fat, and red meat," so they find themselves buying processed foods like sweetened low-fat yogurt and whole-wheat pasta, which leads them to gain weight because those foods further increase insulin secretion, signaling to their bodies to store those calories as fat. Doctors are not trained well on how to have these tougher lifestyle discussions and provide the level of detail patients need to make positive changes.

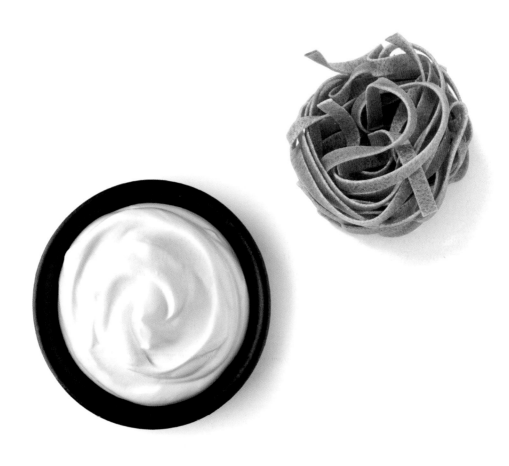

INFLAMMATION, CARDIOVASCULAR DISEASE & PLANTS

Of the leading causes of death and disability, medical evidence connects inflammation most strongly to cardiovascular disease, type 2 diabetes, and metabolic syndrome.[19] We're able to measure some inflammatory biomarkers in the blood, such as high-sensitivity C-reactive protein (hsCRP) and lipoprotein(a), among others. These inflammatory biomarkers can be used alongside data like cholesterol, hemoglobin A1c, fasting insulin, and blood pressure to help discern the risk of developing cardiovascular disease.

A plant-forward lifestyle is key when it comes to controlling cardiovascular inflammation and decreasing your risk of metabolic syndrome (the disastrous combination of high insulin levels and insulin resistance, high cholesterol and triglycerides, and high blood pressure accompanied by abdominal weight gain) and its downstream cronies type 2 diabetes, heart attack, and stroke. The simple science lesson for why a well-balanced, plant-forward lifestyle prevents inflammation comes down to the release of our hormonal friend and foe, insulin. When we eat a diet of mostly vegetables, whole grains, and healthy plant fats and proteins along with well-chosen animal proteins and stay away from ultra-processed foods, our insulin levels stay relatively level.

Lots of research has been conducted that connects a lower risk of cardiovascular disease to a plant-forward diet. The richest research we have is called a *systematic review*, where researchers compile the data from multiple studies into one massive review that identifies the outcomes that were consistent across all of the studies. One review published in 2012 in the *Annals of Nutrition and Metabolism* compiled seven retrospective studies with a total of 124,706 participants and found that vegetarians had a 29 percent lower risk of death due to ischemic heart disease compared to non-vegetarians, as well as a 9 percent lower risk of death from any cause.[20]

We also have prospective research, which is not as robust but, when it involves lots of participants, can be a reliable place to draw conclusions. Prospective population-based research like the Adventist studies looked at over 96,000 Seventh-day Adventists who followed variations on a plant-based diet and showed a link between plant-based diets and lower all-cause mortality and cardiovascular disease.[21] It's important to note that many epidemiological and interventional human studies suggest that plant-based diets are helpful in regard to obesity-related metabolic disease, including type 2 diabetes and chronic low-grade inflammation.[22]

But not all of the evidence out there points concretely to a plant-forward diet when it comes to obesity-related metabolic disease. Prospective studies like the EPIC-Oxford study show conflicting information. In the EPIC-Oxford study, researchers followed a cohort of 48,000 participants in the United Kingdom for eighteen years. The participants were classified into groups that ate meat (regardless of whether they consumed fish, dairy, or eggs), fish eaters (who consumed fish but no meat), and vegetarians (which included vegans). Attempting to control for other important lifestyle confounders (which sounds virtually impossible, doesn't it?), the study found that the fish eaters and vegetarians had a 13 percent lower rate of ischemic heart disease (i.e.,

[19] See note 10 above.

[20] T. Huang, B. Yang, J. Zheng, et al., "Cardiovascular disease mortality and cancer incidence in vegetarians: a meta-analysis and systematic review," *Annals of Nutrition and Metabolism*. 60, no. 4 (2012): 233–40.

[21] M. J. Orlich, P. N. Singh, J. Sabate, et al., "Vegetarian dietary patterns and mortality in Adventist health study 2," *JAMA Internal Medicine* 173, no. 13 (2013): 1230–8.

[22] E. Medawar, S. Huhn, A. Villringer, and A. V. Witte, "The effects of plant-based diets on the body and the brain: a systematic review," *Translational Psychiatry* 9 (2019): 226.

heart attack) compared to the meat eaters. But, interestingly, the vegetarians had a 20 percent *higher* rate of stroke than the meat eaters.[23]

This conflicting information makes things confusing for those who are trying to decide what to eat.

What much of the research doesn't tell us is how other foods come into the mix–like vegetables and whole grains–or how lifestyle factors like exercise and sleep habits affect cardiovascular risk. In the EPIC-Oxford study, where the vegetarians had a 20 percent higher risk of stroke than the meat eaters, were those vegetarians cooking at home or eating out? Were they mindful of the salt in their diet, or were they eating canned soups and preseasoned vegan meat alternatives?

We're left to piece together what we think is the ideal diet for heart health. When I look at the research and expert consensus as a whole, it points to natural plant-forward foods.

INFLAMMATION & CANCER

Almost every patient I see is concerned about decreasing their risk of cancer. To state it simply, cancer is the growth of cells that have gone rogue. For one reason or another, these cells have escaped the body's surveillance system. They generally reproduce at a higher rate than other cells in an uncontrollable way and invade healthy tissue, requiring extra energy from the body at the cost of normal energy expenditures. This is why doctors use symptoms like profound fatigue and unintentional weight loss in combination with localized pain or fullness to guide them toward imaging and biopsy. The body gives signs of something going awry.

Some cancers stay local to the tissue or system they invade. Others are more aggressive and spread throughout the body in the lymphatic system and are called metastatic. Generally, the more widespread a cancer is the more likely it is to take a person's life. Cancer is the second leading cause of death in the United States and around the world, but as we get better about diagnosis and treatment, more people are surviving cancer or living with indolent disease that is not life-threatening.

That said, quality of life plays a role here. Sometimes patients suffer from the side effects and complications of cancer treatment, like chronic underarm pain after a mastectomy, infertility from radiation, or permanent numbness in the feet after chemotherapy. Even if you survive cancer, your life can be forever changed by the treatment, ongoing monitoring and testing, and constant worry that the cancer could return.

Just like for cardiovascular disease, there are certain risk factors for cancer that you cannot change, like your age and family history, but so much is within your control. Getting routine cancer screenings, wearing sunscreen, not smoking, having safe sex, and not drinking too much alcohol are just a few of the interventions that decrease the risk of cancer. Your diet is also a huge factor. And guess what? Plants are important here, too.

---

[23] T. Y. N. Tong, P. N. Appleby, K. E. Bradbury, et al., "Risks of ischaemic heart disease and stroke in meat eaters, fish eaters, and vegetarians over 18 years of follow-up: results from the prospective EPIC-Oxford study," *BMJ* 366 (2019): l4897.

The robust systematic review discussed earlier (see page 43) found an 18 percent decrease in risk of cancer among vegetarians compared to nonvegetarians.[24] Another extensive systematic review of eighty-three studies that combined data from 2.1 million people found that those who had the highest adherence to a Mediterranean diet had the lowest risk of cancer mortality and statistically significant lower risks of colorectal, breast, gastric, liver, head and neck, and prostate cancers as well. The pooled analysis of the data revealed the protective effects of diet appeared to be most attributable to vegetables, fruits, and whole grains.[25]

Still another large systematic review from prospective cohort studies supported an association between healthy dietary patterns and decreased risk of colon and breast cancer.[26] But studies across the board recognize that it's tough to ascertain what else happens in life that makes a "healthy eater" less likely to get cancer. For instance, healthy eaters also tend to exercise more, maintain a normal body weight, and not smoke. All of these factors influence cancer risk.

We also know that inflammation influences cancer risk. One example is the connection between conditions such as chronic liver hepatitis, which can lead to scarring called cirrhosis, and liver cancer. Another example is the connection between chronic inflammation from ulcerative colitis and the increased risk of colorectal cancer: those with ulcerative colitis are twice as likely to get colorectal cancer as those who don't have inflammatory bowel disease. Chronic inflammation wears on the body and can turn good little immune system soldiers into rogue deviants if the inflammation is severe and chronic.

Inflammation directly from the diet also plays a role in cancer. It's been proposed that saturated fats, refined carbohydrates, and red meat may have proinflammatory properties, whereas the phytochemicals and flavonoids in plants like whole soy, whole grains, and legumes may have anti-inflammatory effects.[27]

Again we find ourselves in the situation of not knowing the exact prescription for which foods to eat to prevent cancer, but the research clearly paves a path for a plant-forward diet.

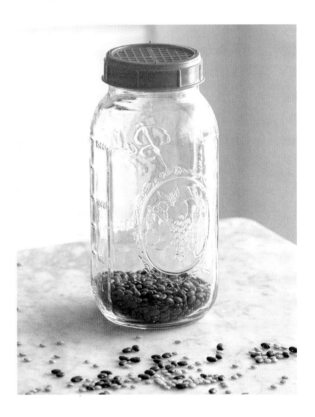

[24] See note 20 above.

[25] L. Schwingshackl, C. Schwedhelm, C. Galbete, and G. Hoffmann, "Adherence to Mediterranean diet and risk of cancer: an updated systematic review and meta-analysis," *Nutrients* 9, no. 10 (2017): 1063.

[26] G. Grosso, F. Bella, J. Godos, et al., "Possible role of diet in cancer: systematic review and multiple meta-analyses of dietary patterns, lifestyle factors, and cancer risk," *Nutrition Reviews* 75, no. 6 (2017): 405–19.

[27] M. Lopez-Alarcon, O. Perichart-Perera, and S. Flores-Huerta, "Excessive refined carbohydrates and scarce micronutrients intakes increase inflammatory mediators and insulin resistance in prepubertal and pubertal obese children independently of obesity," *Mediators of Inflammation* 2014: 849031; A. N. Samraj, O. M. Pearce, H. Laubli, et al., "A red meat-derived glycan promotes inflammation and cancer progression," *Proceedings of the National Academies of Sciences of the United States of America* 112, no. 2 (2015): 542–7; M. A. Islam, F. Alam, M. Solayman, et al., "Dietary phytochemicals: natural swords combating inflammation and oxidation-mediated degenerative diseases," *Oxidative Medicine and Cellular Longevity* 2016: 5137431; H. F. Jheng, M. Hirotsuka, T. Goto, et al., "Dietary low-fat soy milk powder retards diabetic nephropathy progression via inhibition of renal fibrosis and renal inflammation," *Molecular Nutrition & Food Research* 61, no. 3 (2017), epub 2016 Nov 29.

INFLAMMATION & MENTAL HEALTH

Now that I've covered a few of the major causes of death and shown a connection to reducing inflammation with diet, let's move on to some major obstacles to living a high-quality life. As you know, I'm not just about *quantity*, but also about *quality*.

Unaddressed and under-addressed mental health disorders such as anxiety, depression, and bipolar disorder are among the top causes of disability in the United States. Notice that I said unaddressed, not untreated. Doctors don't necessarily have to push drugs on those with anxiety and depression, but if these disorders are left unaddressed without some intervention—including psychotherapy and lifestyle modifications—then the burden on the person and on the greater healthcare system can be astronomical.

Mental health is often overlooked because it's not always physically apparent that a problem exists and because there's a huge stigma attached to diagnosis and treatment. I remember when a close friend of mine was diagnosed with depression when we were in college. She felt so defeated that she had a mental health diagnosis that needed to be addressed—in her case, with a combination of medication and psychotherapy—but I encouraged her to think about it from another point of view. If she had been having shortness of breath while running at the gym or in the context of a respiratory irritant like pollen, she would've gotten a workup for asthma and possibly been treated with an inhaler or antihistamines. The stigma of having asthma is completely different from the stigma of having a mental health issue. I encourage you to be gentle with yourself if you struggle with your mental health.

Emerging evidence is showing the connection of inflammation to mental health, and—just like the other conditions we've discussed—there's a food-based inflammatory component, too.

It turns out that it's not your fault that you crave potato chips when you're feeling sad or worried. The relationship between inflammatory food and mental illness is bidirectional. Not only does eating ultra-processed, calorie-dense, nutrient-deficient foods lead to body inflammation that increases the risk for mental illness like depression, but those who suffer from mental illness, especially depression, bipolar disorder, and schizophrenia, are more likely to reach for these same inflammatory foods compared to the general population, further increasing the body's inflammatory response.[28] New research is more clearly establishing the effect of an anti-inflammatory diet on conditions like depression along with the reduction of inflammation in various pharmaceutical and lifestyle interventions, including consistent exercise habits. Yet another reason for us to put on our walking shoes and go outside for a stroll.

This is an important topic, so I'll come back to caring for our mental health in Chapter 8, which discusses other nondiet healthy behaviors like sleep and exercise that are crucial to a balanced lifestyle.

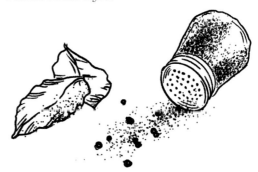

---

[28] J. Firth, N. Veronese, J. Cotter, et al., "What is the role of dietary inflammation in severe mental illness? A review of observation and experimental findings," *Frontiers in Psychiatry* 10 (2019): 350.

INFLAMMATION & DIGESTION

Digestion is a big deal. It is how the body takes the nutrients from what we eat and actually uses them. Digestion also moves out the pollution the body creates and no longer needs.

You may have heard that we are what we eat, but I think that's an incorrect idea. We aren't what we *eat;* we are what we *absorb.* And if we're not absorbing well, we're unable to reap the benefits of the foods we're eating.

How do you know if you're absorbing well? Take a look in the toilet bowl each morning and assess your stool. About once a day, sometimes more often, you get an opportunity to see how your digestion is working. In general, stool should be a uniform medium brown color, relatively smooth with some small cracks, and come out in one long piece. And it should be a relative nonevent in the day, meaning that once you get the urge to go, you head to the bathroom, do your business, and then move on with your life. Even if your stools look normal, if your digestion is accompanied by lots of bloating, gas (either malodorous or noisy), belching, coughing, throat irritation, heartburn, or abdominal pain, then something is not going well and needs to be addressed.

I see so many patients who face the consequences of poor absorption, like vitamin and mineral deficiencies, because their digestion is awry. Sometimes I feel like I should wear a button on my lapel that says, "Loose stools are not normal." Many of my patients have dealt with chronic diarrhea or constipation or uncomfortable bloating for years, especially if they are older or have been diagnosed with irritable bowel syndrome. They just accept that their bathroom difficulties are a fact of life.

Even though functional digestive issues are not listed separately as a major cause of disability in the chart on page 35, in my opinion they should be. When your digestion is off, it can upset your whole day. It's estimated that up to 15 percent of adults have irritable bowel syndrome,[29] and sometimes the symptoms are so severe that they prevent people from living their normal lives, like going to work or school, effectively parenting their children, or engaging in fun activities.

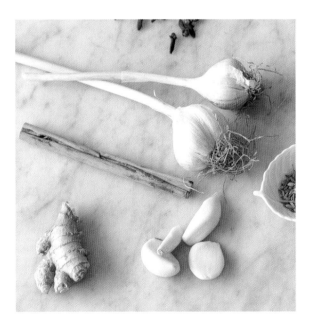

[29] A. C. Ford, P. Moayyedi, B. E. Lacy, et al., "American College of Gastroenterology monograph on the management of irritable bowel syndrome and chronic idiopathic constipation," *American Journal of Gastroenterology* 109, Suppl 1 (2014): S2–S6.

One of my favorite patients, Jim, is a great example of how life can change once digestive problems are addressed. Jim is a fifty-five-year-old father, community volunteer, and high school teacher who happened to have had rip-roaring watery diarrhea several times per day for the last several years, along with abdominal cramping and an inability to gain weight. His symptoms started slowly and progressively worsened over time, becoming so erratic and limiting that he was considering early retirement from teaching because his bowel movements were unpredictable and he felt crummy. Worst of all, he couldn't play golf because he didn't have access to a bathroom at a moment's notice.

Jim saw a gastroenterologist and had a colonoscopy, which showed some inflammation, but otherwise was given a diagnosis of irritable bowel syndrome. We did some investigative testing and started working together to adjust his diet and supplements along with some well-timed antibiotics followed by probiotics. Jim is one of my favorite patients because he is so compliant: whatever I asked him to do, he did in the service of feeling better. And get better he did! In a matter of months, he was having perfectly normal stools a few times per day without urgency or abdominal cramping. And he got back on the golf course, able to enjoy eighteen holes and a post-golf beer with his buddies without any issues.

Your digestive system does more than just absorb nutrients from food. A complex network of nerve fibers works with neurotransmitter signaling, just like in your brain. That's why the gut is called your "second brain" and whole books have been written about the brain-gut connection. Many of the neurotransmitters and hormones that are involved in the central nervous system also play a role in the gut, including serotonin. This is the same serotonin we talk about in regard to depression and anxiety and the target for a whole class of pharmaceutical drugs called selective serotonin re-uptake inhibitors (SSRIs). Serotonin is the "happiness hormone" that regulates moods, the ability to feel joy, sleep rhythms, and the desire for certain foods.

And where is serotonin made? Why, it's made by the gut microbiome.

The digestive tract is home to about 100 trillion harmonious little bacteria known as probiotics. These bacteria make up over two pounds of body weight and outnumber our own cells ten to one. They are crucial to healthy digestive function and carry out important functions like making about 95 percent of the body's serotonin. Yes, you read correctly! Most of our serotonin is not produced in the brain but in our digestive system. Our gut bacteria produce *hundreds* of neurochemicals that the brain uses to regulate basic physiological processes and mental processes like learning and memory in addition to mood regulation.[30]

Our probiotics are happiest when they are eating fiber-rich foods that are also rich in prebiotics. Prebiotics are nondigestible starches that are found in plants in the form of fiber. Fiber-rich foods like asparagus, onions, and garlic are especially yummy to probiotic bacteria. And after they eat those fiber-rich foods, they produce substances called short-chain fatty acids (SCFAs). SCFAs are your best friend because they act as little anti-inflammatory messengers, helping with everything from preserving gut wall integrity to aiding the immune system by preventing tumor growth and infections.[31] This is one way in which our digestive system aids in immune and inflammation surveillance.

---

[30] S. Carpenter, "That gut feeling," *Monitor on Psychology* 43, no. 8 (2012): 50.

[31] J. Tan, C. McKenzie, M. Potamitis, et al., "The role of short-chain fatty acids in health and disease," *Advances in Immunology* 121 (2014): 91–119.

Researchers are discovering new ways SCFAs positively influence our bodies every day, including their effect on lean body muscle maintenance, which ultimately has an impact on our metabolism and ability to maintain a healthy weight.[32] Isn't it interesting the ways in which the body encourages consumption of fiber-rich plants? Probiotics may also help fight obesity by releasing appetite-regulating hormones, further preventing weight gain.[33]

And, to boot, there's emerging evidence that probiotics reduce the calories we absorb from food by increasing dietary fat excretion in the stool.[34] We're getting smarter about connecting the types of probiotics to their direct effects, so stay tuned for more research connecting specific bacteria to weight loss and other beneficial processes in the body. The short story is that probiotics are the best thing since sliced bread!

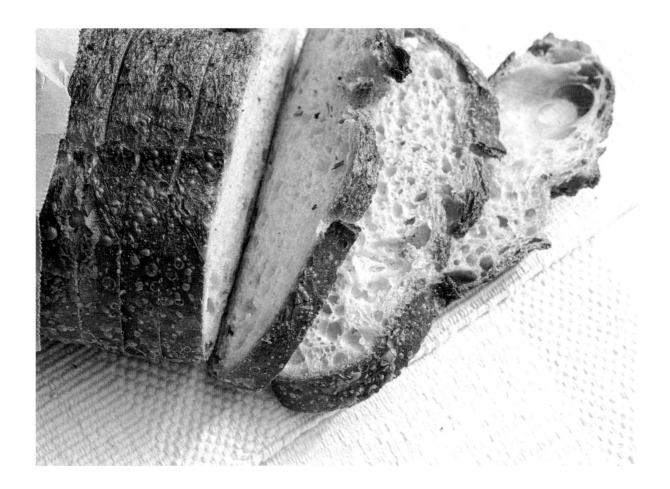

---

[32] J. Frampton, K. G. Murphy, G. Frost, and E. S. Chambers, "Short-chain fatty acids as potential regulators of skeletal muscle metabolism and function," *Nature Metabolism* 2 (2020): 840–8.

[33] M. Wicinski, J. Gebalski, J. Golebiewski, and B. Malinowski, "Probiotics for the treatment of overweight and obesity in humans—a review of clinical trials," *Microorganisms* 8, no. 8 (2020): 1148.

[34] A. Ogawa, T. Kobayashi, F. Sakai, et al., "Lactobacillus gasseri SBT2055 suppresses fatty acid release through engagement of fat emulsion size in vitro and promotes fecal fat excretion in healthy Japanese subjects," *Lipids in Health and Disease* 14 (2015): 20.

OTHER REASONS TO EAT A PLANT-FORWARD DIET

There are a whole host of reasons to consider a plant-forward diet other than the direct effect on your health and longevity. Two of those reasons are cost and environmental impact.

FINDING BALANCE IN YOUR GROCERY BUDGET

Straight up, eating plants is less expensive than eating animal protein, especially if you're opting for high-quality animal products. If you're just buying whatever animal protein is on sale at the grocery store, then maybe the difference in cost isn't apparent yet, but start to pay attention.

One easy-to-see example of the difference between plant and animal products is comparing proteins. I'll get into the details of protein in Chapter 3, but for now, let's look at making a soup with canned beans versus chicken. One can of high-quality organic beans ranges from $2.49 to $3.99 depending on where you live and shop, and one can will easily feed a family of four people. (In the Takayasu household, we buy beans by the case and store them in our basement because they make great weeknight protein additions to many dishes. In addition to ease, buying in bulk is helpful for your wallet.) The same basic pricing applies to tofu: you can feed a family of four with one block of organic tofu, which costs somewhere between $1.99 and $2.99.

Now, let's contrast beans and tofu to organic free-range chicken, which can range from $2.99 to $8.99 or more per pound depending on the cut and whether it's skinless or boneless. Sure, it's possible to find chicken at the supermarket for less than that, but I'd be wary of how it was raised and slaughtered. (I'll talk more about the care of animals in a bit.) Chicken is relatively inexpensive compared to other animal proteins like grass-fed, grass-finished, organic, free-range beef or wild-caught fish, which can cost upwards of $25 per pound. Patients give me a lot of pushback when I talk about buying high-quality animal products because they are so expensive.

One of the best pieces of advice I've heard about finding balance in your food budget is not to worry about spending more for high-quality animal protein because it's offset by the relatively low cost of plant protein. And since we eat a plant-forward diet, the balance is in our favor. It's easier to swallow $30-per-pound wild-caught halibut for dinner when you know your bean soup for lunch that fed four people cost only $10 and provided some leftovers.

Interestingly, our brains are evolutionarily trained to look for efficient sources of nutrition. We are not just drawn to processed foods like Oreos and Doritos because they are "hyper flavored." Our brains recognize that most processed foods are calorically dense, meaning they provide a lot of calories in a small quantity, and for not a lot of money. If you were truly cash-strapped, a package of Chips Ahoy would fit the bill because it gives you a lot of caloric energy for a low price.

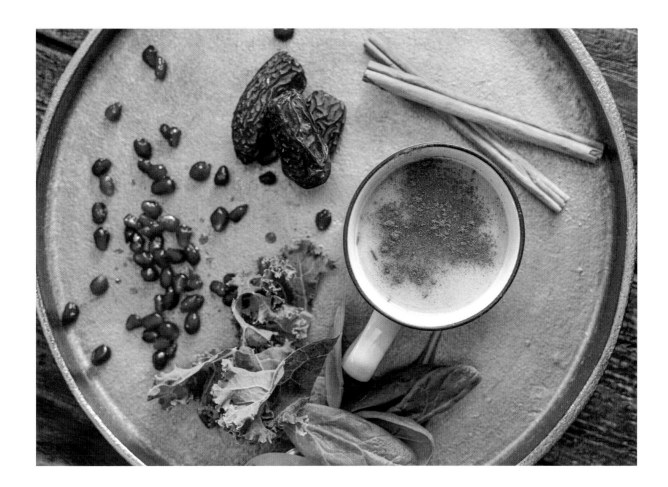

This brings me to food costs overall. Obviously, the point isn't to get as many calories as you can for the lowest cost, but to prioritize foods that meet your energy needs in a thoughtful way. We need to put our money into what really matters. And high-quality food matters a great deal. I'll talk more in Chapter 10 about how to prioritize organic and other important qualifiers that affect price when food shopping, but if you're interested in taking better care of your body, then you'll have to create space in your budget for better food.

Maybe this change in budget is not an overall increase in food spending but more of a reprioritizing of how you spend your money. Maybe you'll decide to eat more home-cooked meals, which are generally a lot less expensive (and healthier!) than prepared meals or take-out and certainly more cost-effective than dining at restaurants with waitstaff.

It's important to recognize, too, that there are ways to buy less expensive produce, including the use of frozen vegetables and fruit, which can go a long way toward improving your health and keeping you on budget.

Ultimately, however, you may need to spend more on food by spending less on something else that doesn't serve your well-being. Could you challenge yourself to find that opportunity? Perhaps it exists in a subscription content service that isn't very fulfilling, or in online shopping for items you don't really need. Leaning into time reading borrowed library books, taking an evening bath, staring into the eyes of a loved one, making a cup of tea, or meal planning how you're going to use all those vegetables you bought could serve you better and be impactful to your budget allowance for healthy food.

FINDING BALANCE FOR THE ENVIRONMENT

Overall, eating plants is better for the environment for two primary reasons: it takes less energy to produce them, and they put delicious oxygen back into the atmosphere naturally through photosynthesis.

Lots of books have been written about the environmental impact of raising animals for food, and I recommend reading them. One of my favorites, Michael Pollan's *The Omnivore's Dilemma,* was a game-changer in the way I viewed the Styrofoam packages of conventional chicken I had been buying at the grocery store.

I read *The Omnivore's Dilemma* as a medical student, and thereafter I found myself shifting my meager budget toward higher-quality animal protein in the service of the environment and my own health. Pollan frequently asserts that we have a "national eating disorder" because we have mass confusion about what to eat, made more difficult because we are omnivores who eat both plant and animal products. He focuses quite a bit of his book on the use of corn in our food system, both to feed industrial-raised livestock and as an additive (mostly in the form of high-fructose corn syrup) that provides sweetness and texture to ultra-processed foods.

In his book, Pollan tells the story of following a specific steer through its life cycle as it's sold to a feedlot in Kansas at six months old and then "grain finished" with a diet of corn to fatten it up quickly.[35] Grain finishing allows for rapid weight gain and produces the kind of marbled meat Americans want. Grain finishing presents a problem because cow stomachs are designed to digest grass. When cows are fed grains, a few bad things happen.

First, because cows lack starch-digesting enzymes in their digestive tracts, feeding them a grain-heavy diet requires farmers to use more antibiotics to prevent the overgrowth of dangerous bacteria and the formation of liver abscesses. (*Abscess* is a nice medical word for pus that develops in places it shouldn't. Gross!) And whatever cows are given is passed to us in the food chain. So if we eat conventional hamburger for dinner, some antibiotics may make their way downstream into our bodies. Passive antibiotics like this are problematic because we have issues with superbugs and antibiotic resistance and because our own microbiomes take a hit. And I just talked about why the microbiome is so important!

Second, grain-finished cattle produce toxic waste products that contain heavy metals and hormone residues. This manure is unsuitable for typical use as fertilizer for crops due to its high nitrogen and phosphorus levels, thus preventing farmers from using the normal life cycle of animals and plants to keep each other going.

Interestingly, Pollan also finds issues with industrial organic farms, which end up using more fossil fuels to balance the inefficiencies of producing large amounts of organic food without chemical pesticides and fertilizers. In his book, he ultimately finds a small, self-sustaining organic farm considered to be a "closed system" where the land is constantly revitalized by the nutrient-dense plants and animals fostered there. What Pollan ultimately advocates for is a deeper connection to our food and an understanding of where it comes from.

If you read the introduction to this book, then you know I grew up among the fields and farms of the rural Midwest. I'm sensitive to smaller animal farmers who do it right, allowing their larger livestock to graze on nutritious, biodiverse, open-grass pastures, where smaller animals like chickens follow and eat the manure and bugs and continue to fertilize

---

[35] M. Pollan, *The Omnivore's Dilemma* (New York: Penguin Books, 2006).

and give back to the land. I'm also aware of the many mass-production farms that give farming a bad reputation and put food into our supply chain that is neither responsibly raised nor good for us.

We all recognize that harmony in the environment serves the human good. My goal for all of life—whether human, animal, or plant—is to be in balance. In my opinion, animal and plant farming done in the right *relationship* to each other on smaller farms that prioritize excellent, nutrient-dense inputs and outputs along with a connection between producer and consumer is the best way to eat well.

I love knowing my spring, summer, and fall produce from the community-supported agriculture (CSA) organization that delivers to our town library each week is grown at a small farm only an hour away. It's not always convenient to get a random rutabaga in my farm share box when I would've preferred carrots, but having locally grown organic produce from a farm I feel connected to is important to me. It reminds me that having asparagus flown in from Argentina in the winter is a luxury. And having some new-to-me produce like fiddlehead ferns, garlic scapes, and purslane has challenged me to be more creative with my cooking and has given me ideas for many new recipes.

> "My goal for all of life—*whether human, animal, or plant*—is to be in balance."

CHOOSING PLANTS MAKES THE MOST SENSE

So why eat plants?

Simply because it makes the most sense. When we look at all of the research on longevity, quality of life, inflammation, cardiovascular and metabolic disease, obesity, cancer, mental health, hormone regulation, and digestion, along with cost and environmental impact, our best strategy is to eat a plant-rich diet that de-emphasizes animal products and nearly eliminates ultra-processed foods and sugar.

So let's talk about how to make that happen.

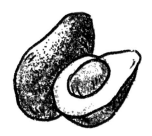

CHAPTER 2

CONCERNS ABOUT A PLANT-FORWARD DIET

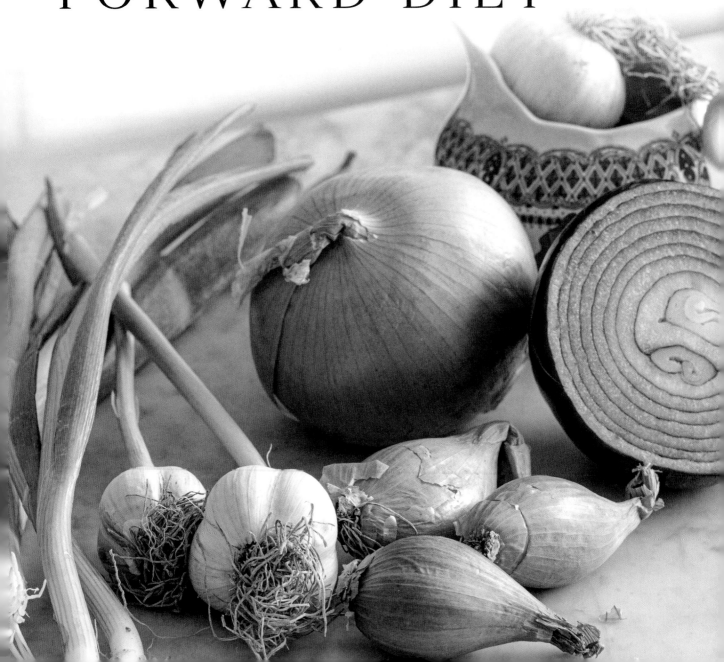

There are a few things to be mindful of when choosing a plant-forward diet. Advocates of other ways of eating may try to dissuade you from eating less animal protein, but I view this as fake news. I don't recommend a 100 percent plant-based diet because I find it too limiting, but I want you to be mindful of five myths about a plant-rich lifestyle.

MYTH #1: YOU CAN'T GET ENOUGH PROTEIN FROM PLANTS

Truth: **Thoughtful plant-forward meals provide the protein we need.**

The most common issue with prioritizing plants in the diet is making sure you get enough protein. I'll talk more about protein in Chapter 3, but for now, let's just get the protein conversation started.

It's entirely possible to get enough protein from plants, but eating plant protein is not as *efficient* as eating animal protein. Because plants are generally a more balanced mix of the macronutrients carbohydrate (including all-important fiber) and protein, they pack a lot of different kinds of nutrition in one package. That's, of course, why I like them! But that can make it challenging to get enough of each macronutrient because you can't simply categorize something like beans as a protein as you can chicken.

For example, one 3-ounce serving of chicken has about 25 grams of protein, which is about one-third to one-half the amount of protein the average person needs in a day. Contrast that to one serving of one-half cup of lentils, which has only about 9 grams of protein, or one-quarter cup of almonds, which has only about 6 grams of protein.

MACRONUTRIENT COMPARISON OF CHICKEN, LENTILS, AND ALMONDS

	Serving Size	Calories	Protein	Fat	Carbohydrate	Fiber
Chicken	3 ounces	204	24g	12g	0g	0g
Lentils	½ cup	140	12g	0.5g	23g	9g
Almonds	¼ cup	220	8g	18g	7g	4g

It's important to point out that lentils and almonds are also significant sources of fiber, the indigestible starch found in plant foods that's your best friend because it helps with digestion, cholesterol and blood sugar control, and satiety and lowers the risk of several types of cancer. While it's true that ounce for ounce, chicken is a more efficient source of protein, it doesn't hold a candle to lentils or almonds when it comes to fiber content.

That said, it's crucial to get both the right *amount* and the right *kind* of protein. I see a lot of patients overeating protein in an effort to eat "low carb." This is a form of orthorexia, a term given to behavior marked by an unhealthy focus on eating in a healthy way, where a person categorically avoids some foods and overeats others. I see many people eating over 100 grams of protein per day when most of us need only 55 to 70 grams if we're of average height and weight. Eating too much protein can be a problem for your kidneys, and it can be stored as body fat if eaten in excess.

The right kind of protein matters, too. Variety is the spice of life, especially when it comes to protein sources. I don't want you to eat beans at every meal. You can't eat any one plant-forward protein exclusively because it won't provide all the amino acid building blocks you need. Twenty different amino acids become the building blocks of protein in our bodies. Some of these we can make on our own, but others we need to consume in our foods. The ones we need to consume are called *essential* amino acids, and it takes a variety of plant-based proteins to create the right balance in the body. For example, beans are missing the essential amino acid methionine. But–guess what?–Nature has a solution. Grains, nuts, and seeds all have methionine, so if you had some steel-cut oatmeal for breakfast this morning, then your dinner of black bean chili would put you in balance for the day.

Animal proteins are said to be complete proteins because they have all of the essential amino acids. But remember, you can be complete if you eat a variety of plant and animal proteins in the right balance. And since I advocate eating a modest amount of animal protein, you'll get all the protein you need in the right balance.

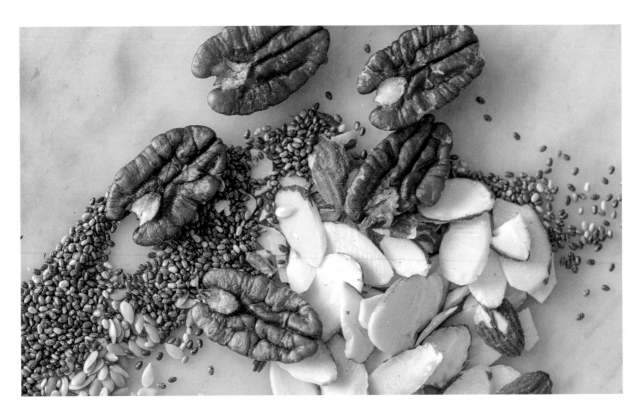

MYTH #2:
YOU'LL DEVELOP VITAMIN B$_{12}$ & VITAMIN D DEFICIENCIES IF YOU DON'T EAT MEAT

Truth: **Most of us need to supplement with vitamins B$_{12}$ and D$_3$.**

Here's the truth: you need vitamin B$_{12}$ in your diet to make healthy red blood cells and support your nervous system, and only a few plant foods, like seaweed, mushrooms, and nutritional yeast, naturally contain B$_{12}$. Vitamin B$_{12}$ is made by anaerobic bacteria in the gut, and animals naturally make it in their gastrointestinal tracts and absorb it. If you eat animal protein, then you naturally get some vitamin B$_{12}$.

So that means people who eat animal protein have sufficient B$_{12}$ levels, right?

Not so fast. Interestingly, I find deficient and insufficient vitamin B$_{12}$ levels in lots of my patients, whether or not they eat meat. How can that be? Just like many other processes in the body, vitamin B$_{12}$ absorption is a complex process that only starts with consuming the vitamin. Absorption of B$_{12}$ is dependent on age, strength of stomach acid, use of pharmaceutical medications like metformin or acid-blockers, history of prior bowel surgery, damage to the gut lining from autoimmune conditions like Crohn's, infections like *Helicobacter pylori,* and bacterial overgrowth, just to name a few.[1]

So you might wonder if you should supplement with vitamin B$_{12}$ regardless of whether you eat plants. The answer is maybe. How do you know if you need to supplement? You can easily check your level with your doctor.

Another vitamin that plant-forward eaters need to be knowledgeable about is vitamin D because it is naturally found almost exclusively in animal products, like the oily fish herring, mackerel, salmon, and sardines, as well as egg yolks, red meat, and liver, especially from lambs. (Porcini mushrooms are a plant-based source.) It's also added to a lot of foods, such as milk (this is why your milk carton says "vitamin A & D fortified") and breakfast cereal, to help the public get more of this essential nutrient.

You may ask the same question about whether vitamin D deficiencies are more common in people who don't eat animal products. Just as with vitamin B$_{12}$, I see a lot of patients with vitamin D deficiencies and insufficiencies. In fact, except in rare cases, I see lower-than-recommended vitamin D levels in almost every patient who is not taking a vitamin D supplement.

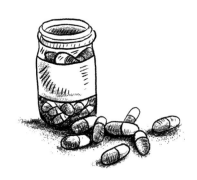

---

[1] R. Obeid, S. G. Heil, M. Verhoeven, et al., "Vitamin B$_{12}$ intake from animal foods, biomarkers, and health aspects," *Frontiers in Nutrition* 6 (2019): 93.

Why are vitamin D levels almost universally a problem? It's not because people are not eating animal products. It's because the best way to get vitamin D is to step outside, and most of us live our lives without spending as much time in the sunshine as we need.

Vitamin D is known as the sunshine vitamin because it's naturally created in our bodies upon exposure to sunlight, and the best way to increase vitamin D levels is to expose a good amount of skin to the sun for at least twenty minutes every day. This presents a problem for many of us, including me. I live in Connecticut, where it's only comfortable to be outside in a tank top and shorts for about three months of the year. And of course, we are all concerned about skin cancer and wrinkles, so we tend to lather up with sunscreen (which is good for us!), but sunscreen doesn't allow our bodies the exposure to sunlight they need.

It's important to get vitamin D because it's crucial to the absorption of other important nutrients like calcium, iron, magnesium, phosphorus, and zinc through the gut. Poor vitamin D levels are associated with all kinds of health problems, including heart disease, cognitive impairment, asthma, cancer, and the bone-softening condition called rickets. So get your bum in the sun for ten to twenty minutes a day in the summer, take a vitamin D_3 supplement in the fall, winter, and spring, and eat some yummy salmon once a week.

For more on supplementing with key vitamins and minerals when eating a plant-rich diet, turn to Chapter 9.

MYTH #3: YOU NEED CALCIUM FROM DAIRY FOR HEALTHY BONES

Truth: **Preventing fractures requires vitamins, minerals, strength, and good balance.**

It's true, calcium is important for bone health. This is because calcium gives our bones the structure and strength they need to support our physical bodies. Interestingly, our bones are the primary storage space for the calcium needed for other crucial functions, like heart and skeletal muscle function and nerve signaling. Our bodies keep blood calcium in a narrow range, storing and using calcium from the bones as needed to maintain that balance. I think it's fascinating to realize that our bones are constantly being remodeled, with new bone forming from osteoblast cells and other bone being broken down by osteoclast cells. If we make as much bone as we break down, our total bone mass remains in check, thus preventing the type of bone loss we see in conditions like osteoporosis.

Where do we get calcium? You may remember the campaigns from the 1980s in which the dairy industry convinced us that milk "does a body good," advocating that we need dairy products to supply adequate calcium. But that's not the whole story. Studies including the Women's Health Initiative, which followed 36,000 postmenopausal women, showed that those who supplemented with calcium and vitamin D$_3$ were no less likely to break a hip compared to women who took a placebo (but were more likely to have kidney stones from the extra calcium), so the jury is still out on the connection of calcium to osteoporosis.[2]

We do know that a certain amount of calcium is needed to keep the body functioning. It probably does not come as a surprise that you can get adequate calcium from plants if you're mindful about it. After all, we are able to get calcium from dairy because cows eat grass. Those powerful grass greens have calcium that is pushed into the cows' milk so that their baby calves get all the nutrients they need to grow big and strong.

The trick is that getting calcium from plant sources is not as efficient as getting it from dairy. Depending on our age and gender, most of us need roughly 1,000 milligrams of calcium per day. Children and women who are pregnant or breastfeeding need more calcium to support growth. Generally, each source of dairy in our diet gives us somewhere in the neighborhood of 200 to 450 milligrams of calcium. A few plant sources, including green vegetables like spinach, Swiss chard, and collard greens, offer a similar amount; it's just that we need to eat a good-sized portion.

PLANT FOODS NATURALLY HIGH IN CALCIUM

Food	Serving Size	Estimated Calcium
Collard greens, frozen	1 cup	360 mg
Sesame seeds, roasted	¼ cup	351 mg
Tofu*	3½ ounces	350 mg
Figs, dried, uncooked	1 cup	300 mg
Spinach, cooked	1 cup	240 mg
Almonds	¼ cup	189 mg
Blackstrap molasses	1 tablespoon	180 mg
Broccoli, cooked	1 cup	180 mg
Kale, frozen	1 cup	180 mg
Bok choy, cooked	1 cup	160 mg
Amaranth, cooked	½ cup	135 mg
Arugula, raw	1 cup	125 mg
Chard or okra, cooked	1 cup	100 mg

*Tofu is high in calcium (one-half cup has a whopping 434 milligrams!) because it's made by curdling pressed soybeans with calcium salts, making it a fortified source of calcium rather than a natural one. You should eat it because it's delicious and because it's a good calcium source.

[2] R. D. Jackson, A. Z. LaCroix, M. Gass, et al., "Calcium plus vitamin D supplementation and the risk of fractures," *New England Journal of Medicine* 354 (2006): 669–83.

DAIRY IS NOT A SEPARATE FOOD GROUP

This brings me to a key piece of advice about dairy: it's not a separate food group. Adults ingrained in me as a kid that I needed to drink milk or have another source of dairy a few times a day. Even today, dairy has its place on the United States Department of Agriculture's MyPlate graphic. In my opinion, dairy should be used as a flavoring for food in the same way that spices are. It creates a depth of flavor that sometimes tastes delicious. But dairy may be obesogenic, meaning that it makes us gain weight, and it's energetically stagnating.[3] Even ancient Chinese Medicine teaches about how dairy creates dampness in the body and that stickiness prevents the free flow of Qi, our vital life energy.

Cows (along with sheep and goats) make milk to feed their babies—to make little cows into big, fat cows. But we are not cows, and we don't want to grow big and fat. Humans drink human milk, and we are weaned from that when we are small children. So let's not eat a lot of dairy. It just doesn't make sense. A little can go a long way in enhancing flavor without all the negatives.

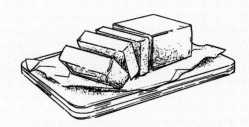

A side note about osteopenia and osteoporosis, because so many of us are given this diagnosis: Osteoporosis is generally not inherently a problem. There are, of course, stories of people with less dense bones suffering fractures while walking or turning their bodies with exactly the wrong torque, but that kind of standing fracture is uncommon. Osteoporosis usually leads to fracture when someone falls, and that fall is usually from a normal height. Anyone can break a bone by falling off a ladder, but most people don't break a bone if they trip and fall unless they have weak bones. So, logically, it seems that not getting yourself into a situation where you can fall is important. If you came to this conclusion, you're right!

So let's talk about my trifecta for fall prevention: we need to be strong, we need to have good balance, and we need to stay safe in our environment. Being strong, having good balance, and preventing safety hazards are imperative to preventing falls, even if our bone density is not perfect. Think about how you can design your life to include activities that build muscle, like squats; train yourself to have better balance, such as by doing yoga; and use rugs with anti-slip mats underneath to prevent trips and falls. (See Chapter 8 for more on movement.)

So here's the take-home on calcium and bone health: eat greens and do some yoga.

---

[3] C. S. Berkey, H. R. H. Rockett, W. C. Willett, et al., "Milk, dairy fat, dietary calcium, and weight gain: a longitudinal study of adolescents," *Archives of Pediatric and Adolescent Medicine* 159, no. 6 (2005): 543–50.

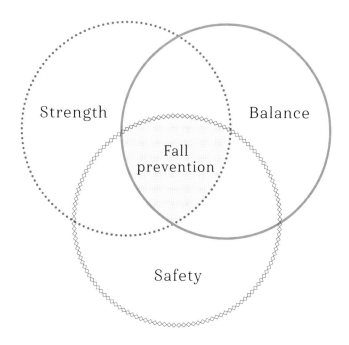

MYTH #4:
YOU NEED IRON FROM MEAT

Truth: **Plants have iron.**

Like calcium, iron is an essential mineral that needs attention if you're following a plant-forward diet. And, just like calcium, it's not that difficult to get iron from plants; it's just a bit more efficient to get iron from animal sources.

Iron is an essential nutrient because it's a building block of hemoglobin, the oxygen-carrying protein in our red blood cells. Iron deficiency anemia occurs when iron is low enough to affect the body's ability to produce normal red blood cells.

Iron is also important to metabolism because it's a component of myoglobin, a protein that provides oxygen to muscles. Iron is necessary for growth and development, which is why young children are routinely checked for anemia.

While iron is important for everyone, it's especially important for growing children (who need from 7 to 15 milligrams of elemental iron per day) and women who are pregnant and breastfeeding (because they are nourishing growing babies, requiring up to 27 milligrams per day). Getting enough iron is extra critical for premenopausal women because of monthly blood loss during the menstrual period, so they require 18 milligrams per day.

The real difference between iron from plants and animals is the type. Many people think of iron-rich foods being exclusively from animal sources like red meat. In truth, dietary iron comes in two forms: heme and nonheme. Plants and fortified foods contain nonheme iron. Iron bioavailability is a bit better from animal sources, but you can increase the amount of iron your body absorbs by consuming it along with vitamin C, which is present in most vegetables and fruits. You can definitely get your daily requirement of iron from plants such as spinach, beans, nuts, apricots, blackstrap molasses, and lentils, but a small amount of animal protein would help you get what you need, too.

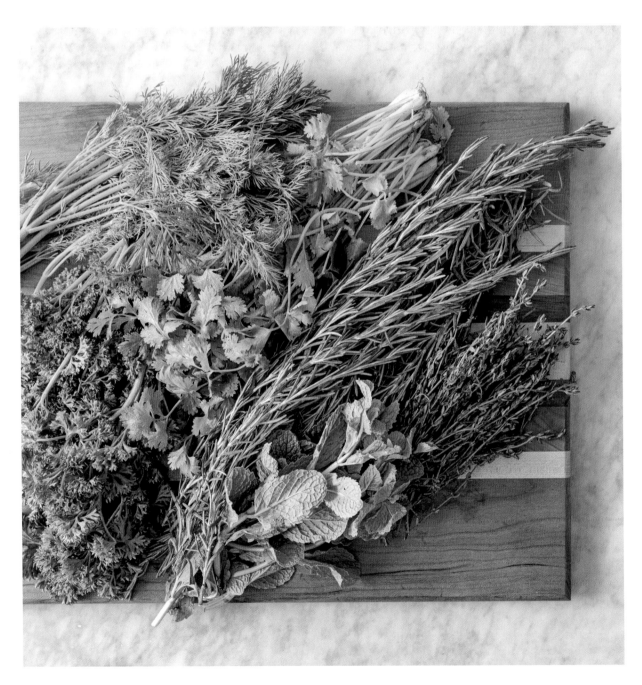

MYTH #5:
YOU DON'T HAVE TIME
TO COOK THIS WAY

Truth: **Creativity in the kitchen equals self-care.**

One of the biggest issues people have with plant-forward eating is the time involved in cooking this kind of food. When we make plants the stars of the mealtime show, the preparation usually takes longer. After all, cleaning and chopping vegetables takes a lot of time and some muscle. I'm a big fan of using shortcuts like pretrimmed and prechopped vegetables, pressure-cooked canned beans, and pre-sprouted grains, but I recognize that making a plant-forward meal generally takes more time than throwing a steak on the grill.

Where does this time come from? We all have the same number of hours in a day. If you want to commit to a plant-forward lifestyle, you will have to spend a little more time in the kitchen and develop some skills with knives and cooking. The good news is that it doesn't require a *lot* more time or skill, just a little. It takes a little reprioritizing and a little elbow grease. When you're tired and busy, this kind of commitment can be hard. And it can seem selfish.

I share some tips with you in Chapter 10 about how to make yourself more efficient in the kitchen so that your time investment is high yield. I want to spend a minute here talking about the fact that investing in yourself in the form of plant-forward eating can seem self-indulgent. We all have unhelpful thoughts that fly through our brains, like "How can I take this much time for myself when I have so much to do at work?" or "I could change my eating habits if I were single, but now I'm a busy mom," but on the precipice of this plant-forward journey, I want you to think about how you treat yourself.

Eating well is a form of self-care. When we eat well, we feel physically, emotionally, and mentally better, and we exist in the world as better humans.

What would it look like if you showed up each day knowing that you're taking care of yourself the best way you can given the resources you have? Even if your plant-forward meals are not ideal, there's benefit to you in *trying* something new and *starting* the shift. And that benefit is knowing you're treating your body the best way you can.

Trust me, the body keeps the score.

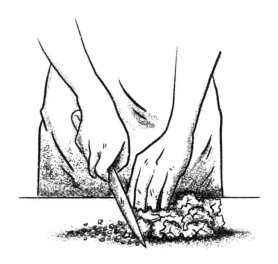

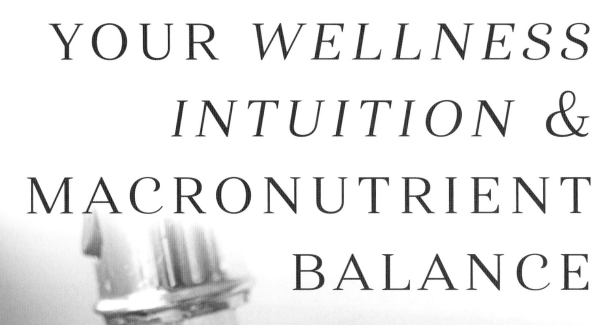

CHAPTER 3

YOUR *WELLNESS INTUITION* & MACRONUTRIENT BALANCE

This is where we put the pedal to the metal—where we take the science and start to make it practical.

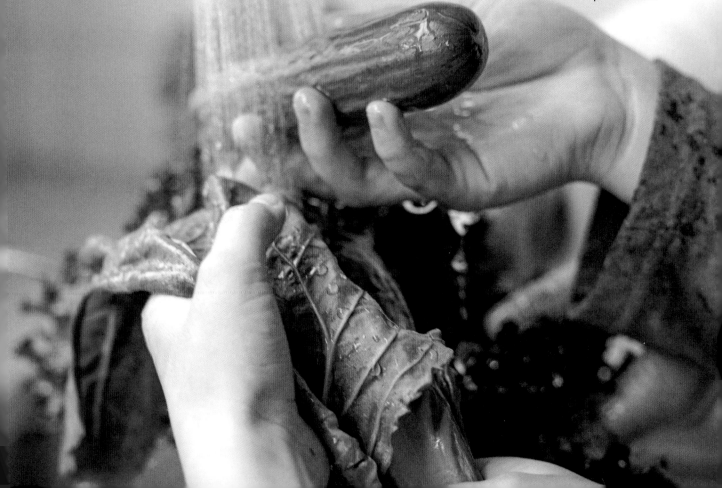

So far I've spent a lot of time digging into the science-backed health, social, and environmental reasons why you should consider a plant-forward diet. And now you know that inflammation is the root cause of so many diseases, disorders, and disabilities that have the potential to affect your everyday life. If you've made it this far, you are not only interested in extending your years on this planet but also invested in making those years matter.

When talking about finding balance on our plates, it's important to point out that we eat food, not isolated protein, carbohydrates, fats, vitamins, and minerals.

We live in a culture of pinpointing the thing that does the thing that does the thing. This reductionist approach is a hallmark of Western medicine and a differentiator in the global approach of Integrative Medicine. The food we eat is a myriad of biochemistry. We are shifting away from focusing on individual nutrients to thinking more holistically about food.

Take, for example, the humble kidney bean. Is it a protein? Is it a carb? The answer to both questions is yes. A kidney bean's calories are about 27 percent protein and 72 percent slow-burning complex carbohydrate, with a nice dose of fiber and a little fat, along with some vitamins like K1 and minerals like folate, iron, and copper. Kidney beans are great, but how do you know if they'll work for you? After all, not every suggestion in this book will work for everyone. This is where your *Wellness Intuition* comes in.

YOUR *WELLNESS INTUITION*

Your *Wellness Intuition* is the unique combination of foods and self-care rituals that makes your body feel great. This is my take on the idea of superfoods being supercharged by lifestyle rhythms, because it takes general recommendations a step further to the individual level. I encourage you to personalize the recommendations in this book to your specific nutritional needs, taste preferences, and lifestyle.

As a nutrient-dense food and balanced lifestyle enthusiast, I think it's important to find which foods and biorhythms feel best in your body. But the only way to know how something feels is to try a modest amount of it and then reflect on its effect.

I encourage you to pay attention to the tiny body signals that we often overlook because we're too busy or it's inconvenient. There's important information to be garnered from the positive and negative signs our bodies give us. The negative signs are generally louder than the positive ones. Most times we don't notice the positive signals and chalk them up to being par for the course.

We tend to pay more attention to negative signs because they're annoying. I mean, unless you're a chronic headache sufferer, how often do you walk around noticing that you *don't* have a headache? Maybe never. We generally don't praise our bodies for the amazing things they do, like *not* having a headache. But how annoyed are you when you *do* get a headache and it wrecks your whole day?

If you have a hard time identifying the positive signals your body is giving you, like increased focus on difficult tasks, a high energy level in the middle of the afternoon, or a perfect poop in the morning, don't give up hope. Start by paying attention to the negative signals. These louder signals range from digestive to neurological to allergy symptoms. Once you've noticed those bigger signals, you can more easily identify the finer details in your body.

Here's a global look at some of the negative signals we tend to notice:

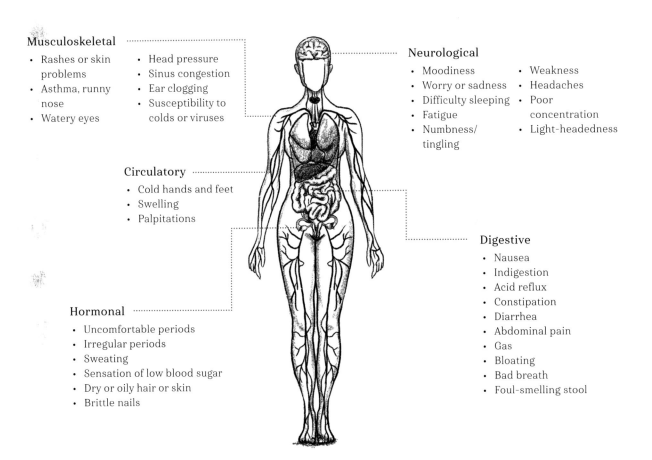

Musculoskeletal

- Rashes or skin problems
- Asthma, runny nose
- Watery eyes

- Head pressure
- Sinus congestion
- Ear clogging
- Susceptibility to colds or viruses

Neurological

- Moodiness
- Worry or sadness
- Difficulty sleeping
- Fatigue
- Numbness/tingling

- Weakness
- Headaches
- Poor concentration
- Light-headedness

Circulatory

- Cold hands and feet
- Swelling
- Palpitations

Digestive

- Nausea
- Indigestion
- Acid reflux
- Constipation
- Diarrhea
- Abdominal pain
- Gas
- Bloating
- Bad breath
- Foul-smelling stool

Hormonal

- Uncomfortable periods
- Irregular periods
- Sweating
- Sensation of low blood sugar
- Dry or oily hair or skin
- Brittle nails

Whew, that's quite a list! And there are likely even more signs to notice if you pay attention.

Sometimes the signs from our bodies are profound and noticeable, like someone banging on the front door. Other times the signs are just quiet knocks. Generally, it takes changing your diet and lifestyle to start noticing these quieter signs. Then you can start to alter your habits to reflect your idiosyncrasies.

One example of someone discovering her *Wellness Intuition* is my patient Jennifer, a forty-seven-year-old teacher and mom of two.

She loves vegetable gardening and experimenting in the kitchen, so she's always been an avid home cook and eaten relatively healthy meals, maintaining a normal weight. But then perimenopause started, and her periods became irregular. Soon she was feeling hot, especially at night, which interrupted her sleep, and she put on a few pounds around her midsection that gave her "a little muffin top," as she liked to call it. She also had chronic low back pain that seemed to be getting worse despite regular acupuncture appointments.

Jennifer decided to do my ten-day *Dr. Katie Detox*, where we spend ten days homing in on nutrient-dense food and the lifestyle habits of joyful exercise, prioritization of rest, and connection to the Spiritual Self. After the detox, she walked into my office and announced that she had never felt better, and she was convinced that dairy was not her friend. After ten days of eating a super clean diet, she decided to treat herself to some yummy cheese from her favorite shop in town. When she woke up the next morning, her back was killing her, but she hadn't done the usual things that caused her back pain, like weeding in the garden or standing too long on the ceramic floor in her kitchen without wearing her supportive slippers. So she tested her theory a few more times, and she was right: consuming any kind of dairy made her back hurt.

So how does Jennifer live authentically in her *Wellness Intuition?* She doesn't eat much dairy, and when she does, she knows she'll feel it in her low back for a few days, but then it passes and she moves on with her life.

Do you have a sign in your body like Jennifer does—something pleasant or unpleasant that you just can't put your finger on? Perhaps you'll discover what it is in the course of reading this book. Or maybe you'll come to find that eating a plant-rich, whole-foods diet combined with mindful self-care practices will help you feel more energetic, prevent the usual winter colds that everyone else gets, and manage your menstrual period without spending the first day in bed in the fetal position wrapped around a heating pad.

That said, it's important for me to state that if I make a recommendation in this book that does not suit you, you should not follow it. If you read about all the amazing benefits of whole organic soy and you know it gives you hives, then I don't want you to eat it. That's your body telling you something, and our bodies have an innate wisdom that is superior to any doctor-advised education. Listening to your *Wellness Intuition* is not about judgment of good or bad, but a recognition of how your external environment affects your internal self.

You can still live an amazing plant-rich life even if you never eat edamame, I promise.

Likewise, in the next section, I give specific recommendations about the ideal balance of protein, fat, and carbohydrate in your diet. If you know that you need more protein to feel satiated, then adjust your macronutrients to reflect your Intuition. I find that I require a certain amount of dietary fat in my meals to feel anchored and satisfied, so I adjust my macronutrients to reflect that need. I also find that if I don't engage in a regular practice of daily movement and yoga, I start to act moody around my husband and boys, so I make sure to build that activity into my life. How did I figure out that I needed more fat in my diet and yoga classes a few times a week? I experimented and listened to the wisdom my body shared with me. Your body will share that wisdom, too. You just have to listen for it.

Alright, now that you've got your *Wellness Intuition* spyglasses on, let's talk about macronutrients, the building blocks of what you're going to eat.

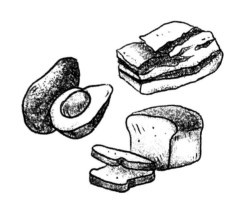

"Listening to your *Wellness Intuition* is not about judgment of good or bad, but a **recognition** of how your external environment affects your internal self."

MACRONUTRIENTS

The macronutrients protein, fat, and carbohydrate are the building blocks of our nutritional habits. Put simply, they are the energy and nutrients we need in large quantities. You can imagine them as large blocks. Next to these large macronutrient blocks are smaller blocks—these are our micronutrients. Micronutrients are the vitamins and minerals that our bodies need in tiny amounts to create magic from the macronutrients we eat. The small micronutrient blocks work together in different combinations to make up the insides of the macronutrient blocks, thus meeting our bodies' individual nutritional needs depending on what we're eating.

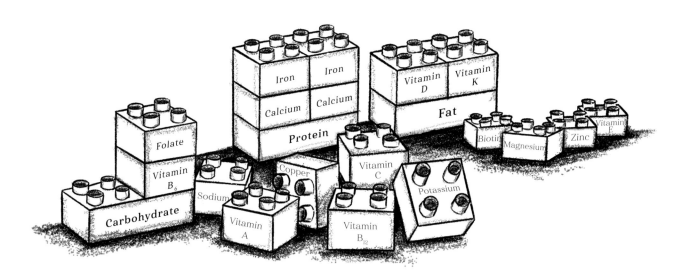

Each macronutrient has multiple functions in the body. Proteins are the backbone of our tissue structures and enzymatic pathways. Fats provide satiety, serve as our energy reserve and insulation, and protect our vital organs. Carbohydrates are converted to sugar that's necessary for meeting our bodies' energy requirements. The three work in harmony to help us feel satisfied and well.

As I've discussed, most plant-forward food choices are not simply carbohydrates or protein or fat. That's the beauty of eating more plants—you hit all of the goals at once when you find the right combination. But it's also harder to figure out what you need because you can't do simple math of 1 + 1 + 1 = 3. In the plant world, it's more like this:

$$0.3 + 0.7 + 0.5 + 0.5 + 0.97 + 0.03 = 3$$

You get to the same answer; it's just a little more convoluted. But that's why you're reading this book. I'm going to talk you through it!

I would like to give you a hard-and-fast rule about how much of your plate should be protein, how much should be fat, and how much should be carbohydrate, but I can't. Why? Because I don't live in your body or know your individual *Wellness Intuition*. But I can give you some general recommendations.

Here's a place to start: your diet should be about 15 percent protein, 30 percent fat, and 55 percent carbohydrates. So, if you're an average lady eating 1,800 calories, start with about 270 calories from protein, 540 calories from fat, and 990 calories from carbohydrates.

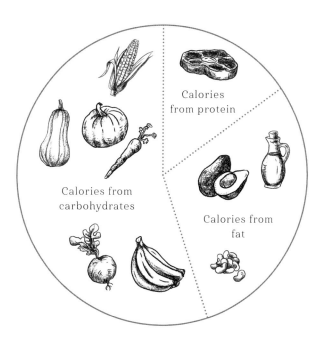

I also offer you a range in which to operate. This goes back to listening to your *Wellness Intuition*. If you need more protein and fat, for example, then decrease your allotment of carbohydrates.

Macronutrient	Range	Suggested Start	Calories per Gram	1,800-Calorie Diet	Grams per Day for an 1,800-Calorie Diet
Protein	10–35%	15%	4	270 calories	68
Fat	20–35%	30%	9	540 calories	60
Carbohydrates	45–65%	55%	4	990 calories	248

FIBER, FAT & PROTEIN

Honestly, I find the macronutrient way of thinking about food entirely too confining. And all the numbers make my head spin a little. I recognize, however, that there are many readers out there who like numbers and specifics.

What makes more intuitive sense to me is thinking about how to construct a plate of food. After all, we don't eat blocks of protein; we eat salmon and beans and edamame. I prefer that you think about finding balance on your physical plate. Each meal should be a mix of fiber, fat, and protein. Notice that I used the word *fiber* instead of *carbohydrates,* since you're looking for fiber-rich carbs, not highly processed ones. (You'll find more on that a bit later.)

Using a visual approach allows for a holistic view of how we build harmony in the body with our food choices.

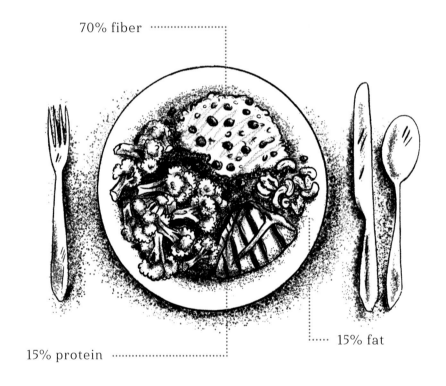

70% fiber

15% protein

15% fat

Think about this graphic in terms of the *real estate on your plate,* not percentages of calories. Just as I don't like counting grams of macronutrients, I don't like counting calories, either. In fact, I haven't counted calories since I revamped my lifestyle at the start of my own plant-forward journey. It took me a long time to figure out, but listening to my hunger and satiety cues has naturally regulated my appetite and my weight and has given me a greater sense of balance and control. Part of that listening is building my plate to look like this graphic at almost every meal.

Another reason I don't like the reductionist view of counting macronutrients is that it silos our thinking about food. After all, you can't sit with a calculator tallying up what you're eating. Doing so can lead to overgeneralizations about vegetables or beans being only carbohydrates or walnuts being only fat. As I talked about at the beginning of this chapter, beans are a beautiful mix of protein *and* carbohydrate, and walnuts are a delicious combination of all three macronutrients. When I construct a salad for lunch, I think about the fact that walnuts are a bit of protein, a fiber-rich carbohydrate, and a healthy dose of omega-3-rich fats, along with essential nutrients my body needs. (In case you're wondering, those essential nutrients happen to be biotin, manganese, molybdenum, and vitamins E and B_6.) The beauty of plants is that they generally cross two or even all three macronutrient categories.

Carbohydrates   Proteins   Fats

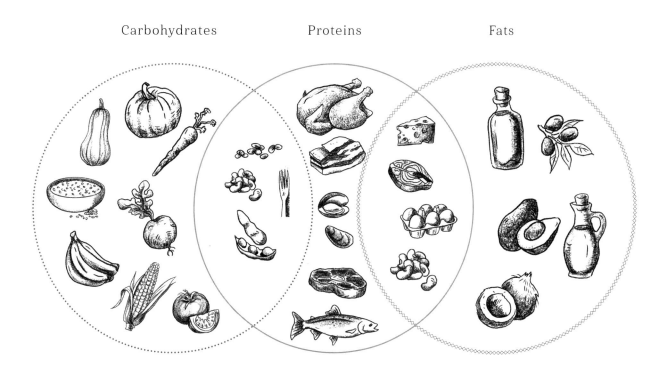

Even though I don't like the silo-thinking of macronutrient *counting*, I do like the idea of macronutrient *balance*. And *balance,* my friend, is the key word here. Finding balance on your plate—either with macronutrient blocks or by visualizing your plate real estate—is the key to unlocking your *Wellness Intuition,* a world where you are not a slave to calorie counting, unplanned weight gain or loss, insurmountable cravings, or feeling unsatisfied after eating. It's a world where you're nourishing your body with what it needs, which makes you feel grounded and confident.

The recipes in this book take macronutrient balance into account very thoughtfully to help you navigate the world of nutrient-dense, whole-food, and plant-forward eating. But after you cook through these recipes, you'll necessarily want more variety, so I'm going to teach you a bit about macronutrients and hormonal signaling to keep you in the game. The secret is that every meal and snack should be a balance of protein, fat, and fiber-rich carbohydrates.

PROTEIN

Protein provides nutrients to build bones, muscles, and connective tissue like cartilage and collagen. It is the backbone of your body's structural integrity and allows you to physically move through the world. Some proteins become active enzymes, which assist in various biochemical processes, including digestion, DNA-to-gene translation, and energy metabolism, while others are messengers involved in hormonal signaling or are part of the immune surveillance team. Basically, proteins do all the work in your cells.

Proteins are made up of smaller units called amino acids. There are twenty amino acids—some of these we can make on our own, and some we need to consume. The ones we need to consume are called *essential* amino acids.

Proteins from animal sources are very efficient because they are *complete* proteins, meaning they have all of the essential amino acids that our bodies can't make. There are a few plant-based proteins that are complete as well, including quinoa and whole organic soy. If you're eating some animal protein along with lots of plant-based protein from a variety of sources, you'll almost assuredly get the amino acid balance you need.

It's entirely possible to get enough protein from plants, but eating plants is not as *efficient* as eating animal protein because plants are generally a more balanced mix of macronutrients. If you're following a 100 percent vegan diet, you'll want to watch your protein intake carefully to ensure you consume enough total protein and essential amino acids.

Proteins have four calories per gram. Most of us need 55 to 70 grams of protein per day, but remember that—as with many things in life—nutritional requirements are a bell-shaped curve, so some of us need less and some of us

need more. I recommend that you start with 15 percent of your total calories from protein. If you're an average lady eating about 1,800 calories per day, then you'll aim for 270 calories' worth of protein, which equates to 68 grams.

I see a lot of patients overeating animal protein in an effort to be "low carb." This is its own form of orthorexia, an unhealthy view of eating that restricts certain foods in the name of a healthy diet. I see many people eating over 100 grams of protein per day when they don't need to, which can be hard on the kidneys and the body as a whole.

We need more protein in our diets when we are young and after we reach age sixty-five due to protein's effect on the growth hormone IGF-1. IGF-1 promotes growth and development through adolescence and young adulthood. After the age of sixty-five, IGF-1 levels naturally trail off, so we need more protein to fend off fragility and decline from loss of muscle mass, called sarcopenia. I can't tell you how many pediatric patients I see who are total "carb-hounds" and eat only processed carbohydrates and how many elder patients I see who eat little to no protein, following what doctors call the "tea and toast" diet.

What's interesting is that during midlife, too much protein in our diets can unnecessarily stimulate IGF-1, which can contribute to premature aging and DNA damage, leading to an increased risk of cancer, diabetes, and overall mortality. What's even more interesting is that this increase in death and disability applies only to animal proteins, not plant proteins. In a study of over 6,300 adults using data from a national-representative dietary survey in the US (called NHANES III), researchers found that the associations of increased protein intake and mortality in respondents ages fifty to sixty-five were "abolished or attenuated" if the proteins were plant derived.[1] This is fascinating for those of us who love plants. We don't know from the study why that correlation exists, but I'm willing to put my money on the amazing phytonutrient effects that plant-based proteins have on our whole being, not just their proteins.

I'll get into how to balance animal- and plant-based protein sources in the coming chapters.

FAT

Fats provide satiety, aid in energy storage and insulation, cushion vital organs, form essential hormones in the body, maintain cell membrane integrity, and help the body absorb fat-soluble vitamins like A, D, E, and K.

Fat is energetically dense. It packs nine calories into each gram (which is why it's efficient storage for extra energy in the body), which is more than twice the calories per gram in carbohydrates or protein. That means fat is not going to take up a lot of real estate on your plate. Just compare one-half cup of avocado to four cups of chopped cauliflower: both have 100 calories, but the cauliflower is not as calorically dense.

Dietary fat does not make us fat unless we eat way too much of it. I'm a proponent of a healthy dose of fat at every meal and snack because it's satiating and makes food taste good. After all, what would roasted vegetables be without the delight of extra-virgin olive oil?

I recommend you get about 30 percent of your calories from fat. If you're an average lady eating an 1,800-calorie diet, you'll get about 60 grams of fat per day, to the tune of 540 calories. Woohoo!

Fat is made up of smaller units called fatty acids. There are three main categories of fatty acids: trans fats, saturated fats, and unsaturated fats.

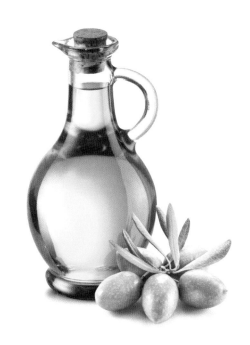

---

[1] M. E. Levine, J. A. Suarez, S. Brandhorst, et al., "Low protein intake is associated with a major reduction in IGF-1, cancer, and overall mortality in the 65 and younger but not older population," *Cell Metabolism* 19, no. 3 (2014): 407–17.

TRANS FAT

Trans fat should not exist in your diet. Most of this type of fat comes from food companies processing good fats by adding hydrogen molecules to them, which makes them more solid at room temperature. They were designed to replace saturated fats in foods to make those foods more healthy and shelf-stable, but we've since discovered that trans fats are toxic. This engineered fat is found in shortening, margarine, fried foods, and many baked goods. Read labels and avoid these bad actors at all costs.

The other types of fats—saturated, polyunsaturated, and unsaturated—are fine to consume in the right combination and in the right quantities.

SATURATED FAT

Saturated means that the carbon-hydrogen bonds in the fats don't have bends in them, so they lie more compactly together. For this reason, saturated fats are more likely to be solid at room temperature.

Not all saturated fats are created equal. There's a debate about whether plant-based saturated fats like those found in dark chocolate and coconut are as inflammatory as saturated fats from animal sources like beef, lamb, pork, poultry, lard, and dairy. It may come down to the amounts of saturated fat consumed at one time and how those fats are metabolized next to other nutrients.

Eating too much saturated fat can alter your cholesterol, increase your risk for heart disease, and be inflammatory no matter where it comes from. For this reason, while I include a bit of butter, ghee, and coconut oil in my diet, I primarily eat and cook with the unsaturated and polyunsaturated fats predominant in avocado oil, extra-virgin olive oil, and other plant-based foods.

About 10 percent of your daily calories should come from saturated fat. For the average person, this means 150 to 200 calories' worth, which—amazingly—is the amount found in a nice serving of extra-dark chocolate. Let that coincidence sit with you for a hot second. Maybe it's Nature telling us to enjoy a little chocolate every afternoon.

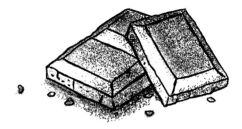

UNSATURATED FAT & OMEGA-3 FATTY ACIDS

Unsaturated fats are molecularly not as easy to stack, so they are usually liquid at room temperature. There are two main types: mono-unsaturated fatty acids (MUFAs) molecularly have one double bond between their carbons, while polyunsaturated fatty acids (PUFAs) have multiple double bonds.

MUFAs are known to be healthier in the diet because multiple studies have shown their ability to lower blood pressure, improve insulin sensitivity, and lower LDL cholesterol (especially the sticky kind that adheres to blood vessel walls to create plaque and hardening of the arteries).[2] Most plant-based fats fit into the category, including avocados and avocado oil, olives and extra-virgin olive oil, nuts and nut butters, and seeds and seed butters.

PUFAs are a little more complicated, but the two most important types are omega-3 and omega-6 fatty acids. You need both, but in the right balance. Most Americans eat way more omega-6 fats, which are found in inflammatory foods like refined vegetable oil and in processed foods, so we tend to talk about prioritizing omega-3-rich fats because of this imbalance.

Omega-3-rich fats are your best friend because they're like medicine on your plate. In fact, to date, the research on the anti-inflammatory effect of omega-3 fats is so robust that eating oily fish like salmon, halibut, sablefish, mackerel, sardines, tuna, and herring is a universal recommendation I make to patients unless they have an allergy to fish.

The anti-inflammatory effects of omega-3s stretch across multiple organ systems, including promoting cardiovascular health; protecting the brain from Alzheimer's, dementia, and attention deficit and hyperactivity disorder (ADHD); maintaining mental health, including management of depression and anxiety; and preventing metabolic syndrome (the disastrous combination of high blood pressure, high triglycerides, and elevated blood sugar); along with a whole host of other chronic diseases.[3] I recommend taking a modest dose of omega-3 in pill form if you don't get oily fish in your diet once or twice weekly, especially if you're at risk for any of the conditions mentioned here, but talk with your doctor before starting it on your own.

You can also find omega-3 fats in plants, including whole organic soy, walnuts, and chia, flax, sunflower, pumpkin, and hemp seeds and their butters and milks. The problem is that the form of these omega-3 plant fats, alpha-linolenic acid (ALA), is not very efficient in the body. Our bodies generally use omega-3 fats in the form of docosahexaenoic acid (DHA) and eicosapentaenoic acid (EPA), which is the kind found in wild fatty fish. ALA has to be converted to DHA and EPA before it can be used, and only 7 percent of our intake makes it through the conversion process. So, unfortunately, while eating ground flax seeds on your oatmeal each morning might be good for many other reasons, flax seeds are not an efficient source of omega-3 fats.

---

[2] L. G. Gillingham, S. Harris-Janz, and P. J. Jones, "Dietary monounsaturated fatty acids are protective against metabolic syndrome and cardiovascular disease risk factors," *Lipids* 46, no. 3 (2011): 209–28.

[3] S. Lorente-Cebrián, A. G. Costa, S. Navas-Carretero, et al., "Role of omega-3 fatty acids in obesity, metabolic syndrome, and cardiovascular diseases: a review of the evidence," *Journal of Physiology and Biochemistry* 69, no. 3 (2013): 633–51; M. Loef and H. Walach, "The omega-6/omega-3 ratio and dementia or cognitive decline: a systematic review on human studies and biological evidence," *Journal of Nutrition in Gerontology and Geriatrics* 32, no. 1 (2013): 1–23.

CARBOHYDRATES

Carbohydrates provide the most available energy to our bodies and come in the form of sugars, starches, and fiber. Complex carbohydrates like starches are broken down during digestion into glucose that is essential for our bodies' function, whereas simple sugars don't require as much digestive power. Without starches and sugars, your body would have to work really hard to come up with fuel.

Unlike sugars and starches, dietary fiber from plants is not broken down during digestion and provides the roughage that makes up stool. The more fiber you eat, generally, the easier it is for you to have a daily bowel movement.

I recommend you get about 55 percent of your calories from carbohydrates. For the average lady who eats an 1,800-calorie diet, that amounts to almost 1,000 calories per day. It's important that those carbohydrates be in the whole-food form of fiber-rich vegetables, fruit, whole grains, and plant proteins like beans, lentils, and whole organic soy, and not in the form of sugar and processed foods.

FIBER IS YOUR BEST FRIEND

Fiber is present in all plant foods in varying amounts, and it's magical. You can think of it as fertilizer for your helpful gut bacteria, a plunger for your digestion by supporting regular bowel movements, a squeegee for your blood vessels by binding cholesterol and thus preventing plaque formation, and an anchor for your appetite and blood sugar by slowing the rate at which carbohydrate sugars are released into your bloodstream, which makes and keeps you full.

Most of us get just a sliver of the fiber we need. Our ancestors ate upwards of 100 grams of fiber a day, but the average American today gets only about a tenth of that. I ask patients to aim for 20 grams of fiber per 1,000 calories in their diet. For most of us, that means 30 to 40 grams of fiber per day. That's a lot, but it's certainly not impossible, especially with the serving recommendations I make in Chapter 4.

Fiber comes in two types:

- **Soluble fiber** is found in most fruits, some vegetables, oatmeal and oat bran, nuts, seeds, and beans. When soluble fiber mixes with the water in the digestive tract, it becomes thick and gelatinous. Soluble fiber is known to decrease cholesterol and keep blood sugar stable.

- **Insoluble fiber** is found in most vegetables, fruits, and whole grains and is not absorbable. Its role is to keep waste moving through the digestive system and provide food for the probiotics in our microbiome.

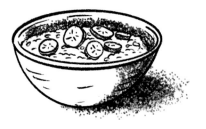

The reason the type of carbohydrate matters comes back to how quickly it's absorbed into the bloodstream, which is affected by its sugar complexity and the amount of fiber it has. The more fiber a food contains, the slower its sugars are absorbed. And slow is the name of the game because sudden spikes in blood sugar trigger bigger releases of our fat-storage hormone, insulin. Your goal is to keep your blood sugar relatively even throughout the day with slow-burn carbohydrates in combination with fat and protein to prevent the literal roller coaster of ups and downs in blood sugar that trigger weight gain, cravings, energy crashes, mood swings, and crabby or "hangry" feelings (a disastrous combination of being angry because you're so hungry).

You want a nice, smooth ride on the blood sugar train.

EFFECTS ON BLOOD GLUCOSE OVER TIME

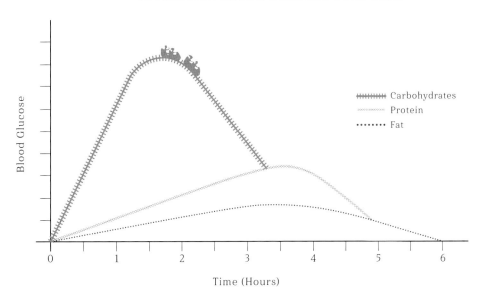

HORMONES OF DIGESTION

A lot of complex processes happen in our bodies to make digestion possible, but I want to focus on one key hormone: insulin.

Insulin is necessary for life. It is the hormone secreted from the pancreas that drives glucose from the bloodstream into our cells so that the cells can use it for energy production. This is all fine and good when you're consuming sugar in combination with fiber, protein, and fat and in an amount that suits your body's needs. But a big problem ensues when you start to push the envelope by consuming too much sugar, or in the wrong forms, or in the wrong combinations with other foods.

When you eat a lot of sugar at one time, your blood sugar shoots through the roof, and your body necessarily releases a huge dose of insulin to bring the blood sugar back to normal. To boot, the body often overcorrects with insulin, leading to drastic drops in blood sugar that can make you feel relatively hypoglycemic. Take a look at the roller coaster graphic above. What happens when you get into that relatively low blood sugar zone? You start to feel weak or light-headed or nauseated, and your body wants you to eat more sugar.

When insulin doesn't work as it should, diabetes develops. Type 1 diabetes is an auto-immune disease that destroys the cells of the pancreas that make insulin, so those with type 1 diabetes have to give themselves injections of insulin to manage their blood sugar. Type 2 diabetes is a metabolic disease in which the pancreas is capable of secreting insulin, but the body is so tired of the constant ingestion of sugar and resulting release of insulin that it becomes resistant to insulin. That's why the precursor to type 2 diabetes is called *insulin resistance*.

How do you know if you have insulin resistance? Sometimes you don't know.

Occasionally I see this "invisible" insulin resistance in strapping young male patients. It's found in their laboratory tests only when we specifically test for it, usually spurred by a significant family history of diabetes or of someone who died young from a massive heart attack or stroke.

Other times I see insulin resistance in young female patients who notice they are gaining weight around the midsection, developing acne, or growing dark hair from their chins, along with having irregular menstrual periods (signifying irregular ovulation). Usually these women seek my help because they want to get pregnant. In the course of their workup, I diagnose both polycystic ovary syndrome (PCOS) and insulin resistance.

Most often, however, I make a diagnosis of insulin resistance in middle-aged patients who complain that no matter what they do, they can't seem to lose weight. And they are hungry all the time. Just *looking* at dessert makes them gain weight. They feel bloated and lethargic, and their sugar cravings are off the hook. They notice "low blood sugar" symptoms like light-headedness, fatigue, and nausea. Their primary care doctors can't find anything wrong and simply tell them to "eat less and move more." But often doctors don't order the right tests because they weren't taught to test for these biomarkers. When I discover the hormonal imbalance of elevated insulin levels and a borderline three-month blood sugar test (called a hemoglobin A1c), the patients are relieved to have an answer but annoyed that they couldn't get the diagnosis sooner.

This exact scenario happened with my patient Jane, a fifty-five-year-old who had noticed that since menopause, she had started to put on weight around her midsection. She had always been trim when she was younger and had been able to lose the baby weight after her children were born without much effort. She exercised regularly and had a decent diet—until about 4 p.m. In the late afternoon, she would start to feel really tired but knew that she needed to continue working for a few more hours, so she would reach for gummy bears, milk chocolate, and Skittles. By the time she got home from work, she was ravenous and would eat anything she could get her hands on. She would then feel extremely guilty and shame herself into cycles of "being good" with her diet until she fell off the rails again and went for the sugar. And of course, all that sugar made it difficult for her to sleep, which just furthered her exhaustion and frustration.

Jane's reliance on late-afternoon sugar is very innocent. She's tired, her brain is overwhelmed, and she needs to find a way to power through until she can go home. So she reaches for sugar. It's not her fault. Our brains are hardwired to look for the simplest energy source possible, and easily absorbed glucose from candy fits the bill.

The problem with consuming sugar and processed foods is that it causes your blood sugar to skyrocket, and your body releases a large amount of insulin. In the case of insulin resistance, the body needs an even *larger* dose of insulin to get the same amount of blood sugar lowering, and this surge of insulin often overcorrects blood sugar to be lower than we want it to be. The bigger problem is that this sugar-insulin response is a continuous feed-forward cycle, meaning that the more insulin your body releases in response to the sugar you've eaten, the hungrier you are. So you eat more sugar and processed food because your body wants easy-to-digest calories. And you

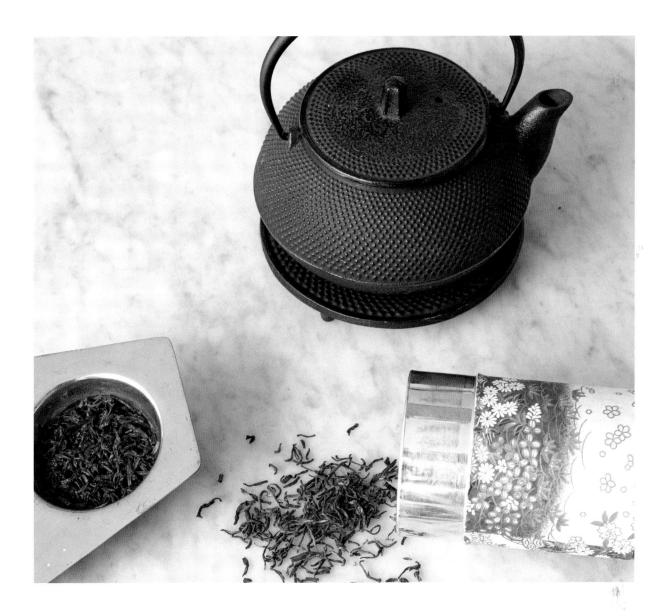

release more insulin. Do you see how this is a game you can never win?

The only way to stop the cycle is to stop eating and drinking those foods that are designed to make us fail. Generally, those foods are the ones that have been lab-engineered or come in plastic packaging with more than a few ingredients on the label. It's the soda, diet drinks, and other sweet beverages. It's the packaged chips, cookies, and crackers. It's the bread and pasta, even if it's made from something that sounds wholesome, like quinoa, because the whole grains have been processed. It's any food that you look at and can't trace back to Mother Nature.

So what should you do after being armed with this information about sugar, insulin, and the no-win game of consuming processed foods?

The answer is to stop eating them.

And that's really hard...for a few days. Then the cravings will lessen, your taste buds will start to rebound to appreciating the natural sweetness of real food, and you will start to feel amazing. And then you can start actually enjoying all those vegetables I want you to eat! This is the philosophy of my *Dr. Katie Detox*, which we'll walk through in Chapter 12.

HORMONAL CONTROL THROUGH GLYCEMIC LOAD

You're probably at a place where you want to understand the blood sugar response one step deeper. That's where glycemic load comes in.

Glycemic index and *glycemic load* are measures used to help us understand the rate at which carbohydrates are converted to sugar in our bodies. The higher its glycemic index, the more a food will raise your blood sugar when you eat it. It's a scale based on glucose, which has a glycemic index of 100. Glycemic load takes our understanding of a food's sugar absorption one step further by accounting for the actual amount of that food that you might eat at one time. This allows you to compare carbohydrate foods more thoughtfully. Here's a general guideline:

	Low	Medium	High
Glycemic index	≤55	56–69	≥70
Glycemic load	≤10	11–19	≥20

Many vegetables don't even register on the glycemic load scale because they don't significantly raise blood sugar.[4] Hooray for that!

But a starchy vegetable like butternut squash—which is inherently sweet-tasting—has a relatively higher glycemic index of 51 compared to something like kale, which sits at a whopping 2. (Recognize that 51 is still low on the GI scale!) However, when you consider how much butternut squash you might eat at a time—I recommend about one-half cup as a serving—the glycemic load is only 4.

I've talked so much in this chapter about finding balance among the three macronutrients, and understanding how plate balance affects glycemic load is important to your success. Recognize that adding fat and protein to a meal that includes a higher-glycemic load carbohydrate matters immensely. That's one reason I recommend being generous with the healthy oil in which you roast your squash. The addition of fat not only makes the squash incredibly delicious, but it slows the rate of absorption into your system. (Interestingly, the way you prepare a vegetable changes its glycemic index. Because roasting allows for caramelization of a vegetable's sugar, it raises the glycemic index a little.) And if you combine that roasted squash with some protein and healthy fat, as in my delicious Almond Furikake Crusted Halibut recipe on page 268, you've got yourself a slow-burn meal that will keep your blood sugar stable.

---

[4] K. Foster-Powell, "International table of glycemic index and glycemic load values: 2002," *American Journal of Clinical Nutrition* 76, no. 1 (2002): 5–56.

This idea of balance is also why my patient Jane found herself in a downward spiral every afternoon when she reached for candy. One of the first things she and I worked on together was choosing a better, more balanced snack. In fact, in that first visit, I didn't mention changing anything else in her diet because I knew the candy was the real problem. And, boy, did she fight me on the candy! But once she substituted those empty calories with real food—even something easy, sweet, and satisfying, like an apple along with some almonds or almond butter—she had much more control over her appetite. And, no surprise, she had lost a few pounds by the time she returned. Some of that was real fat loss, but most of it was just the loss of the extra fluid her body was hanging on to. Because, adding insult to injury, too much insulin also causes water retention. So, as soon as Jane's insulin levels went down, her body let go of that extra bloat. You can bet she was a happy camper!

You might be wondering why I spent time talking about the balance of macronutrients and understanding glycemic load when choosing carbohydrates. It's because these pearls are the secret to stabilizing your blood sugar and insulin levels, finding a weight that feels good in your body, and preventing diabetes and metabolic disease. They're the secret to feeling satiated and anchored instead of always wanting to pick at more food. They're the secret to having amazing energy throughout the day and restorative sleep at night.

Choosing slow-burn, fiber-rich carbs in balance with fat and protein in the right combination on your plate and in alignment with your *Wellness Intuition* is the most important thing I can teach you.

"As soon as Jane's *insulin levels went down,* her body **let go of that extra bloat.**"

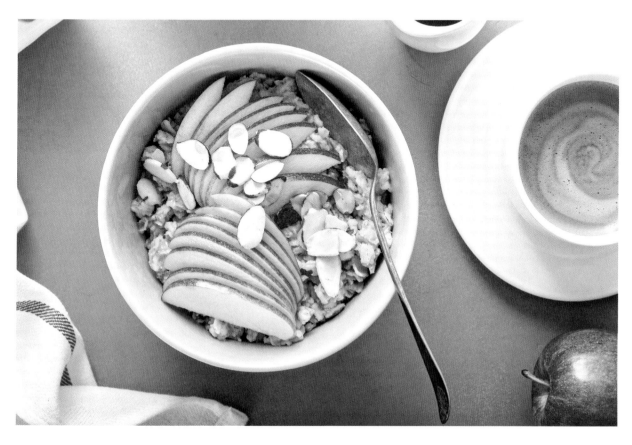

CHAPTER 4

APPRECIATING FOOD & SATIETY

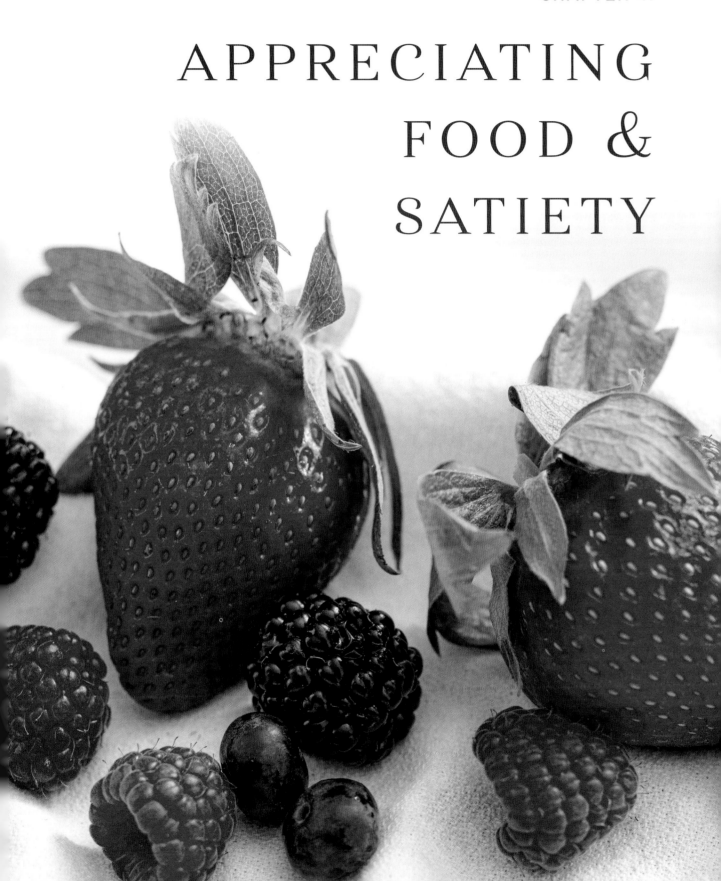

Food signifies so much. Food is nourishment in the best way possible—it's a combination of biological, social, emotional, and spiritual energy from the outside in. Nothing else in our culture physically provides nourishment while also anchoring us to friends, family, and community.

But food can also be wrapped up in not-so-great things. It's often used punitively—as in the case of a child being sent to bed without dessert after misbehaving. It's also a reward—as in the case of treating yourself to something divine after finishing a difficult task. It's addictive—as in the case of sugar—and impossible to abstain from, in contrast to other addictive substances. And it's often used to self-soothe in an effort to rectify uncomfortable feelings such as guilt, shame, worry, sadness, or boredom.

I'm sure you've noticed that I haven't said much about calories when discussing the need for food as energy. That's because I don't personally count calories or encourage my patients to do so. Instead, I encourage you to listen. Listening to your body is the hallmark of understanding your *Wellness Intuition,* your internal guide to making well-balanced decisions for yourself.

I didn't really have an appreciation for my own body's hunger and satiety signals until I was pregnant with my twin boys in my early thirties. For the first time in my life, I knew what it meant to be full, mostly because near the end, the babies took up so much space in my belly that there was literally nowhere for more food to go. I distinctly remember making a delicious wholesome meal a few weeks before delivery. I took about three bites and then couldn't eat any more. (Thankfully, I had heeded the sage advice of another twin mom and gained weight earlier in the pregnancy, so I was able to continue nourishing my little people adequately until delivery.) But I also recall waking up in the middle of the night with pangs of true physiological hunger that a drink of water didn't resolve, so I found myself enjoying my favorite healthy snack at the time—a bowl of plain full-fat yogurt topped with fruit and a little honey. I realized during pregnancy that my body literally told me what to do. I ate when I was hungry and stopped when I was satiated. And I put on exactly the amount of weight my doctor recommended for twins. I am grateful to have been pregnant for so many reasons, but tapping into my *Wellness Intuition* sticks with me as an unexpected pearl of that privilege.

The key to listening to our bodies' signals starts with feeding ourselves nourishing food. Our hardworking bodies need fuel, and eating real food leads to satisfaction and optimal function. Eating real food can also help us feel a *sense of indulgence* for doing what makes us feel amazing. Having been overweight for much of my childhood and young adulthood, being on and off diets, and worrying incessantly about my weight from morning to night, I realize now that I didn't know how to listen to my body.

This chapter is designed to help you listen to your body in the spirit of deepening your *Wellness Intuition.* Our bodies have so much to teach us.

HUNGER, FULLNESS, APPETITE & SATIETY

Hunger and satiety are regulated by a symphony of hormones, including insulin, cortisol, leptin, and ghrelin, and involve delicate signaling between the brain and belly.

Hunger is a normal sensation that makes us want to eat. It is controlled by the part of the brain called the hypothalamus, which is involved in everything from hunger and thirst signaling to body temperature regulation to endocrine and hormone function. But hunger is also influenced by our blood sugar levels and how empty our stomachs and intestines are. Hunger is a physical sensation, usually accompanied by stomach growling and uncomfortable feelings in the belly known as hunger pangs.

Satiety is the opposite of hunger; it's a feeling of being satisfied. Notice that I used the word *satisfied,* not *full.* Satiated does not equate to full. In my mind, fullness is a physical sensation of having a certain volume of food in the stomach that activates the stomach stretch receptors to signal to the hypothalamus and tell us to stop eating. We can be physically full but still not feel satiated, mostly due to appetite.

Appetite is the desire for food. Satiety and appetite are closely linked because choosing the right foods allows for their alignment. If out of sync, the desire to eat can outpace satiety and fullness, and we continue to eat long after we've physically had enough. Conversely, appetite can work against us and stop us from eating. A poor appetite was what I experienced in medical school when I was so anxious that I couldn't eat, even though I was physically hungry.

Feeling satiated comes down to your *Wellness Intuition* and the fiber, fat, and protein combination that makes you feel your best. When you find the right balance, your body knows how much to eat and when. It was my goal when writing the recipes for this book to develop a realistic starting point to discovering your own *Wellness Intuition.*

FAT IS THE KEY TO SATIETY

I personally and professionally find that the key to satiety is dietary fat intake. While all three macronutrients are important, it's the right ratio of fiber and protein to fat that tells your brain you're full. A meal rich in healthy plant-forward fat will leave you feeling satisfied, well nourished, and balanced in your appetite, hunger, and satiety signals. What's more, fat just tastes good. It's a vehicle for flavor and nutrients, allowing for the absorption of many vitamins and minerals necessary for life. Best of all, it talks directly to your brain and tells it that the meal or snack you just ate hit the spot.

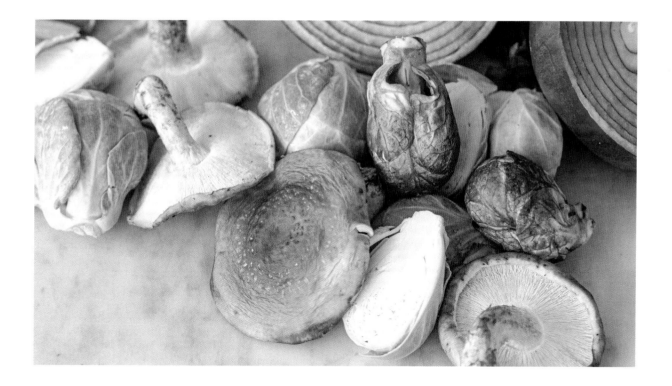

APPRECIATING FOOD

The experience of eating involves all of our senses. It includes the visual appeal of how food looks and the satisfying sound we hear when unwrapping something delightful or taking that first bite of something crunchy, but most of our enjoyment actually happens through our sense of smell.

The full appreciation of food's sensuousness and flavor combines smell and taste. The tongue's taste buds allow us to experience the basic texture of food along with the familiar sweet, salty, sour, bitter, and umami tastes (the Japanese word for "savory" or "meaty"), but the aromatic compounds of smell account for at least 70 percent of flavor, and maybe as much as 90 percent.[1]

Trauma to the olfactory sense can wreak havoc on a person's ability to enjoy food. I have a lovely young patient named Sarah who suffered a severe concussion that left her with chronic headaches and hyposmia, or the inability to smell anything except very strong odors. She doesn't mind the loss of smell as much as she hates her newfound problem of being unable to really taste food. She came to me as a patient both for help with the headaches (which a combination of herbs, magnesium, and acupuncture has greatly improved) and to lose weight, because when she lost her ability to taste, she leaned into highly processed foods because of their hyper-flavored components. Over time, we've talked about the other senses that go into enjoying food—including sight and hearing—and about texture. And while Sarah loves cooking with the bright color of chard or hearing the snappy crunch of celery, she doesn't derive much satisfaction from eating, and that makes me feel sad for her.

---

[1] Bill Bryson, *The Body: A Guide for Occupants* (New York: Penguin Random House, 2019): 106.

MANAGING THE TIME LAG

Once the first bite of food goes down the hatch, it takes about twenty minutes before your brain starts to recognize satiety and fullness signals. If you're eating too quickly, you can blow right by these signals and find yourself stuffed, which feels uncomfortable both physically and mentally because so many of us beat ourselves up for overeating.

Here are a few strategies to help your body digest and recognize your food:

- **Ask yourself if you're really hungry.** Get curious about whether you are experiencing physical hunger or are eating to self-soothe due to procrastination, boredom, worry, or sadness. It's okay to soothe yourself with food occasionally, but using food to numb feelings is not a helpful coping strategy. Try taking a few deep breaths, taking a drink of water or a short walk, or calling a friend to see if the sensation of hunger is fake and passes.

- **Chew your food twenty times before swallowing.** Doing so allows you to properly grind and hydrate your food, allowing for the release of digestive enzymes that starts in the mouth. Proper chewing also releases the flavors in food so that your nose and taste buds can appreciate what's in front of you. Plus, chewing your food twenty times takes a considerable amount of time. You may even need a break in the middle of your meal to give your chompers a rest.

- **Eat just enough.** I'm sure you've heard the saying "stop when you're 80 percent full," but what does that mean? I like to think of hunger and satiety on a scale of 1 to 10. A hunger cue of 1 is being so hungry that you'd eat your arm, and a fullness signal of 10 is being so full that you can't move. It's best to operate in the optimal zone of 3 to 8, meaning that you don't wait to get so hungry that you can't make good choices and don't eat past the point of feeling satiated. Twenty minutes after you stop eating at being 80 percent full, reassess your desire for more food. You will probably find that the desire to eat has passed.

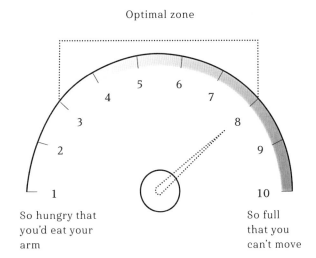

Optimal zone

So hungry that you'd eat your arm

So full that you can't move

MINDFUL EATING

Another scale exists in my mind when it comes to feeling satiated, and that's the one that encompasses emotional eating and mindful eating. Emotional eating often comes from a place of scarcity, fear, lack of safety, or rebellion either inherently about food or manifesting in food because of those feelings being present in other areas in our lives. Food is an easy target for emotional escape because it's a tool within reach of almost everyone.

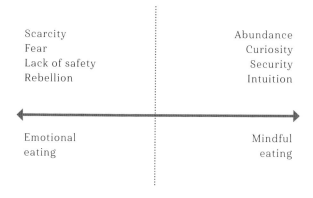

Scarcity	Abundance
Fear	Curiosity
Lack of safety	Security
Rebellion	Intuition

Emotional eating — Mindful eating

"**Mindful eating** is the practice of *being present with ourselves* while we are eating."

Mindful eating is based in mindfulness, the idea of being present without judgment, letting go of a right and wrong way to do something. Mindful eating is the practice of being present with ourselves while we are eating. It helps us tune into our bodies' physical hunger and satiety cues so that we can respond effectively. Mindful eaters cultivate curiosity toward food while being grounded in the awareness of the present moment combined with feelings of abundance, security, and intuition.

In short, mindful eating is hard. Even the best of us forget to do it or just plain refuse to do it because it takes effort, and sometimes at the end of the day, when you've had enough of life, you just want to dive into your dinner and wash it down with a glass of wine.

It's okay not to eat mindfully all the time. Again, come back to the 80/20 rule. You don't need to be perfect. I've recognized over time that when I eat alone, with just my food and centered thoughts, those meals and snacks not only gift me with immense pleasure, but I reach the point of satiety much sooner. Mindful eating is an important part of our *Wellness Intuition*, our ability to listen to our bodies, minds, and spirits that leads us to inherently know how to take care of ourselves.

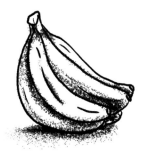

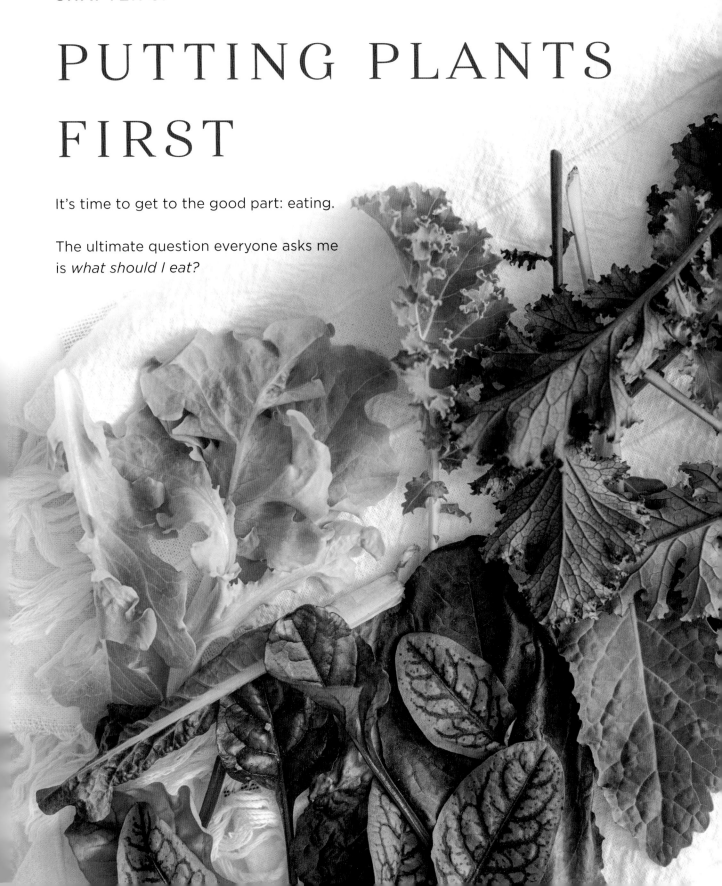

CHAPTER 5:

PUTTING PLANTS FIRST

It's time to get to the good part: eating.

The ultimate question everyone asks me is *what should I eat?*

When I see a new patient in the office and we talk through their concerns about cholesterol and weight management or about lessening the burden of chronic headaches, our conversations inevitably come back to food. After we review everything that person eats and drinks in a typical day, including portion sizes and brands of products and how they feel after eating, almost every patient will tilt their head, look at me with deer-in-the-headlights bewilderment in their eyes, and then meekly ask, "So, Dr. Katie, what *should* I eat?"

FOOD IS NOT JUST FUEL, IT'S INFORMATION

We know that food provides our bodies with the calories and nutrients they need to function. But ultimately, food is *information.*

Food tells our bodies what to do. I think about food almost like software. Computer software tells the hardware what to do and how to function so that when you type, the computer magically puts the words on the screen. In order to make that happen, a lot of complex actions have to occur behind the scenes.

What you put in your body three times a day, plus or minus a snack, programs your hard drive. Literally every bite you take leads you down one pathway or another.

Some foods—like vegetables—lead you down the soothing pathway of harmony, quelling inflammation and signaling to your body that everything is hunky-dory. Other foods—especially processed foods—are like throwing lighter fluid on a fire.

Just imagine what it might look like in your body when you eat some Cheetos. Upon that first taste, the delicious combination of sugar, salt, and fat lights up your brain, and your body fires up its inflammatory cascade. This cascade causes a roar of cellular signaling that further scares your body into high gear, and it revs up its engine and prepares for battle. Except there's no battle to be fought. You just wanted to eat some Cheetos.

Can you go your whole life never eating Cheetos? Maybe. But it's unrealistic to think that you'll never ever again eat unhealthy or processed food. That's where balance comes in.

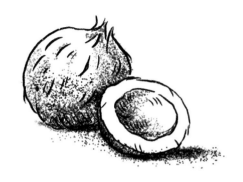

EAT MOSTLY PLANTS

I love the genius words of whole-food activist and bestselling author Michael Pollan: "Eat food. Not too much. Mostly plants."

Sounds simple, right? It actually *is* simple, but most of us get sidetracked by all the confusing information out there. The key words are *mostly plants.*

If you eat a plant-forward diet, even if it's not perfect (and honestly, I don't want your diet to be perfect because perfection is not fun, flexible, or attainable), you will balance the inflammatory cascade that's fired up by some occasional Cheetos with the soothing anti-inflammation of all the gorgeous, nutrient-dense, natural foods you eat.

There's a lot of noise in the diet industry, and it's confusing for a consumer to know what to eat. The best nutrition advice I can give you is to look at where all the reasonable, non-fad, whole-food diets overlap. These areas of overlap suggest that the optimal diet includes vegetables, fruit, plant-based protein, occasional high-quality animal protein, monounsaturated fats, whole grains, omega-3-rich foods, and fermented foods.

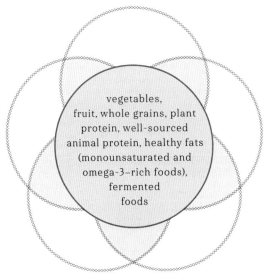

vegetables, fruit, whole grains, plant protein, well-sourced animal protein, healthy fats (monounsaturated and omega-3–rich foods), fermented foods

You know from the title of this book that I encourage people to eat a plant-forward diet. But what does plant-forward mean? I advocate for at least 80 percent plants. A plant-forward diet emphasizes foods like vegetables, fruit, whole grains, nuts, seeds, legumes, whole organic soy, and chocolate (hooray!) and has fewer foods like beef, pork, poultry, fish, dairy, and eggs.

How do you eat mostly plants? As a girl who grew up in Ohio eating animal protein at almost every meal, I did not find shifting to a plant-forward diet easy. But in my years as an

Integrative physician, a mom to two growing and energetic boys, a wife whose husband loves carbs and genetically tends toward metabolic issues with triglycerides and high blood sugar, a woman who wants to be strong and live a full life, and a steward of general good vibes for the Universe and my community, I have learned so much about why changing to a plant-forward diet is important and how to practically make it happen. That's why I wrote this book for you. Consider it the shortcut that took me over ten years to put into practice!

BEING AN OMNIVORE WHO FOLLOWS THE 80/20 RULE

I'm all about the 80/20 rule. I don't recommend eating a diet that is 100 percent plants—also called a vegan diet, which about 2 percent of the adult population in the US follows[1]—unless that's what you want for yourself based on your own feelings about the environment or about eating animals. I don't recommend that you be a vegetarian, either, unless that's what you want for philosophical reasons. Even though I don't recommend vegan or vegetarian diets, it's possible to get the nutrition you need with a vegan or vegetarian diet if you're mindful of a few important caveats, including amino acid balance and vitamin intake.

There's a wide range of what vegetarians eat or don't eat, so I've included this graphic[2] to make it easier for you to understand what your friends might be doing or what you might be reading about as you venture into the world of plant-forward eating.

I have quite a few patients who identify as pescatarians who eat eggs and limited dairy, so we spend time during their visits talking about how to prioritize and find balance.

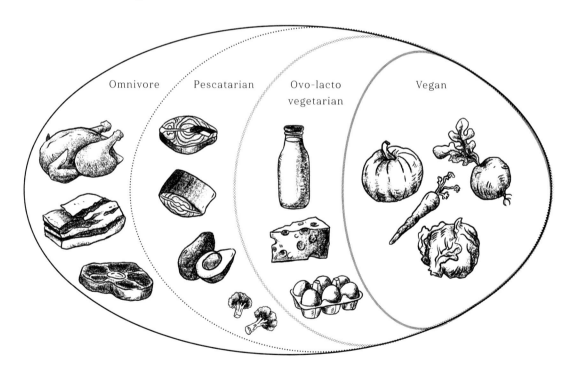

[1] G. Sebastiani, A. H. Barbero, C. Borras-Novell, et al., "The effects of vegetarian and vegan diet during pregnancy on the health of mothers and offspring," *Nutrients* 11, no. 3 (2019): 557.

[2] E. Medawar, S. Huhn, A. Villringer, and A. V. Witte, "The effects of plant-based diets on the body and brain: a systematic review," *Translational Psychiatry* 9 (2019): 226.

To be clear, I recommend being an omnivore, which means that you eat both plants and animals. I encourage you to eat and enjoy every whole food on the face of the planet. I personally don't categorically avoid any food. Variety is the spice of life!

In general, if a food comes from Nature, meaning you recognize it as a whole food that Mother Nature made, and it comes to your plate in a similar way to how it appeared in its untouched, natural form, then generally it's okay to include in your diet. I'm okay with eating lobster, pork, red-skinned potatoes, and corn on the cob. All of these foods are natural and whole. What I urge you to limit are impostors like imitation crab meat, processed flavored sausage patties, potatoes fried in palm oil, and high-fructose corn syrup.

There are only a few things in the American diet that I recommend ditching almost 100 percent of the time, and that's sugar-sweetened beverages and noncaloric sweeteners (which I'll talk about in a little bit). There's no good reason to drink or eat these types of foods unless you want the smallest of small tastes.

I recommend eating a plant-forward diet 80 percent of the time, so there's a bit of wiggle room. That 20 percent could be high-quality animal products, with a special emphasis on omega-3-rich wild-caught fish (like salmon), organic grass-fed red meat and dairy, and pasture-raised poultry and eggs along with minimal amounts of processed or unhealthy foods that don't have any redeeming value other than simply making you happy. (I would argue—do those ultra-processed, unhealthy foods really make you happy? I don't think so. But that's a question for another book!)

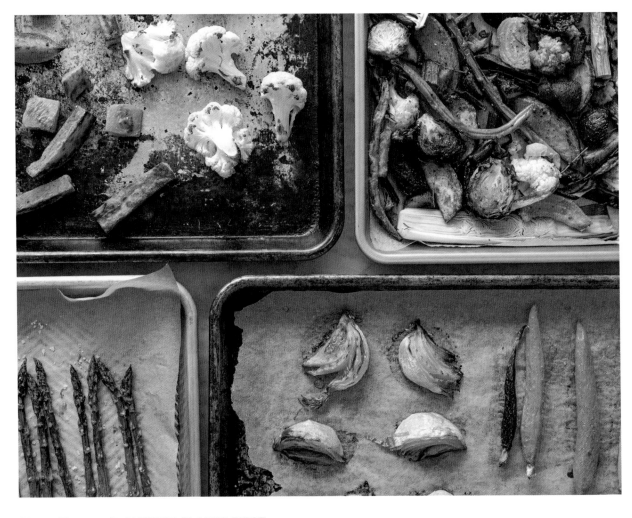

EAT REAL FOOD

The most important thing for me to tell you is that when all else fails, you should simply eat real food.

Many Americans rely on factory-made, ultra-processed fake foods for calories and energy. These fake foods contain disastrous foodlike components in the form of high-fructose corn syrup (HFCS), monosodium glutamate (MSG), noncaloric sweeteners, and preservatives and are invented by food scientists using laboratory genetic engineering. These scientists are experts in identifying what investigative journalist Michael Moss calls out as the "bliss point" of a food. The bliss point is the perfect combination of salt, sugar, and fat that hijacks our brain's dopamine reward circuit, making it almost impossible to say no to more of that food.[3]

Ever notice that you can't have just one Pringle chip when you peel open that familiar canister? Simply peeling open the can releases a delicious smell of salt, sugar, and fat. Most engineered foods follow a similar recipe of combining salt, sugar, and fat in ways that lead your taste buds to heaven. This ultra-processing tricks your taste buds into wanting more and more and ruins your taste for other foods. Ever notice how bitter a raspberry tastes after you eat ice cream? But take that same raspberry and put it on your morning steel-cut oatmeal with some sliced almonds and it's a whole different story.

In fact, I recently challenged a patient on her observation that raspberries are "sour and bitter" in the context of her highly processed food diet. She came into my office saying that every joint in her body hurt, with chronic constipation and bloating and a feeling of "heaviness" that she just couldn't shake. No surprise, her diet was riddled with factory-made fake foods. I didn't tell her what to eat on that first visit. I simply asked her to start limiting the foods in her diet that didn't look like what Mother Nature provides and let her figure out some simple changes on her own. And then I told her to eat raspberries again after a few days of implementing these changes. She came back and said that for the first time in her life, she understood why I described raspberries as sweet. It's because they *are* sweet. After all, fruit is Nature's candy. She just couldn't tell because the fake foods she'd been eating had been polluting her taste buds. And wouldn't you know, her joints felt better too after just a few weeks of more whole foods.

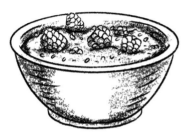

---

[3] M. Moss, *Salt Sugar Fat: How the Food Giants Hooked Us* (New York: Random House, 2013).

LOOK AT INGREDIENT LABELS

Even if you use my "Did Mother Nature make this?" question to decipher whether a food is healthy, sometimes we are left scratching our heads about how natural something is. This is where ingredient labels come in.

Obviously, some foods don't need ingredient labels. When we pick a bunch of celery off the shelf at the grocery store, we know it contains just one ingredient: celery. That's one reason I love shopping in the produce section—there's almost no label reading! You can pick up what appeals to your eye and place it in your cart without much thought and know that it's healthy.

But once you head down the aisles at the grocery store, the ease of shopping starts to diminish because you have to start looking at labels, which takes time and some knowledge.

Some packaged foods are brilliantly obvious to decipher. A bag of dried quinoa is just going to be quinoa. Same thing with a bag of dried lentils or beans. But then it starts to get a little more complicated.

Once a food is cooked or prepared in some way, you have to spend time looking at the label. Even a can of beans requires this detective work to make sure it doesn't contain too much salt or something mysterious like "natural spices" or "natural flavors." (Who even knows what that means? If the ingredients are "natural spices," why wouldn't the food company just say that the spices are nutmeg and cinnamon? Consider why they want to hide that information from you. In my estimation, the reason can't be good.)

When we look at the labels of many packaged foods, we notice they tend to contain a lot of ingredients, many of which are difficult to pronounce. If you can't tell what something is, then my rule is that you shouldn't eat much of it.

Let's look at an example. Imagine you're at the store and you come across a newfangled food that all of your healthy friends are serving at their summer barbecues. Imagine flipping over the package and reading this list of ingredients:

Water, Pea Protein*, Expeller-Pressed Canola Oil, Refined Coconut Oil, Rice Protein, Natural Flavors, Cocoa Butter, Mung Bean Protein, Methylcellulose, Potato Starch, Apple Extract, Pomegranate Extract, Salt, Potassium Chloride, Vinegar, Lemon Juice Concentrate, Sunflower Lecithin, Beet Juice Extract (for color)

Hard to tell what it is, right?

This is the label from Beyond Beef, a relative newcomer to the meat-alternative market. But is it a real food? I don't think so. Let's compare it to the mushroom burger on page 276. Do you recognize all the ingredients in that yummy plant-forward meat alternative? Of course you do. Because they're all real foods.

What's the major difference between a Beyond Beef burger and a homemade mushroom burger? Well, the most obvious one is that the mushroom burger can't be bought at a store. If you want to enjoy it, you have to make it at home. And herein lies the secret to better health: you need to get into the kitchen.

"That's one reason *I love shopping* in the *produce section*— there's almost **no label reading!**"

HOME COOKING
IS YOUR FRIEND

There's no nice way to say this: you need to get out of the habit of total convenience and get your hands dirty in the kitchen. After all, there's a reason food that someone else makes for us tastes amazing . . . and most times it's because they're adding stuff to the food that we wouldn't add for ourselves, mostly in the form of unnecessary fat, salt, and sugar.

I know you're busy. I'm busy, too. We all have demands on our time that are both within our control and outside our control. But you're reading this book because you want something different in your life. Maybe you want to go a day without stinky gas or heartburn. Or you want to stop having headaches. Or you want to avoid the midafternoon slump so you can finish your work earlier and have more free time for a hobby. Or you want to avoid being crabby and in the fetal position in bed on the first day of your period. You just want to feel better.

Which means that something has to shift.

If you're already spending time in the kitchen, then your shift to a healthier way of eating is going to be focused on choosing more anti-inflammatory foods. But if you're buying most of your food already prepared–dining in restaurants, picking up takeout, eating from the food bar at your local Whole Foods, or buying all the interesting preseasoned foods at Trader Joe's that require only heating–then you're going to have to make two changes. The first is to choose real, whole foods when you're grocery shopping, and the second is to get a little more comfortable in the kitchen.

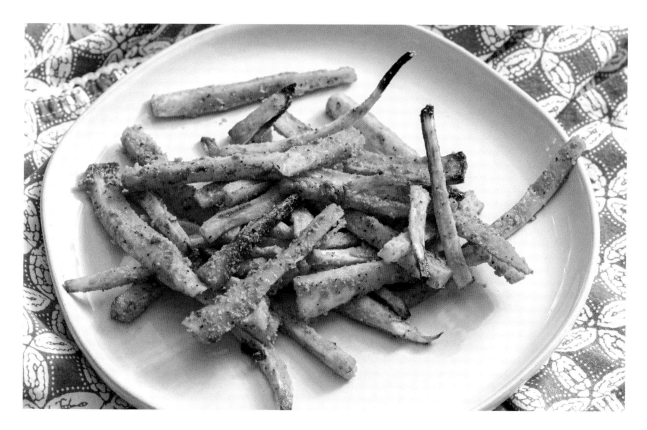

Don't worry; just because I want you getting your hands dirty doesn't mean I expect you to spend all day in the kitchen. I'm not against shortcuts like prechopped vegetables or canned beans already pressure cooked with kombu (which, as I'll talk about later, helps with the digestion of plant proteins). I'm not suggesting that you buy whole heads of lettuce instead of boxes of greens that are already washed and cut into perfect bite-sized pieces. Those types of shortcuts can save you major time (and a cramp in your chopping hand) in the service of making wholesome, nutrient-dense meals.

I also recognize that we have constraints on what food is available to us. My mom often laments that in rural northwest Ohio, she doesn't have ready access to shiitake mushrooms or bok choy like we do in suburban Connecticut. Conversely, I don't have access to home-grown, freshly picked summer strawberries or crisp green beans from a farmer who lives just down the road like she does. No place is perfect. It all evens out because there are workarounds. My mom buys celery when she wants bok choy, and I buy cartons of strawberries when I can't get the local ones. Just do the best you can.

It's important to note that real food generally costs more than processed food. This is another way in which processed foods are designed to make us fail. They appeal not only to our palates but to our wallets, too. After all, if you were cash-strapped and needed calories, you could get the most caloric bang for your buck with something from the snack-food aisle, like chips, cookies, or snack cakes.

Americans don't spend as much on food as people in other countries do. Europeans spend more than twice what Americans do on food. If we don't put the money in up front, we're going to be putting it in on the back end in the form of medical bills.[4] I'm confident our poor nutritional habits as a nation are part of the reason we spend almost 18 percent of gross domestic product on healthcare. That crazy number is estimated to reach almost 20 percent by 2028 given that our healthcare expenditures are growing faster than the GDP itself.[5]

In addition to the barriers of time, availability, and cost, there's an educational piece. Most of us aren't learning how to cook, and we're not teaching the next generation how to cook, either. As Dr. Mark Hyman writes in his book *Food: What the Heck Should I Eat,* we've essentially "handed over the act of cooking, this unique task that makes us human, to the food industry. We have become food consumers, not food producers or preparers, and in doing so, we have lost our connection to our world and to ourselves."[6]

The importance of reconnecting to your *Wellness Intuition* is why I'm writing this book. It's why I chose to practice medicine, and it's why I started the *Dr. Katie Detox.* I want to share with you what I've learned so that you can educate yourself and teach the next generation how to do the same.

Now that I've addressed what constitutes real food (and what we should avoid because it's not natural) and why real food needs to be prepared in a real kitchen, let's dive into the specifics about which foods to include and in what quantities. To do that, I'll use *Dr. Katie's Anti-Inflammatory Diet,* otherwise known among my patients and Detoxers as the *Dr. Katie Pyramid.*

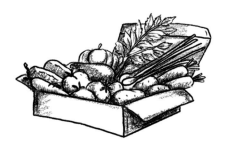

[4] M. Hyman, *Food: What the Heck Should I Eat?* (New York: Little, Brown, 2018): 17.

[5] "NHE Fact Sheet," available from: https://www.cms.gov/Research-Statistics-Data-and-Systems/Statistics-Trends-and-Reports/NationalHealthExpendData/NHE-Fact-Sheet

[6] Hyman, *Food:* 18.

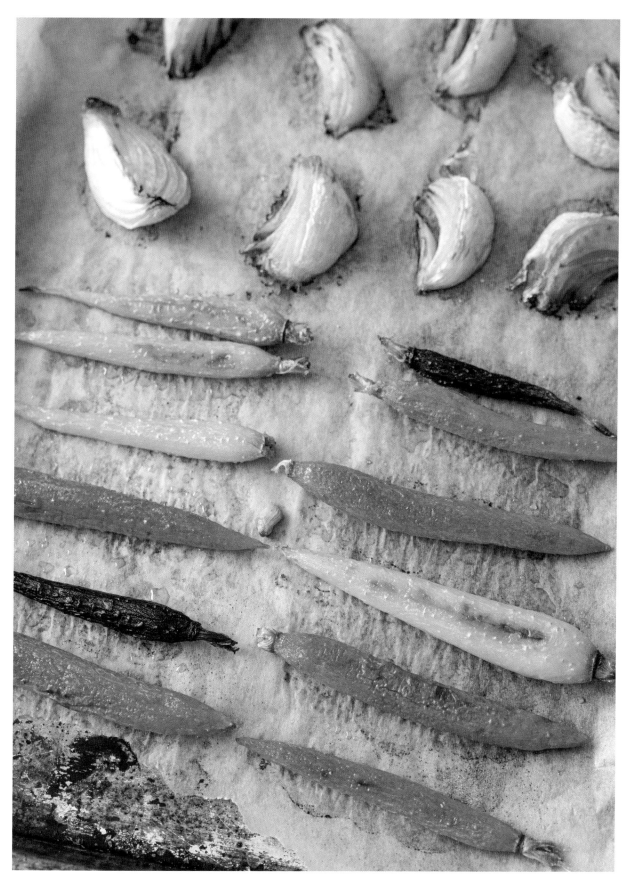

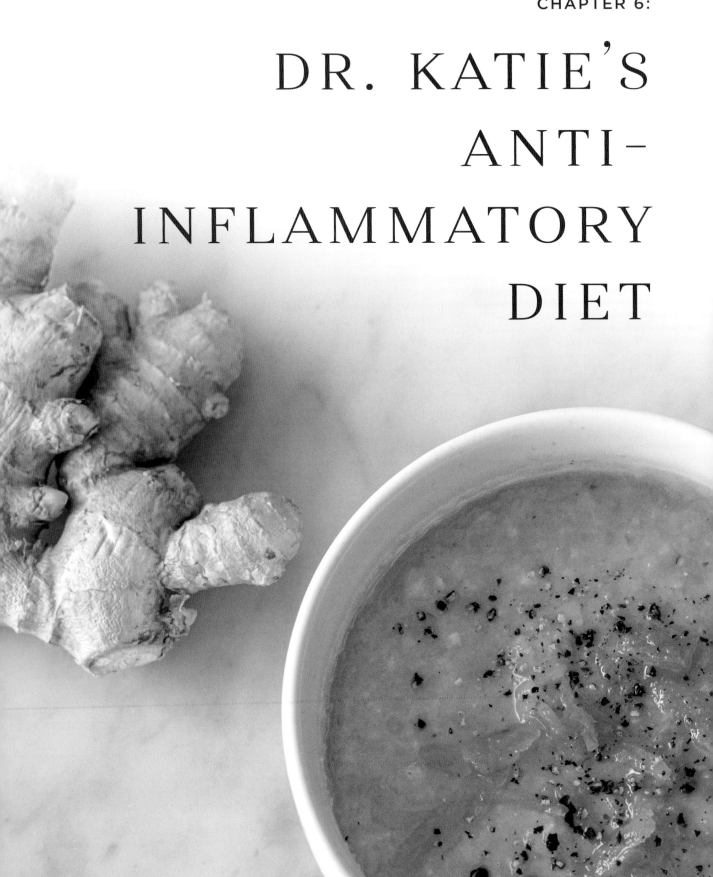

CHAPTER 6

DR. KATIE'S ANTI-INFLAMMATORY DIET

Dr. Katie's Anti-Inflammatory Diet is my approach to eating a well-balanced plant-forward diet. It came into being because I couldn't find a graphic that explained all the important components of a harmonious existence on one page. So I did what any person who is invested in guiding others toward health and authenticity would do: I created my own graphic on a paper napkin, took a picture of it with my phone, and sent it to a fantastic graphic designer to make magic.

Instead of focusing on what to cut out and what *not* to eat, this pyramid focuses on what you *should* build into your diet on a daily and weekly basis. If you hit most of these blocks on most days, you'll be following the 80/20 rule and doing a pretty good job. And, as you know, you just have to find the individual balance that allows your body to take your inputs and transform them into great outputs.

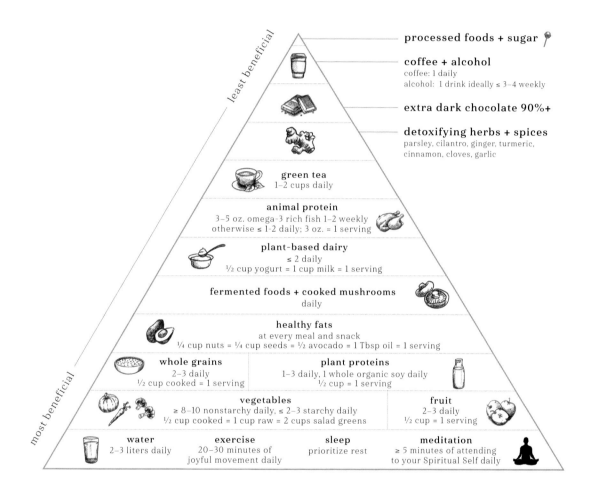

least beneficial

processed foods + sugar

coffee + alcohol
coffee: 1 daily
alcohol: 1 drink ideally ≤ 3–4 weekly

extra dark chocolate 90%+

detoxifying herbs + spices
parsley, cilantro, ginger, turmeric,
cinnamon, cloves, garlic

green tea
1–2 cups daily

animal protein
3–5 oz. omega-3 rich fish 1–2 weekly
otherwise ≤ 1–2 daily; 3 oz. = 1 serving

plant-based dairy
≤ 2 daily
½ cup yogurt = 1 cup milk = 1 serving

fermented foods + cooked mushrooms
daily

healthy fats
at every meal and snack
¼ cup nuts = ¼ cup seeds = ½ avocado = 1 Tbsp oil = 1 serving

whole grains
2–3 daily
½ cup cooked = 1 serving

plant proteins
1–3 daily, 1 whole organic soy daily
½ cup = 1 serving

vegetables
≥ 8–10 nonstarchy daily, ≤ 2–3 starchy daily
½ cup cooked = 1 cup raw = 2 cups salad greens

fruit
2–3 daily
½ cup = 1 serving

water
2–3 liters daily

exercise
20–30 minutes of
joyful movement daily

sleep
prioritize rest

meditation
≥ 5 minutes of attending
to your Spiritual Self daily

most beneficial

My patients call this the *Dr. Katie Pyramid* because it's not just about food. In fact, the foundation of the pyramid is not food at all.

The *Dr. Katie Pyramid* is my approach to finding harmony and balance in the body, and we can't make music the way it was composed if we're missing an entire section of the orchestra. The foundation of my pyramid is adequate hydration, joyful movement, time for rest, and connection to your Spiritual Self in the form of meditative activities or any other pursuit that allows you to tap into the real you. I put these components at the base of my pyramid because they're important, and—wait for it—there's a *whole chapter* coming up on movement, rest, and meditation.

But since we're deep into diet, let's focus on the food first.

MOST IMPORTANT: VEGETABLES

No surprise, the biggest section of the *Dr. Katie Pyramid* is dedicated to vegetables. That's because vegetables are, hands-down, the most nutrient-dense foods we eat on a daily basis. Of all foods, vegetables pack the most vitamins, minerals, fiber, antioxidants, phytonutrients, and anti-inflammatory compounds in the most calorically lean way. Even though they are mostly carbohydrates, they don't spike your blood sugar because they contain the magical indigestible substance called fiber that I talked about in Chapter 3.

Most people should eat at least eight servings of vegetables per day, with a serving being equal to ¹/₂ cup of cooked or 1 cup of raw vegetables, or 2 cups of raw salad greens.

When I share these numbers with patients, many of them look at me meekly, swallow hard, and ask, "Well, um, Dr. Katie, if I'm eating all those vegetables, then what else am I eating?" To which I reply, "That's the whole point—a diet that is plant-forward is mostly vegetables!"

I make a point of suggesting at least eight servings of nonstarchy vegetables a day and three servings or fewer of starchy vegetables. Most of the vegetables we eat should be nonstarchy green ones like artichokes, asparagus, bok choy, broccoli, Brussels sprouts, cabbage, cauliflower, cucumbers, green beans, kale, and kohlrabi, along with others like cauliflower, mushrooms, and onions, just to name a few. In fact, you can go to town on nonstarchy vegetables. Eat as much as you want. (Just don't increase your overall fiber content too quickly, or all that fiber will give you bloating and constipation. Remember, slow and steady wins the race.)

The amount of starchy vegetables you should consume is based on your activity level and how many whole grains you eat. The more active you are—imagine a kid who runs around on the soccer field—the more starchy vegetables and whole grains you need to maintain your energy. As an illustration of how much more active kids are than adults, I gave my son my step tracker one day when he went to sports camp. By three o'clock in the afternoon, he had already taken 20,000 steps! Unfortunately, most of us are not getting that much activity, so we need only about ¹/₂ cup of starchy vegetables or whole grains one to three times a day.

How do you know if a vegetable is starchy? The simple way to tell is by its taste. A starchy vegetable has a sweeter flavor. Think about beets, carrots, green peas, jicama, parsnips, potatoes, squash, and sweet potatoes. They are all on the sweeter side, especially when you compare them to nonstarchy vegetables like broccoli, cauliflower, and green beans (though I would argue that these veggies have their own innate sweetness) or to bitter greens like arugula, collards, kale, and Swiss chard.

Of course, a lot of that starchiness depends on whether the vegetable is raw or cooked. This is why roasted carrots taste much sweeter than raw carrots—because cooking changes the chemical structure of a carrot. The dry, intense heat of the oven caramelizes the natural sugar in the vegetables along with forming new aromatic compounds, and this is what makes roasted vegetables so irresistible. In fact, if you're trying to persuade someone that vegetables are delicious, I definitely recommend leading with your best hand. Roast those carrots for dinner using the Easy Roasted Vegetables recipe on page 286.

What? You don't think carrots are sweet? Just wait, my friend. If you're not on the "vegetables are sweet" train, you will be soon.

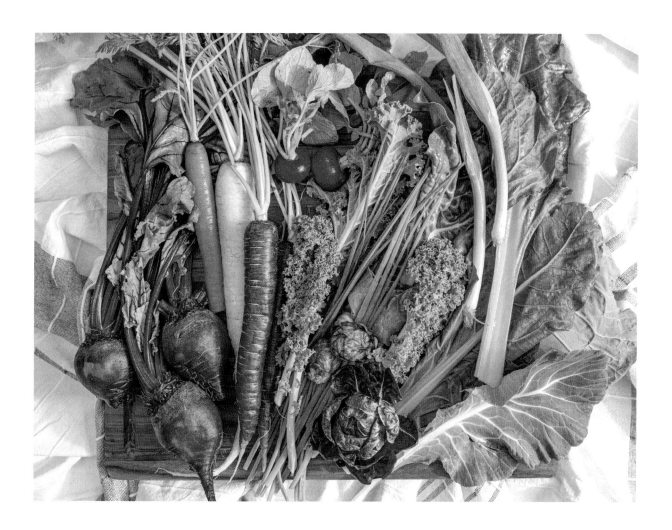

"I DON'T LIKE VEGETABLES"

I have patients who tell me they don't like vegetables. My immediate response is a sly smile and the reply, "What? You don't like vegetables? I'm not sure we can be friends." It's my belief that if someone doesn't like vegetables at all, then they probably haven't had the right vegetables prepared in the right way. If vegetables have been canned or boiled to death or under-roasted, making them rubbery; or over-roasted and burned; or—worst—processed into something that doesn't even resemble the original vegetable, then it's possible that they'll taste bad.

If you have a hard time loving vegetables, start by roasting them with some extra-virgin olive oil and tasty spices along with salt and pepper. Then dress them up with a drizzle of a yummy dressing, like my Lemony Basil Cashew Cream (page 300), or a healthy sprinkle of dukkah from the Spiced Nut Mix recipe (page 326). Even a dash of store-bought teriyaki sauce will do the trick for vegetable haters. Plain vegetables might be boring, but consider making them the backdrop for some kitchen creativity!

VEGETARIANS WHO DON'T EAT MANY VEGETABLES

One of the pitfalls I find my vegan, vegetarian, and ketogenic diet friends succumbing to is not eating enough vegetables. If you've ever been to a vegan restaurant, you won't find a lick of animal protein, but you'll find a lot of sugar in various forms. I'm always a little wary of going to a vegan restaurant, especially when people who are not baseline healthy eaters have told me that the food is *ah-mazing*. I often find that vegan and vegetarian restaurants and cookbooks replace the flavor of animal protein with more salt, fat, and sugar than is necessary, especially sugar in processed forms.

Likewise, I find that many of my patients who are "vegetarian" are not actually eating that many vegetables. Instead, they're just avoiding meat, making up the calories with ultra-processed foods that just happen not to contain animal protein.

SLOW CARB, NOT LOW CARB

Conversely, I often find that my patients following keto diets skimp on vegetables in exchange for foods with more animal protein because they are trying to keep themselves in ketosis. Ketosis is a metabolic state that results from carbohydrate restriction that forces the body to burn fat for energy, which leads to the production of ketone bodies.

Our bodies are not designed to exist in a constant state of ketosis. Remember, it's quick-burning carbohydrates that are the enemy. Slow-burning carbohydrates in the form of vegetables are good for you. The name of the game is *slow carb, not low carb*.

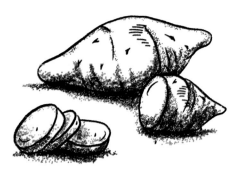

CRUCIFEROUS VEGETABLES

I make a point of eating cruciferous vegetables every day because they are probably the most important group. Cruciferous vegetables are rich in indoles and isothiocyanates (ITCs), which protect against cancer by helping our bodies make protective enzymes. This helps prevent cancer cell growth, block blood vessel formation to new tumors (called *angiogenesis*), and increase detoxification in the body.[1] Cruciferous vegetables also regulate the inflammatory response by supporting the protein complex NF-κB, which fires up our innate and adaptive immune response.

Some of these naturally occurring compounds are starting to be sold as separate bottled supplements, especially the indoles indole-3-carbinol and 3.3'-diindolylmethane (known as DIM) and the ITC sulforaphane.[2] Most people don't need a supplement of these compounds; they just need to eat cruciferous vegetables.

I recommend eating at least one serving per day of a cruciferous vegetable. Here are some examples to inspire you:

- Arugula
- Bok choy
- Broccoli
- Broccoli sprouts
- Brussels sprouts
- Cabbage
- Cauliflower
- Collard greens
- Daikon
- Horseradish
- Kale
- Kohlrabi
- Mustard greens
- Radishes
- Rutabaga
- Turnips
- Wasabi
- Watercress

Interestingly, one of the best sources of the anti-cancer compounds in cruciferous vegetables is broccoli sprouts. Research done at Johns Hopkins shows that three-day-old broccoli and cauliflower sprouts contain up to 100 times more glucoraphanin (the precursor to sulforaphane) than their mature plant counterparts.[3] Broccoli sprouts also have more vitamin K than broccoli. Don't replace all of your broccoli with sprouts, however. Broccoli is a better source of vitamins A and C. This is Nature's way of suggesting we find balance. I love sprouting my own broccoli and cauliflower seeds on my kitchen countertop. All you need is a sprouting kit, some seeds, and a few days of patience.

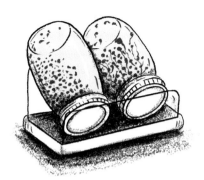

[1] H. Wang, T. O. Khor, L. Shu, et al., "Plants vs. cancer: a review on natural phytochemicals in preventing and treating cancers and their druggability," *Anti-Cancer Agents in Medicinal Chemistry* 12, no. 10 (2012): 1281–305.

[2] F. Fuentes, X. Paredes-Gonzalez, and A. T. Kong, "Dietary glucosinolates sulforaphane, phenethyl isothiocyanate, indole-3-carbinol/3,3'-diindolylmethane: anti-oxidative stress/inflammation, Nrf2, epigenetics/epigenomics and in vivo cancer chemopreventive efficacy," *Current Pharmacology Reports* 1, no. 3 (2015): 179–96.

[3] J. W. Fahey, Y. Zhang, and P. Talalay, "Broccoli sprouts: an exceptionally rich source of inducers of enzymes that protect against chemical carcinogens," *Proceedings of the National Academy of Sciences of the United States of America* 94, no. 19 (1997): 10367–72.

SEA VEGETABLES

I need to give another quick shout-out in our vegetable party to seaweed. Sea vegetables are among the most nutrient-rich foods we can eat, providing essential minerals that are rarely found in the standard American diet. Seaweed is a natural source of iodine, which is essential for thyroid function and hard to come by for those of us who are using fancy sea salts that are not fortified with iodine like traditional iodized table salt. Seaweed is also rich in manganese, vitamin C, and iron and is an important part of an anti-inflammatory diet.

I didn't eat sea vegetables before I became a Takayasu. When my husband and I moved in together, I started to find strange foods in my pantry, including wakame flakes, strips of kombu, and sheets of nori. I knew of nori because I had eaten maki at sushi restaurants, but the others were new to me. I saw him use these dry, dark-green and black foods in a lot of his cooking, but I never tried to incorporate them into my own recipes—that is, until I started to eat a plant-forward diet. That's when I recognized Japanese genius. Now I keep a shaker of dulse on my countertop and sprinkle it on almost every dish. And I've convinced one of my sons that roasted salted seaweed is a perfect snack. You'll see these sea vegetables sprinkled into my recipes.

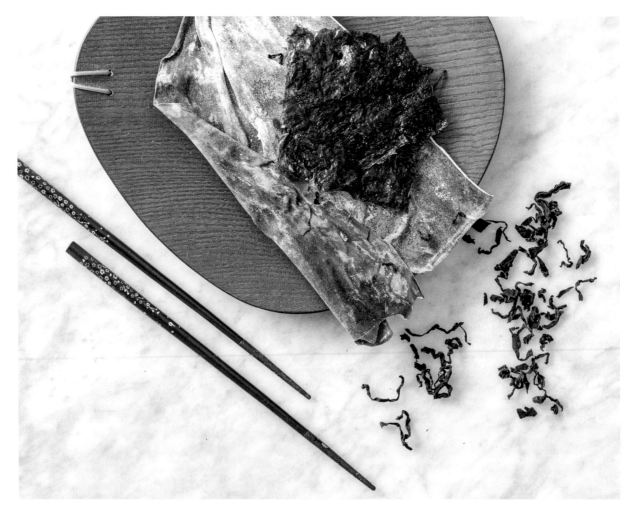

EAT THE RAINBOW

I encourage you to eat a rainbow of plant colors. In fact, finding the rainbows on our plates was one of my favorite food activities with my kids when they were younger. And who doesn't love a little ROYGBIV action on a white plate?

There's a reason we are drawn to the vibrant red color of beets and radishes and the gorgeous purple color of Japanese eggplant and the spectacular look of rainbow chard or rhubarb with vibrant green leaves. All those colors signify different phytonutrients that your body needs. Let your eye be your guide. If it's pretty to look at, then it's probably good for your body (assuming it was made by Nature and not in a laboratory).

But while we are drawn to color, don't let white vegetables like onions, garlic, leeks, and cauliflower fool you. They're just as nutritious as their colorful friends. Here's a little guide to get your rainbow connection flowing.

COLOR	PHYTONUTRIENT COMPOUND(S)	EFFECTS OF PHYTONUTRIENT IN THE BODY	VEGETABLE SOURCES
Red	Lycopene	Protects against heart disease and cancer	Tomatoes, bell peppers
Orange	Alpha-carotene and beta-carotene	Protect against cancer, preserve vision and skin	Carrots, pumpkin, sweet potatoes, winter squash
Yellow-green	Lutein and zeaxanthin	Protect against heart disease	Spinach, collard greens, mustard greens, turnip greens, sweet corn, green peas, avocados
Green	Sulforaphane, isocyanates, indole-3-carbinol	Protect against cancer by inhibiting carcinogens, preventing oxidative damage, and supporting detoxification	Cruciferous vegetables like arugula, bok choy, broccoli, kale, and watercress
Blue-purple	Anthocyanins	Protect against blood clots and cellular aging, preserve integrity of brain and nerve cells	Eggplant, beets, purple cabbage, purple potatoes
White	Allicins, quercetin, kaempferol	Protect against cancer and infection	Alliums like garlic, onions, leeks, and shallots

ORGANIC & FROZEN VEGETABLES

I recommend prioritizing your supermarket spending on organic vegetables that you eat without peeling, like celery and spinach. That said, I have found that organic vegetables generally taste better, so I tend to buy organic whenever I can.

I fully support the purchase of frozen vegetables, since they may be even more nutritious than fresh and certainly make life easier and more wallet friendly. Unless you're in a big pinch, don't buy canned vegetables, which tend to be laden with salt.

For more on buying and preparing vegetables, check out Chapter 10, where I share my high-yield *Life Kitchen* tips.

VEGETABLES IN YOUR *WELLNESS INTUITION*

Of course, there are some idiosyncrasies to this recommendation based on your personal constitution. Not everyone is made to eat every food. Do cruciferous vegetables like broccoli and cauliflower give you terrible gas no matter how you prepare them? Then maybe those aren't the best choices for you, at least until you figure out why that's happening. Look for guidance in the conversation about food aversions on page 227 and the discussion of eating to your individual constitution on pages 150 to 152. But good news, my friend: even if you don't like eggplant, there are a lot of other delicious vegetables to enjoy!

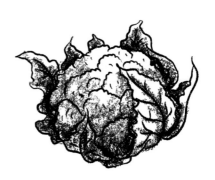

FRUIT

Many of my healthy patients overdo it with fruit. Sure, fruit is healthy, but it's also a natural sugar. What makes whole fruit perfect is that Nature combines the natural sugar with fiber, so the release of insulin in the body in response to the fructose is slowed. At my house, we call fruit Nature's candy. And it is exactly that—a natural form of sugar wrapped up in a delightful little package.

FRUCTOSE & YOUR LIVER

Fructose, or fruit sugar, can be a disaster in the body if it's not consumed with fiber because it's processed almost entirely by the liver, where it's metabolized into fat. Fructose consumption also correlates to high triglycerides. You probably remember from page 41 that high triglycerides are a part of the disastrous triad of metabolic syndrome along with prediabetes. Fructose derivatives, like high-fructose corn syrup, are especially bad for us, which is why I don't recommend drinking soda at all except in the rarest of circumstances. The liver's ability to metabolize fructose into fat leads not only to weight gain around our midsections but also to fatty deposits in the liver, which could result in needing a liver transplant in severe cases. I don't have a problem with fruit in moderation because the fructose is accompanied by soluble fiber, which slows its absorption and gives your liver a little more time to metabolize it.

It's important to remember that you need *at least four times* as many servings of vegetables on a daily basis compared to fruit. That's why I always say, "Eat your vegetables and fruit" instead of "Eat your fruit and vegetables." Reword that phrase to remind yourself of your priorities.

Colorful low-glycemic fruits like berries are the best fruits to eat. Who can argue with something that's Nature-made and bright red or blue? Wild fruits, especially berries, pack the most antioxidants and fiber with the least sugar, making them an important part of an anti-inflammatory diet. In fact, many wild berries are used medicinally because of their antimicrobial and anti-inflammatory properties, including barberries, which are bottled and sold as berberine. I use berberine all the time in my practice to help those with intestinal infections or dysbiosis (an imbalance of good and bad probiotics that leads to bacterial overgrowth and malabsorption, along with stool irregularities, gas, bloating, and abdominal pain).

I recommend spending at least one of your two fruit servings per day on some kind of wild berry. Here's a list to inspire you:

- Acai berries
- Bilberries
- Blackberries
- Cranberries
- Elderberries
- Goji berries
- Mulberries
- Raspberries
- Strawberries
- Wild blueberries

Note that some of these berries are available only in dried form. If you're eating dried fruits, keep your serving size to a tablespoon or less due to the concentration of sugar in dried fruit compared to its fresh or frozen counterpart. A study published in the *Journal of Biomedicine and Biotechnology* looked at the effects of freezing and drying on the antioxidant anthocyanin content of fresh blueberries.[4] When the researchers measured and compared the anthocyanin activity among the fresh, dried, and frozen berries, they found no significant difference.

Fortunately, this shows that dried fruit is still anti-inflammatory, which makes it a great way to add natural sweetness in small amounts, but it doesn't address the underlying concern of sugar. One cup of dried blueberries has more than three times the calories and twice as much sugar as the same amount of fresh or frozen blueberries.

Speaking of sugar, many of my patients say they avoid bananas or grapes because they have too much sugar but then go on to consume sugar in other processed forms, like lentil pasta. That doesn't make much sense! Yes, it's better to consume bananas when they are on the green-yellow side, but trust that Nature has made you some delicious dessert options and enjoy two half-cup servings of fruit per day. Maybe an apple a day does keep the doctor away!

To know which fruits to consume on the regular, you can use glycemic load to help you. Note that as fruits are dried, their glycemic load increases. For example, the glycemic load of grapes is 11, while the glycemic load of raisins is a whopping 28. It's better to consume fruits with a glycemic load of no more than 11.

As with vegetables, I recommend prioritizing your spending for organic on the fruits you eat without peeling, like apples and plums. You can buy conventional bananas if you want to save a bit of money. I have found that organic fruit generally tastes better. For more on eating organic, see page 193.

As with vegetables, I'm also okay with frozen fruit, since it may be even more nutrient-dense than fresh. But please don't buy canned or packaged fruit in syrup. Fruits in syrup are just sugar bombs.

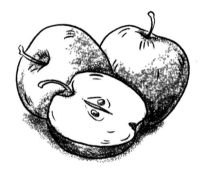

---

[4] V. Lohachoompol, G. Srzednicki, and J. Craske, "The change of total anthocyanins in blueberries and their antioxidant effect after drying and freezing," *Journal of Biomedicine and Biotechnology* 2004, no. 5 (2004): 248–52.

DON'T DRINK YOUR FRUIT

One last point on fruit: fruit juice is not the same as fruit. Fruit juice is just the extrapolated sugar and water from the fruit without all the natural fiber. This makes fruit juice akin to drinking sugar water with some vitamins and minerals.

Drinking fruit juice is also not natural. It takes about five medium oranges to make one 8-ounce glass of orange juice, but when would you ever sit down and eat five oranges at one time? You wouldn't. Same thing with the juice: it's just too much sugar at one time. (Many of my patients have juice every day when they take their medications, vitamins, and supplements. Just wash your pills down the hatch with water. It's so much better for you!) Be careful of green juices, too. If it's not a truly savory (read: almost salty) juice, then it's not good for you.

Likewise, be careful when making smoothies at home or buying them from your local juice bar. Sometimes my patients use way too much fruit, which basically turns their smoothies into milkshakes with vitamins. Aim for a 2:1 ratio of vegetables to fruit to keep yourself in check. That means for every cup of kale, you can have one-half cup of frozen raspberries. If the smoothie doesn't taste sweet enough at first, then allow yourself more fruit and slowly cut back over the course of a few weeks until you're at a 2:1 ratio. You can use my Recovery Smoothie recipe (page 248) to get started.

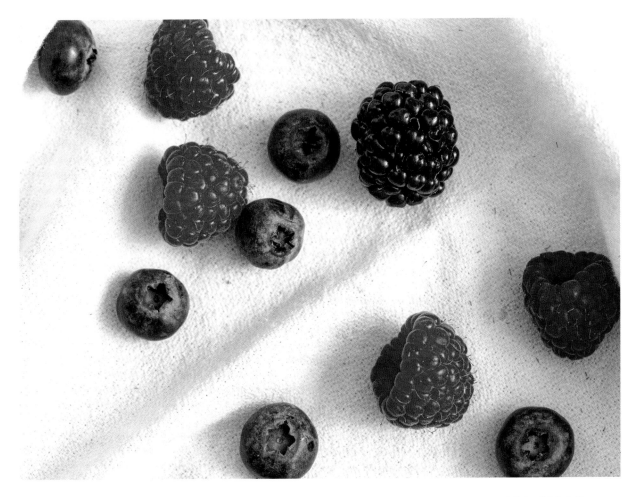

WHOLE GRAINS

I love talking about whole grains with patients because this is where a lot of those "aha" moments come in.

Whole grains are the seeds of grasses cultivated for food. They come from the ground and appear on our plates in pretty much the same form; they haven't been processed into anything else.

Eating whole grains preserves their intrinsic fat and fiber to help make the release of sugar in our bodies slow and steady, which has a more positive effect on our blood sugar than processed grains, which are converted to sugar almost instantaneously. In our bodies, there's almost no difference between eating a spoonful of sugar and a highly processed grain like pasta, crackers, chips, or bread. So consider those processed starches as treats and make them less prominent in your diet.

CHEERIOS DON'T GROW ON TREES

Whole grains are a super confusing subject because "whole grain" seems like it's written on every package these days as a way to convince consumers that the product is healthy.

Take Cheerios, for example. Right there across the middle of the box, it says "made with 100% whole grain oats." But Cheerios don't grow on trees. They aren't real whole grains. They are whole grains in sheep's clothing. General Mills—and all the other breakfast cereal companies—take the goodness of a real whole grain and process it into something that doesn't look remotely like it did in Nature. And that, my friend, is where the problem lies. Once a natural whole grain is processed into something else, it becomes an impostor, a fake food. And our American diets are littered with fake foods.

When I explain this to patients, one of the most common replies I hear is, "But Dr. Katie, Cheerios has only one gram of sugar, so I thought it was good for me. And it's supposed to lower cholesterol." Therein lies another problem with the marketing of whole-grain impostors.

It's true that Cheerios and many of its friends on the breakfast cereal shelf have only a few grams of sugar, but when you look at the nutrition label, you see a whole lot of carbohydrates. This quick-burning starch is pretty much like sugar except that food companies don't have to list it as sugar on the label. And if you look at the list of ingredients, you'll see that the rest of the ingredients after "whole grain oats" are other forms of sugar or additives to preserve freshness, along with a bunch of vitamins and minerals that were added because the milling process stripped them away from the oats.

PROCESSED GRAINS ARE BAD NEWS

Let's talk about why the processing of whole grains is troublesome. To do that, we have to examine the anatomy of a whole grain.

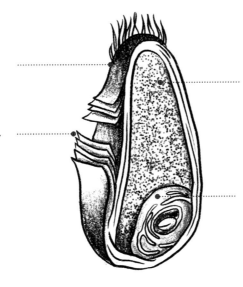

Hull
Inedible protective layer removed during processing

Bran
The skin of the kernel, rich in

- Antioxidants
- Phytonutrients
- Minerals
- B vitamins
- Fiber

Endosperm
Provides food for the germ, containing

- Starchy carbohydrates
- Some protein
- Some B vitamins

Germ
The grain's embryo, rich in

- B vitamins
- Vitamin E
- Antioxidants
- Phytonutrients
- Unsaturated fats

There are nearly two dozen edible grains:

- Amaranth
- Barley
- Buckwheat
- Bulgur
- Corn
- Einkorn
- Farro
- Fonio
- Freekeh
- Kamut
- Kaniwa
- Millet
- Oats
- Quinoa
- Rice
- Rye
- Sorghum
- Spelt
- Teff
- Triticale
- Wheat
- Wild rice

There are four parts to a whole grain, and each has a role. With a true whole grain, only the indigestible outer shell is removed before the grain is packaged.

With processed grains, like white flour, bread, and white rice, the milling process removes most of the bran and germ to give the grains a finer texture and improve their shelf life. Unfortunately, the bran is where you find nutrients and most of the fiber, and the germ is where you find nutrients and most of the fat. Processing leaves only the easy-to-chew endosperm that's rich in starch but not much else. Processed grains don't have much fiber, iron, or B vitamins, so food companies generally add them back in.

I recommend that you eat whole grains and stay away from refined and enriched grains.

Whole Grains	Refined Grains	Enriched and Fortified Grains
Sold in whole form with only the indigestible outer shell removed	Milled to remove the germ and bran, which gives refined grains a finer texture and extends their shelf life	*Enriched* means that some of the nutrients lost during processing are artificially replaced, most notably B vitamins (including folate or folic acid) and iron. *Fortified* means nutrients that don't occur naturally in the food have been added to artificially increase its nutritional value.
Good sources of fiber and other important nutrients, such as B vitamins (including folate or folic acid), iron, selenium, potassium, and magnesium	The refining process removes many nutrients, including fiber.	Removed nutrients are artificially re-added to make the refined grain more nutritious.
Examples: amaranth, barley, buckwheat, bulgur, whole corn, einkorn, farro, fonio, freekeh, kamut, kaniwa, millet, oats, quinoa, rice (brown, red, black), rye, sorghum, spelt, teff, triticale, wild rice	Examples: flour, white rice, breads, breakfast cereals, crackers, pastries	Examples: flour, breads, breakfast cereals, crackers, pastries

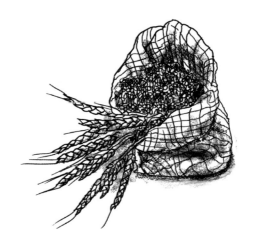

GLUTEN IS NOT INHERENTLY EVIL, BUT GLUTEN-FREE PRODUCTS CAN BE

It's important to talk about gluten. Gluten is not inherently evil, but the way it enters our diet often is.

Gluten is a family of proteins called prolamins found in wheat, rye, barley, farro, and triticale. It's got a gluelike function, holding grains together when heated due to its elastic structure. This makes for optimal leavening and maintenance of moisture in baking. It's what makes bread fluffy and cookies chewy. Gluten is also frequently used in processed foods to improve texture and promote moisture retention so that packaged goods can sit on store shelves longer and stay fresh. If you read labels, you'll find gluten all over the place.

Unless you have an allergy to gluten called celiac disease or a sensitivity to gluten (often called NCGS, or non-celiac gluten sensitivity), you can certainly enjoy gluten in small amounts. But let's talk about where gluten makes its way into our diets. It usually appears in the form of processed foods, like breads, pastas, crackers, and desserts, or as an additive to "helpers" in the kitchen, like gravies, sauces, salad dressings, and spice blends. These gluten-containing products are not good for anyone, regardless of an allergy or sensitivity to gluten.

Gluten-free products are all the rage these days, but most of us don't need them. I definitely recommend modest consumption of gluten-containing whole grains if you're not gluten sensitive. However, processed foods containing gluten, like crackers and pasta, are not good for anyone because sugar is not good for anyone.

Likewise, just because a product is gluten-free does not mean it's healthy. Pasta is unhealthy regardless of whether it's made from lentils, brown rice, or whole wheat. The same is true for crackers or any other processed product. It doesn't matter if your crackers are made from chickpeas or any other seemingly healthy food. Once a whole food is processed into something that doesn't exist in Nature, it is by definition less healthy—it's a treat and should be consumed as such. If our great-great-grandmothers wouldn't recognize it, then we shouldn't eat it very often.

That said, there are newer products on the shelves that are processed but have only one or two ingredients, like flaxseed crackers and one-ingredient pasta. I buy these products occasionally because I like to have something crunchy with my lunch salad, and my children like pasta with their primavera sauce. But it's not an everyday occurrence. Tread lightly with these types of gluten-free products and pay attention to the way you feel after you eat them. You might be better off eating toasted flax seeds and zucchini noodles!

Oats are a naturally gluten-free whole grain, but oats are often processed on machinery that has come into contact with gluten-containing grains, so you may want to buy gluten-free oats if you are gluten sensitive. That said, the oat protein avenin is similar to gluten, and some research suggests that those with an intolerance to gluten could also be sensitive to avenin.

How do you know if you're gluten or avenin sensitive? Well, this goes back to decoding your *Wellness Intuition* as discussed in Chapter 4. Try eliminating gluten-containing grains from your diet and see how you feel. I recommend a trial of gluten elimination for anyone with an underlying autoimmune disease or vague body symptoms such as fatigue, headaches, digestive woes, moodiness, or achiness. Generally, you have to avoid a questionable food for at least three weeks to decipher whether you're sensitive. I'll talk more about this in Chapter 12 because I advocate for a break from gluten during the *Dr. Katie Detox*.

I hope you understand after reading this section that the reason to avoid processed carbohydrates–whether they originate from whole grains or contain gluten–is because they have a high glycemic load, which quickly raises blood sugar and necessitates a quick rise in insulin. That quick rise not only forces storage of those calories as fat but inherently makes us hungrier. On top of that, the body often overshoots the blood sugar target, making us relatively hypoglycemic, which leads us to reach for those same foods that will quickly raise our blood sugar.

In short, those high-glycemic, quick-burning carbohydrate-rich foods that cause drastic ups and downs in blood sugar are designed to make us fail. Your success will come from choosing slow-burning whole grains in moderation.

WRAPPING UP WHOLE GRAINS

My ultimate whole-grain advice: eat only the whole grains found in Nature. The preservation of nutrients, fiber, and fat is what makes real whole grains like barley, brown rice, farro, millet, quinoa, and steel-cut oats nutrient-dense, slow-burn carbohydrates. And by now you know our motto is *slow carb, not low carb.*

I'm happy to recommend a modest amount of whole grains in *Dr. Katie's Anti-Inflammatory Diet* because I find that regular consumption of whole grains actually *decreases* sugar and processed carbohydrate cravings for many of my patients. Many people cut out carbohydrates of all types in an effort to be healthy, which stems from rhetoric about keto and Atkins-type diets that carbs are dangerous. As you now know, it's true that processed carbs are not good, but modest amounts of whole carbs are fine.

So how much whole grain can you have? I recommend one to three half-cup servings of whole grains per day depending on how active you are and how much starchy vegetables you are eating.

Going back to our plate real estate on page 69, you'll notice that a portion of the daily meal is dedicated to either whole grains or starchy vegetables. I would try to do a mix of both to satisfy the space of healthy starch in your diet. So maybe you have a whole-grain porridge like my Slow Cooker Apple Pie Oatmeal (page 236) at breakfast, some roasted sweet potato on your salad at lunch, and some Harvest Wild Rice (page 284) for dinner. You'll see that I sometimes allow for both a starchy vegetable and a whole grain in the same meal, like the Almond Furikake Crusted Halibut recipe (page 268), which includes both forbidden rice and kabocha squash. It's okay to do that as long as you keep the real estate on your plate in balance.

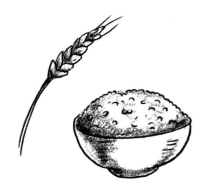

PLANT PROTEIN

Getting adequate protein is usually the biggest concern in a plant-forward diet, but you know from Chapters 2 and 3 that you can get adequate protein from a plant-forward lifestyle if you're mindful of what you're eating.

There are so many delicious sources of plant protein that provide the essential amino acids we need for lean body mass maintenance, digestion and energy metabolism, gene translation, hormonal signaling, and immune surveillance. The trick is getting a mix of plant proteins and mixing in some healthy animal protein along the way. (I'll talk about animal proteins a little later in this chapter.) And you already know the reason to prioritize plant-based protein: its natural mix of fiber along with many vitamins and minerals makes it anti-inflammatory in the body.

To make it easier for you, I've categorized plant protein sources into higher and lower amounts based on how much a person might eat at one time. For example, nutritional yeast is a complete source of protein (meaning it has all of the essential amino acids your body cannot make on its own), but most of us only eat about a tablespoon at a time, which gives us 3 grams of protein, so nutritional yeast is not an efficient source of protein.

Higher Amounts of Protein	Lower Amounts of Protein
Beans—black beans, black-eyed peas, chickpeas (aka garbanzo beans), cannellini beans, navy beans, kidney beans, pinto beans, adzuki beans	Nutritional yeast
Lentils—red, black, green, yellow, brown	Quinoa
Other legumes—peanuts	Spelt
Nuts—any type	Teff
Seeds—chia, hemp, sunflower, pumpkin	
Whole organic soy—tofu, tempeh, edamame, soy nuts, miso, natto	

I recommend one to three half-cup servings of plant protein per day depending on how much protein your body needs and how much animal protein you're eating. Returning to our ideal plate balance, you'll want a bit of real estate at every meal and snack to be dedicated to protein so that you meet your body's protein needs.

BEANS, LEGUMES & LECTINS

Beans and other legumes like lentils are great sources of plant protein that come in a beautiful package of fiber, B vitamins like folate and B_6, and minerals like iron, zinc, potassium, and magnesium. They're inexpensive and widely available. They are agriculturally robust because they can grow in relatively nitrogen-deficient soil, absorbing nitrogen directly from the atmosphere (which contributes to their high protein content). And eating beans is correlated with longevity and weight management and decreased risk of heart disease, diabetes, cancer, and general inflammation.[5]

But of course, no food is perfect.

Lectins are proteins that bind to the carbohydrates present in uncooked legumes. Their purpose is to protect plants in Nature. They have gotten a lot of press recently due to some fad-type diet books that connect them to obesity, chronic inflammation, and auto-immune disease. Lectins are found in all plants, but dried legumes like beans, lentils, peas, soybeans, and peanuts (along with shellfish and grains like wheat) contain the highest amounts.

Lectins may cause problems with digestion because they resist being broken down in the gut and are stable in acidic environments. Animal and cell studies have found that lectins can interfere with the absorption of essential minerals like calcium, iron, and zinc by binding to the cells that line the digestive tract.[6] Additionally, they can injure the integrity of the gut lining, letting harmful bacteria and lipopolysaccharides into our bodies and leading to a toxic inflammatory response.

But lectins aren't really a problem for most plant-protein eaters because of that word *uncooked.* When would you ever eat uncooked black beans? Um, never. Cooking, especially wet high-heat methods like boiling, stewing,

and pressure cooking, or even soaking for a few hours will inactivate most lectins. Fermentation is another great way to decrease the potentially harmful effects of lectins because during the fermentation process, beneficial bacteria break down and digest the lectins. Consider adding a fermented bean like natto to your diet.

If you have digestive woes like gas or bloating or worries about lectins that limit your desire to eat more beans, see page 220 for my tips on making them easier to digest.

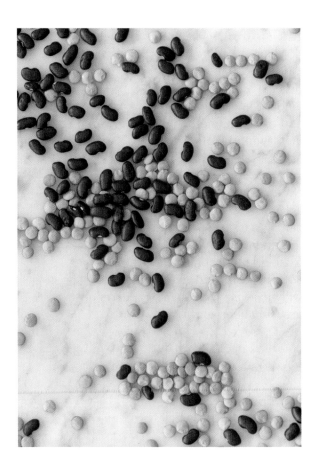

---

[5] V. Miller, A. Mente, M. Dehghan, et al., "Fruit, vegetable, and legume intake, and cardiovascular disease and deaths in 18 countries (PURE): a prospective cohort study," *The Lancet* (London, England) 390, no. 10107 (2017): P2037–49.

[6] D. L. J. Freed, "Do dietary lectins cause disease? The evidence is suggestive—and raises interesting possibilities for treatment," *British Medical Journal* 318, no. 7190 (1999): 1023–4.

WHOLE ORGANIC SOY
(IT WILL NOT GIVE YOU MAN-BOOBS)

Many of my patients are afraid to eat soy because they think it will raise their risk of breast cancer or give them man-boobs, but you don't have to be afraid. There are, however, a few points that warrant our attention.

I advocate for whole organic soy because it is rich in vitamins and minerals and is a natural source of polyphenols, a type of antioxidant that can help protect the body against inflammatory processes like cell damage and heart disease, increase the good cholesterol HDL, and lower the bad cholesterol LDL and triglycerides, as well as help with blood sugar and insulin regulation.[7] I recommend soy to my perimenopausal patients because regular modest consumption has been shown in a large meta-analysis of nineteen studies to reduce hot flashes by 20 percent compared to placebo.[8] This modest amount is equal to one-half to three-quarters cup of edamame per day. And have no fear: a dietary intake of about one-half cup of whole organic soy per day has been shown in studies to decrease the risk of *recurrence* of breast cancer in survivors with estrogen-receptor and progesterone-receptor positive breast cancer and those receiving adjuvant endocrine treatment with the aromatase inhibitor anastrozole.[9] Modest amounts of whole organic soy not only will *not* give you breast cancer, but will decrease your risk of recurrence if you're a breast cancer survivor.

Those words *whole* and *organic* are the differentiators between good and bad soy. Whole organic soy has the right ratio of a subclass of polyphenols called isoflavones that make it anti-inflammatory. Isoflavones are nonsteroidal soy building blocks and bind to estrogen receptors. Whole soy contains approximately equal parts of the isoflavones genistein and daidzein, whereas processed soy has four times more daidzein, which is inflammatory. I consider tempeh and edamame to be the two best sources of whole organic soy, with tofu as a close third. Even though tempeh and tofu are processed, they still approach the right ratio of soy isoflavones, making them anti-inflammatory, unlike processed soy, such as soy protein isolates. It's important to buy organic soy because organic soy is not a genetically modified organism (GMO). You want to avoid GMO soy because it may be less nutrient-dense and contain more herbicide residue than organic soy.

Consider consuming one half-cup serving per day of whole organic soy like edamame, soy nuts, tofu, or tempeh. Fermented soy like tempeh, miso, and natto is especially good because the fermentation process makes it easier to digest and absorb its nutrients. I feel confident about this and serve whole organic soy to my sons as part of our family's diet.

The soy I want you to stay away from is the soy found in ultra-processed foods and other foods that shouldn't have soy in them. Take a look at the back of your granola bar. Does it have soy protein isolates on the ingredient list? Or what about those vegan meat substitutes at the grocery store? Widely available products like Clif Bars and Boca Burgers contain soy proteins, as do soy protein powders, soy hot dogs, and soy baby formula. These types of products have the wrong ratio of isoflavones and are inflammatory. I recommend avoiding them.

[7] K. Fang, H. Dong, D. Wang, et al., "Soy isoflavones and glucose metabolism in menopausal women: A systematic review and meta-analysis of randomized controlled trials," *Molecular Nutrition & Food Research* 60, no. 7 (2016), 1602–14; D. Malenčić, J. Cvejić, and J. Miladinović, "Polyphenol content and antioxidant properties of colored soybean seeds from central Europe," *Journal of Medicinal Food* 15, no. 1 (2012): 89–95; O. A. Tokede, T. A. Onabanjo, A. Yansane, et al., "Soya products and serum lipids: a meta-analysis of randomised controlled trials," *British Journal of Nutrition* 114, no. 6 (2015): 831–43.

[8] K. Taku, M. K. Melby, F. Kronenberg, et al., "Extracted or synthesized soybean isoflavones reduce menopausal hot flash frequency and severity: systematic review and meta-analysis of randomized controlled trials," *Menopause* (New York) 19, no. 7 (2012): 776–90.

[9] X. Kang, Q. Zhang, S. Wang, et al., "Effect of soy isoflavones on breast cancer recurrence and death for patients receiving adjuvant endocrine therapy," *CMAJ: Canadian Medical Association Journal* 182, no. 17 (2010): 1857–62.

NUTS & SEEDS HAVE PROTEIN, TOO

Nuts and seeds are a mix of fiber, fat, and protein, which makes them ideal in my book because they satisfy several parts in our effort to find balance on our plates. If you're thinking about protein, some of my favorites are hemp, sunflower, chia, flax, and pumpkin seeds along with almonds, pistachios, and cashews. I'll discuss all of these in the next section on healthy fats.

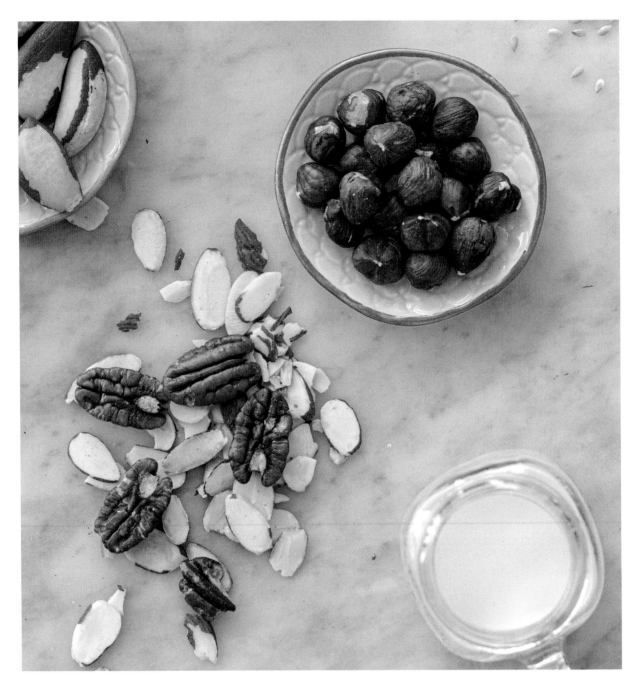

HEALTHY FATS

By now, I hope you know that eating fat will not make you fat. In fact, it may keep you lean because it's the key to satiety—to telling your brain you've had enough food. And we know the right amount of anti-inflammatory fat in the diet doesn't cause heart disease. In fact, it was the low-fat, higher-sugar diet touted in the 1990s that increased obesity and diabetes—two inflammatory conditions strongly linked to heart disease. And over and over again, when we compare the plant- and fat-forward Mediterranean diet to a low-fat diet, we see a decreased risk of heart disease and stroke, lower fasting glucose, lower blood pressure, decreased inflammatory markers, and overall lower mortality.[10] We need fats in our diets for healthy cell membranes, for making hormones like estrogen and testosterone, for metabolism regulation, and for making immune cells, which impacts inflammation downstream.

But we have to distinguish between healthy and unhealthy fats. While I love fat and find it helpful for satiety, blood sugar balancing, and taste, it's important to choose the right kind. There are lots of inflammatory fats in our food system.

THE RIGHT & WRONG KINDS OF FATS

Most of your dietary fat should be monounsaturated, combined with appropriate amounts of saturated fat, omega-3 fat, and medium-chain triglycerides (MCTs). While all of these fats are important, finding the right balance is key. Prioritizing monounsaturated fats like olives, olive oil, nuts, seeds, avocados, and avocado oil, along with smaller amounts of other fats, like those found in extra-dark chocolate, coconut, coconut oil, butter, and ghee, is the way to go.

One easy way to incorporate more healthy fat into your diet is to roast your vegetables with extra-virgin olive oil. I grew up in the 1990s when low-fat was all the rage, and my mom loved to steam vegetables. I rarely steam vegetables these days because it's not as flavorful or interesting, and because it misses the opportunity to add healthy fats.

When thinking about the right fats to include, it's important to consider an oil's smoke point, which tells you how to use the oil. For instance, you know I love extra-virgin olive oil, but it's not a great choice for searing meat or fish over high heat because it has a relatively low smoke point. As soon as an oil starts to smoke, you know you've gone too far. The smoke is a sign that the fat is decomposing and generating toxic fumes along with free radicals that are dangerous to the body. Plus, it makes food smell and taste bad. You don't need to memorize the smoke points of oils. I make it easy by using avocado oil when I'm planning to use a higher heat for searing; otherwise, I use extra-virgin olive oil and occasionally coconut oil or ghee (clarified butter).

[10] M. Gwynne and A. Mounsey, "Mediterranean diet: higher fat but lower risk," *Journal of Family Practice* 62, no. 12 (2013): 745–8; G. De Pergola and A. D'Alessandro, "Influence of Mediterranean diet on blood pressure," *Nutrients* 10, no. 11 (2018): 1700.

As discussed in Chapter 3, you should stay away from trans fats and partially hydrogenated fats found in processed foods. Thankfully, trans fats are rare because the FDA took them off the "generally recognized as safe" list and ordered food companies to phase them out of products.

Likewise, you should avoid using refined, bleached, and deodorized vegetable oils like sunflower, soybean, safflower, palm, canola, corn, cottonseed, and grapeseed oils because they oxidize easily and increase inflammation in the body. These oils are generally found in processed foods and are extracted from plants using a chemical solvent or oil mill, and they can be chemically altered compared to the original plant.

Refined oils—even from sources like avocados, coconut, and olives—are not so helpful because they too are made by chemical extraction. Not only are these refined oils less natural compared to the unrefined versions made from crushed or pressed plants and seeds, but they also increase inflammation, which can play a role in downstream health conditions.

Helpful Fats		Not-So-Helpful Fats	Unhelpful Fats	
Not Highly Processed and Not Refined		Refined or Not as Healthy	Polyunsaturated (Refined, Bleached, Deodorized)	Trans (Hydrogenated)
All-purpose	Use caution with heat (better for dressing and finishing)	Limited use	Use only sparingly	
Extra-virgin olive oil, avocado oil, ghee/butter, virgin (unrefined) coconut oil and MCT oil, macadamia oil	Most nut and seed oils (almond, flax, sesame, walnut)	Refined avocado oil, refined coconut oil, refined olive oil, peanut oil, tallow, lard, duck fat	Canola (rapeseed) oil, corn oil, cottonseed oil, grapeseed oil, palm oil, safflower oil, soybean oil, sunflower oil	Processed foods (margarine, shortening, chips, crackers, mayonnaise, salad dressings)

SATURATED FAT

Saturated fat is not evil. In fact, we need saturated fat in our diet to make hormones and cell membranes. I advocate that we get about 10 percent of our daily calories from saturated fat, but I find that a lot of otherwise healthy eaters skimp on saturated fat because of misinformation.

Saturated fat has gotten a bad reputation in the last fifty years, stemming from a time when scientists were convinced that heart disease was caused exclusively by high cholesterol. Saturated fat does increase "bad" LDL cholesterol, but it also raises "good" HDL cholesterol, the kind that protects you from heart disease. I liken HDL to Pac-Man because it goes around like a scavenger and eats up all the bad cholesterol in our arteries. While saturated fat is increasing our LDL, it's *simultaneously* making the particles less sticky and more fluffy. If you're going to have "bad cholesterol" circulating, then you want it to be fluffy because fluffy particles are less likely to make plaque than the smaller, denser, stickier LDL particles from processed foods. Newer research shows that developing heart disease is so much more complex than having high cholesterol, and the causes include inflammation, elevated insulin levels, high triglycerides, and obesity.

Saturated fat comes from both plant and animal sources. You're probably familiar with the animal sources of saturated fat, including beef, bacon, sausage, and eggs, but plant-based saturated fats are found in extra-dark chocolate, avocados, coconut, and nuts. How do we make sense of what type of saturated fat to eat?

A lot of it comes down to the difference between what animal- and plant-based saturated fats do in your system. Plant-based saturated fat comes from fatty acids, and many of those fatty acids are an anti-inflammatory dream. Take dark chocolate, for example. When you read the nutrition label, you can see that its macronutrient makeup is primarily saturated fat. What the label doesn't tell you is that this type of saturated fat from stearic acid is converted in the liver to oleic acid, a monounsaturated fatty acid. Stearic acid does not raise LDL levels. It's a bit different from getting your saturated fat from salt-, sugar-, and nitrate-laden processed bacon.

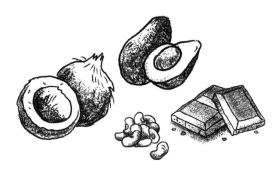

Nutrition Facts

3 servings per container

Serving size	1/3 bar (28g)

Amount per serving

Calories	180

	% Daily Value*
Total Fat 13g	17%
Saturated Fat 7g	35%
Trans Fat 0g	
Cholesterol 0mg	0%
Sodium 0mg	0%
Total Carbohydrate 11g	4%
Dietary Fiber 4g	14%
Total Sugars 4g	
Includes 4g Added Sugars	8%
Protein 3g	
Vitamin D 0mcg	0%
Calcium 19mg	2%
Iron 1mg	6%
Potassium 200mg	4%

*The % Daily Value tells you how much a nutrient in a serving of food contributes to a daily diet. 2,000 calories a day is used for general nutrition advice.

But what about natural bacon from a reputable pork farmer? Could that be okay for you to eat? Absolutely. But in the right amount and as a flavor-enhancing sideshow on a plate bursting with vegetables. Unfortunately, many food authorities, including the American Heart Association, don't make that distinction. They don't tell you about all the good saturated fats that exist; they just tell you not to eat much saturated fat because it will raise your LDL. Further, they tell you to replace saturated fats with polyunsaturated oils, which for most people means corn and soybean oil. These harmful oils have been shown to increase mortality rates even though they lower LDL cholesterol.[11]

Even though saturated fat is not as evil as we once thought, you shouldn't eat it with abandon. We know that the saturated fat in plant-based foods like coconut oil and responsibly farmed animal products can be fine in moderation and alongside other healthy foods (as opposed to being accompanied by sugar, like in an Oreo), but I recommend prioritizing natural plant-based sources like avocados.

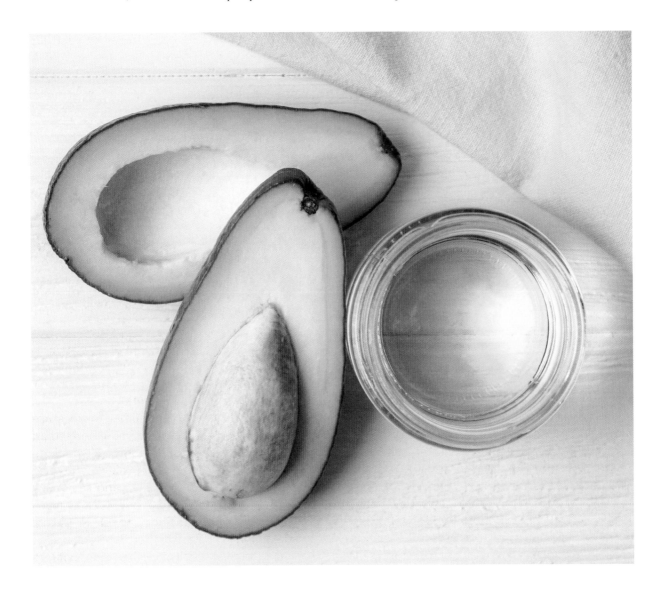

[11] C. E. Ramsden, D. Zamora, S. Majchrzak-Hong, et al., "Re-evaluation of the traditional diet-heart hypothesis: analysis of recovered data from Minnesota Coronary Experiment (1968–73)," *British Medical Journal* 353 (2016): i1246.

OMEGA-3 FATS

The polyunsaturated fat omega-3 gets a lot of attention because it's hard to get in the diet unless you're purposeful about it. Omega-3 is important because of its anti-inflammatory effect on carcinogens through the down-regulation of inflammatory enzymatic pathways, neuropsychiatric disease like developmental delay and mental health, and cardiovascular disease, including metabolic syndrome.

The typical American diet leads to an imbalance of omega-3 and omega-6 fats. We need both, but generally, omega-3s are good, and omega-6s are not-so-good because they increase inflammation and oxidative stress. Omega-6 fats are found in refined corn and soybean oils, so keeping your omega-6-to-3 fats in balance should be pretty easy if you are smart about the oils you cook with and follow a whole-foods diet that includes natural omega-6-rich foods like chicken, edamame, and nuts. Our prehistoric ancestors consumed an omega-6-to-3 ratio of close to 1:1, but Americans who eat a lot of processed food approach a ratio of 20:1.

The most important omega-3s are EPA (eicosapentaenoic acid), DHA (docosahexaenoic acid), and ALA (alpha linolenic acid). EPA and DHA, which are prominent in animal sources, are more potent because the body can readily use them in their native form. Unfortunately, plant-based ALA has to be converted to DHA in the body, and the conversion rate is a measly 7 percent, so it's not nearly as efficient. This is one reason I recommend that vegetarians and vegans consider supplementing with omega-3 fish oil pills or eating fish once weekly.

Omega-3 fatty acid deficiencies are a problem for some people. One of my longtime patients, Diane, a lovely woman in her fifties who's been following variations on a vegetarian or vegan diet for about twenty years, recently saw me for a mysterious tingling sensation she'd been having in her hands and feet for a few months. She had seen multiple doctors, including her primary care doctor, neurologist, and physiatrist, and had endured several comprehensive lab tests, MRIs, and an uncomfortable EMG (electromyography), a diagnostic procedure in which long needles are placed in certain muscles to see if the nerve-muscle connection is intact. Her other doctors couldn't find anything wrong with her and offered her nerve-modulating medication to treat her symptoms. In the course of our visit, she mentioned she was taking a vegan omega-3 supplement made from flax oil. We discussed the poor conversion of omega-3s from plant sources, and I recommended she make one exception to her vegan diet and take a fish oil-based supplement instead. At our follow-up visit three weeks later, she said the omega-3 pills–an equivalent dose to eating salmon twice weekly–had worked miracles: the numbness and tingling had completely resolved.

Even a modest amount of omega-3 fats in the diet produces positive effects in the body. Just one or two 3½-ounce servings of fatty fish like wild salmon, black cod, herring, sardines, or halibut per week (generally equivalent to a daily fish oil supplement) is enough. Fortunately, it doesn't matter whether the fish is fresh, frozen, or canned. Tuna and mackerel are also rich in omega-3s but can be sources of mercury if overconsumed. What's nice about choosing omega-3-rich fish is that they are also an amazing source of protein (which I'll talk about later in this chapter).

While omega-3s from animal sources are more bioavailable (i.e., usable in the body) than plant-based omega-3s, it's important to include plant-based omega-3s in your diet in the form of whole organic soy and nuts and seeds like walnuts, ground flax seeds, and chia seeds because of their high fiber and other phytonutrient content. Be wary of foods like eggs that are "omega-3 enriched," as they contain only a small amount. Omega-3 fats can vary considerably from 30 to 125 milligrams per egg. Compare this to a serving of wild salmon, which has 1,500 to 2,000 milligrams of the usable omega-3 fats DHA and EPA.

Animal omega-3s (DHA and EPA)

Cod liver oil

Herring

Krill

Oysters

Sardines

Tuna and mackerel (take care with amount due to mercury)

Wild Alaskan black cod (aka sablefish, butterfish)

Wild Alaskan salmon

Wild halibut

**Plant omega-3s
(only 7% conversion of ALA to DHA)**

Chia seeds

Flax seeds (ground)

Hemp seeds

Pumpkin seeds

Sunflower seeds

Walnuts

Whole organic soy—tofu, tempeh, edamame

OTHER TYPES OF FAT: MCTs, BUTTER & GHEE

I'm in favor of modest use of medium-chain tri-glyceride (MCT)-rich oils like coconut, as well as butter and ghee. While I recommend pri-oritizing monounsaturated fats as discussed earlier, it may make sense to incorporate these fats based on your individual tastes and health goals.

MCT-rich oils have gotten a lot of press with the advent of bulletproof coffee, ketogenic diets, and fitness recommendations targeted at athletes. MCTs are a type of saturated fat nat-urally occurring in coconut oil, palm oil, breast milk, and full-fat dairy. In fact, more than 50 percent of the fat in coconut oil comes from MCTs. The use of MCT oil has been associated with improved memory, weight loss, enhanced microbiome health and gut barrier protec-tion, and increased athletic endurance, but we need more research to support more robust use in the diet. I use coconut oil occasionally when cooking but rely much more routinely on monounsaturated fats like avocado oil and extra-virgin olive oil.

Likewise, I incorporate a bit of organic grass-fed butter and ghee into my diet. Ghee is a type of clarified butter that's more concen-trated in fat than traditional butter because the water and milk solids have been removed, which also makes it tolerable for people who have sensitivities to the milk sugar lactose or the milk protein casein. Unlike traditional but-ter, ghee can be kept at room temperature. It's used most often in Indian and Pakistani cuisine and has been a part of Ayurvedic medicine since ancient times. I choose ghee over but-ter for stovetop cooking because of its higher smoke point. Butter and ghee are among the few foods that naturally contain butyric acid (also called butyrate), an anti-inflammatory short-chain fatty acid normally produced by the gut microbiome when you eat fiber-rich food, as discussed in Chapter 2.

That said, ghee is not significantly more healthy than butter, so if you enjoy a pat of butter on your baked potato, go for it! A bit of butter and ghee go a long way toward satiety and enjoyment and round out a well-lived life. As celebrity chef Paula Deen says, "Everything's better with butter!"

SERVING SIZE OF FAT

It's difficult to put a number on how much healthy fat should be included in each meal because it can vary from person to person. Some people feel great when they eat a quarter of an avocado; others like a half. See what feels good in your body and trust your *Wellness Intuition.* Generally, you can start by thinking of a serving being 1 tablespoon of oil, 1 tablespoon of nut or seed butter, one-quarter cup of nuts or seeds, one-quarter cup of coconut, or a quarter to a half of a medium Hass avocado.

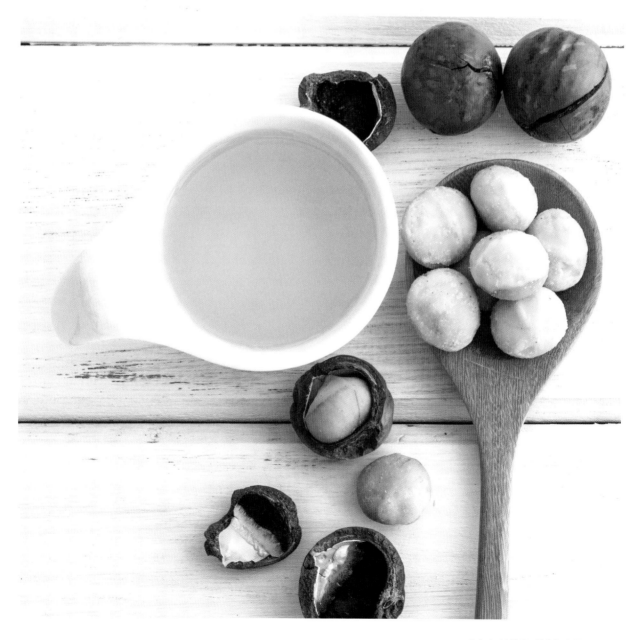

FERMENTED FOODS

Fermented foods are high in probiotics, the natural bacteria that live in our digestive systems and keep us healthy. In fact, each of us has around a kilogram of bacteria hanging out in our system right now!

Probiotic-rich foods include miso, kimchi, sauerkraut, tempeh, kefir, yogurt, kombucha, and natto. I'm of German ancestry, so I grew up eating sauerkraut and generally love sour stuff, and I don't mind fermented foods at all; however, I recognize that this is not true for everyone. Do your best to have one probiotic-rich food per day.

You know what probiotic bacteria munch on in your digestive system? Prebiotics. Prebiotic-rich foods are high in fiber and contain indigestible resistant starches, especially onions, garlic, leeks, sunchokes (Jerusalem artichokes), and asparagus. In fact, every time you eat something that's high in fiber, your probiotics eat some of the calories you consume. This is a great example of how "calories in" does not necessarily equal "calories out" and how mixing a variety of foods into one meal can be helpful in multiple ways.

Although I don't love the effect of dairy on our bodies, I do make an exception for fermented dairy like plain full-fat yogurt and kefir if it agrees with you. It's important to buy plain yogurt products so that you don't drown the good guys in sweetness and outdo the good of the probiotics with inflammation from sugar. I often wonder how probiotic bacteria can stay alive when swimming in a sugar bath. My advice is to buy plain yogurt and sweeten it yourself.

Interestingly, fermentation can also enhance the body's absorption of certain phytochemicals. One good example is the fermentation of cabbage, like in sauerkraut or kimchi. In addition to the innate benefit to the gut from all that healthy bacteria, the fermentation process increases the bioactivity of several anti-cancer compounds, making the work of digesting and utilizing these phytonutrients easier for the body.

You can easily ferment food at home on your countertop. All you need is a jar, water, spices, and some patience. Just don't use vinegar (or, for that matter, buy store-bought fermented vegetables that have vinegar in the ingredient list) because vinegar acts like an antiseptic in this case and kills the live bacteria you're trying to help proliferate.

When buying fermented food, be sure to read the labels to avoid large doses of sugar or salt. Kombucha is especially tricky because it's made by fermenting tea and then sweetened with fruit juice. Choose a kombucha that has less than 8 grams of sugar per 8-ounce serving, and preferably less than 5 grams of sugar. I recommend keeping kombucha to about 8 ounces per day to avoid unwanted digestive side effects and to keep sugar intake low.

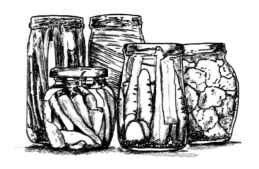

COOKED MUSHROOMS

Mushrooms are amazing, and we're still discovering the extent of their medicinal power.

Mushrooms are a natural, plant-based source of vitamins B_{12} and D, which are vital for plant-forward health. Mushrooms contain a lot of fiber, especially in the form of beta-glucans, which have been linked to improving cholesterol and cardiovascular health along with regulating blood sugar. There's also evidence that mushrooms may boost our immunity and have antimicrobial properties, which means that they protect us from bacteria and viruses and prevent illness. And varieties like Lion's Mane may improve outcomes when it comes to neurological decline from stroke, Alzheimer's, Parkinson's, and depression by increasing nerve growth factor.[12]

I place a special emphasis on Asian mushrooms like shiitake, maitake, and oyster—basically all of the irregular-looking varieties at the grocery store—which are the fiber-rich, phytonutrient-packed, anti-cancer mushrooms. Even though I prioritize Asian mushrooms, it's important to say that even the humble white button mushroom—once thought to be short on nutrition—has been shown to have anti-cancer compounds similar to aromatase inhibitors, a type of breast cancer treatment.[13] Who knew that eating mushrooms could be so good for us?

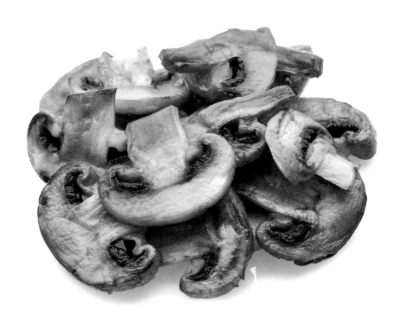

[12] I. C. Li, L. Y. Lee, T. T. Tzeng, et al., "Neurohealth properties of *Hericium erinaceus* mycelia enriched with erinacines," *Behavioural Neurology* 2018: 5802634.

[13] B. J. Grube, E. T. Eng, Y. C. Kao, et al., "White button mushroom phytochemicals inhibit aromatase activity and breast cancer cell proliferation," *Journal of Nutrition* 131, no. 12 (2001): 3288–93.

The most important part about eating mushrooms is to eat whole, cooked mushrooms, stems included. Not only do cooked mushrooms taste better, but cooking them protects you from potentially cancer-*causing* toxins present in the raw fungi. Some people eat raw mushrooms on sad-looking salads or pizza, but I don't recommend it.

I recommend building cooked mushrooms into your diet once a day. Here's a list of common edible mushrooms to try:

· White (includes button, portobello, and cremini)
· Beech
· Chanterelle
· Enoki
· Hen of the Woods
· Lion's Mane
· Morel
· Oyster
· Porcini
· Shiitake
· Turkey Tail

"Not only do *cooked mushrooms taste better,* but *cooking them* **protects you** from potentially cancer-causing toxins present in the raw fungi."

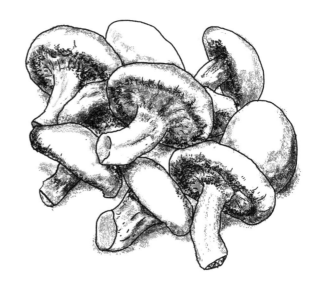

PLANT-BASED DAIRY ALTERNATIVES

In order to talk about plant-based dairy alternatives, we have to start with dairy from cows and other animals. It's not good for us to eat dairy in large amounts. Don't get me wrong—I love me a little high-quality cheese and ice cream. Dairy gives food a flavor and richness that is unparalleled in vegan cooking, though there are many flavors that approximate it. The problem is that as Americans, we have put dairy in its own food group, and old-school food guidelines suggest that we consume it at every meal.

DAIRY IS NOT ITS OWN FOOD GROUP & WON'T PROTECT YOUR BONES

Let's start with why dairy exists. Milk from a cow, for example, is meant to nurse a baby calf into a big, fat grown-up cow. But we are humans, not cows. You have to admit, it's weird that humans drink the breast milk of cows, sheep, and goats, right? In fact, cow dairy has more than sixty naturally occurring bovine hormones that can cause cancer and lead to weight gain.[14] And most of us don't want to gain unnecessary weight. Animal dairy is also allergenic, meaning that it revs up our immune response unnecessarily, leading to rashes and other inflammatory reactions. We don't need dairy on the regular.

The evidence shows that dairy does not promote healthy bones or prevent fractures even though it appears to be a good source of calcium, phosphorus, and protein.[15] Dairy is a naturally poor source of vitamin D (and devoid of vitamin D if it's nonfat or low-fat because vitamin D is a fat-soluble vitamin that gets removed when fat is removed), so milk is fortified with vitamin D to increase its nutritional value.

Of all dairy products—including milk, cheese, butter, ice cream, yogurt, and kefir—I make an exception for modest amounts of grass-fed butter and ghee and fermented dairy products like plain unsweetened yogurt and kefir because the fermentation process aids in its digestion. As previously discussed, it's important to buy unsweetened yogurt and kefir so that you don't have the sugar equivalent of a soda for breakfast!

After experimenting without dairy, I can honestly say that I feel better when I don't eat much of it. It pains me to say that because no one loves ice cream more than this girl. In fact, ice cream is my number two favorite delight after dark chocolate...but when I eat dairy, it's a big treat for me, and one I take very seriously. I do my best to find full-fat, organic, grass-fed dairy that's worth the indulgence.

[14] Hyman, *Food: What the Heck Should I Eat?*: 263.

[15] H. A. Bischoff-Ferrari, B. Dawson-Hughes, J. A. Baron, et al., "Milk intake and risk of hip fracture in men and women: a meta-analysis of prospective cohort studies," *Journal of Bone and Mineral Research: The Official Journal of the American Society for Bone and Mineral Research* 26, no. 4 (2011): 833–9.

Over 70 percent of the world's population has issues digesting dairy, mostly due to difficulties metabolizing the milk sugar lactose but possibly due to sensitivities to dairy proteins.[16] Dairy is generally stagnating for everyone, but most times we are too busy to notice the effect. It is heavy, both energetically and calorically, and weighs us down. According to the philosophy of Chinese Medicine, dairy leads to stagnation in the body, a stickiness that often translates to bloating, gas, constipation, diarrhea, or other digestive problems. If you're chronically constipated, it may behoove you to try going without dairy for a few weeks. This is a good example of tapping into your *Wellness Intuition* to find a life rhythm that suits your constitution.

Dairy from goats might be a bit easier to tolerate compared to cow dairy because it has only A2 casein proteins, which are less inflammatory than the A1 casein of our modern cows. Goat milk also has medium-chain triglycerides (MCTs), which can be helpful for metabolism and brain function, but recognize that goat dairy still exists for baby goats, not humans.

If you do eat dairy, use it in the way it was intended: to make the rest of your food taste better. Consider sprinkles of dairy in your diet instead of giving it prime real estate on your plate, such as a little half-and-half in your coffee, a tablespoon of cheese on your salad, or a spoonful of whipped cream on your oatmeal apple crisp.

PLANT-BASED DAIRY ALTERNATIVES ARE BETTER

These days, there are so many great plant-based dairy alternatives that you don't have to feel deprived or deal with the side effects of maldigestion. Check out full-fat, unsweetened coconut, cashew, or almond yogurt. Consider full-fat coconut milk, which is rich in MCTs and satisfying, or try oat, hemp, or macadamia milk, or make your own nut or seed milk. (Check out www.DrKatie.com for an easy recipe for homemade nut milk; it's really no more complicated than soaking nuts and seeds in water, squeezing them through a piece of cheesecloth, and then adding some flavor with vanilla and anything else you desire.) There are even beautiful cheeses made from cashews that can be enjoyed in small amounts, but recognize that those types of dairy alternative products often contain additives to make them shelf-stable.

It's important to buy plant-based dairy substitutes that don't have gums or additives added to them to make them more like traditional animal dairy products. One such additive, carrageenan, is a thickening agent that's commonly used in both animal and plant-based dairy. Carrageenan is derived from seaweed, which makes it sound pretty harmless, but carrageenan is bad for us. It is an irritant associated with digestive problems in humans and causes cancer in lab rats.[17] I recommend steering clear of all thickeners in dairy products, including gums like xanthan gum, guar gum, and locust bean gum and anything else that doesn't sound like Mother Nature made it.

I recommend that you consume two or fewer one-half cup servings of plant-based dairy substitutes per day.

---

[16] M. B. Heyman and the Committee on Nutrition, "Lactose intolerance in infants, children, and adolescents," *Pediatrics* 118, no. 3 (2006): 1279–86.

[17] J. K. Tobacman, "Review of harmful gastrointestinal effects of carrageenan in animal experiments," *Environmental Health Perspectives* 109, no. 10 (2001): 983–94.

ANIMAL PROTEIN (INCLUDING OMEGA-3-RICH FISH, DAIRY & EGGS)

Animal protein is not evil. In fact, in my book, it's delicious.

You know that I grew up on the farmlands of Ohio, and oh, does this girl love a good steak now and then. But those words now and then are the key to animal protein–especially if the animal protein is naturally higher in inflammatory fats.

A plant-forward diet does not kick out all animal protein; it just categorizes it as less prominent compared to the normal American diet. In their quest for weight loss, a lot of my patients get into the habit of overeating animal protein because it's satiating and doesn't have any carbohydrates, and they are convinced that carbohydrates are the enemy. As you know, the enemy is not carbohydrates, but *processed* carbohydrates, so finding balance on our plates with fiber, fat, and protein is important.

I put all animal protein in the same group, including beef, pork, chicken, turkey, dairy, eggs, and our beloved omega-3-rich fish. As you know, omega-3-rich fish like wild salmon, black cod, sardines, and halibut are in a special class and deserve to be eaten at least once weekly because of the anti-inflammatory properties inherent in omega-3 fats. I've already discussed limiting dairy, so we're left with meat, poultry, and eggs.

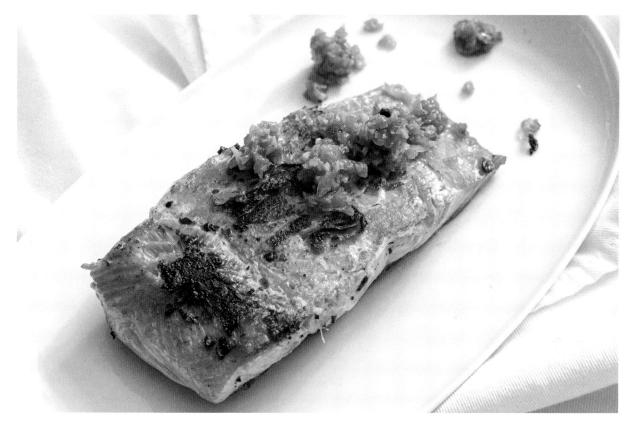

ANIMAL PROTEIN IN THE RIGHT AMOUNT IS IMPORTANT FOR HEALTH

I think it's important to include animal protein in the diet because it is an efficient source of protein and essential vitamin B_{12}, and, as discussed in Chapter 3, we need protein to live. If you are vegan—meaning you abstain from animal protein altogether—you have to work really hard to get all your protein and have to supplement with vitamin B_{12}. Just one 3-ounce serving of chicken has about 24 grams of protein, which puts you well on your way toward your daily goal. You'd have to eat over a cup of lentils or 1½ cups of black beans to get about the same amount of protein.

Animal protein is also a natural source of vitamin E, vitamin D, and other B vitamins, as well as essential minerals like zinc, selenium, magnesium, and iron. The heme iron in animal protein is more bioavailable, or usable, than the nonheme iron found in plants.

Generally, I recommend limiting animal protein to one or two servings a day. What I'd really like to see you do is make *at least one* of your meals with a plant protein. So, if you decide to have eggs for breakfast and you're planning on chicken for dinner, I want you to get your lunchtime protein from nuts, seeds, lentils, beans, or whole organic soy. Ideally, you might transition to having only one meal per day that includes animal protein. The idea is to avoid consuming animal protein at every meal. Think less about *limiting* animal protein and more about *prioritizing* plant protein. This mindset shift is the key to any substantial dietary change that may take longer to incorporate. Our quest is not deprivation, but prioritizing health.

Let's hit a few of the animal protein highlights.

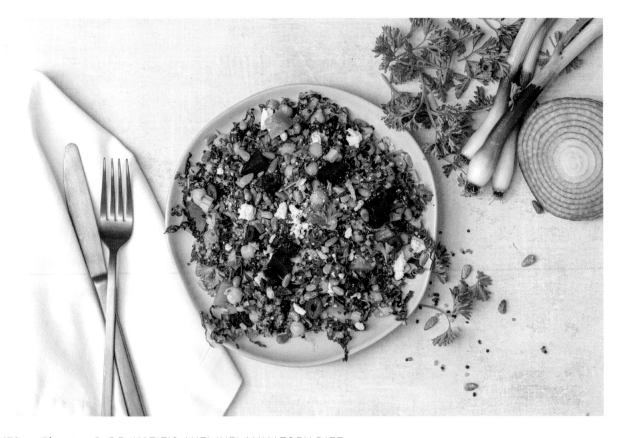

MEAT

Red meat encompasses all of the mammal muscle meats we eat, including beef, veal, bison, pork, lamb, mutton, goat, and wild game like venison. Red meat used to be demonized because its cholesterol and saturated fat content was linked to heart disease, but we don't need to remove it from our diets altogether; we just need to proceed with care. We know that heart disease is a complex condition that involves not only cholesterol but also inflammation, blood sugar, and triglycerides, which were discussed in Chapter 2. It's neither helpful nor correct to boil down a discussion of heart disease to avoiding meat. That said, I don't recommend eating meat with abandon, either.

Grass-fed, organic, pasture-raised meats are worth the extra cost. You want to stay away from the less expensive factory-farmed animals because they are generally eating mass-produced, genetically modified grains treated with pesticides and given hormones and antibiotics in an effort to fatten them up quickly and on the cheap. Remember, what they eat, you eat. And none of us needs those dangerous compounds in our body. As discussed on page 52, factory farming is not great for the environment, either. Animals like cows and goats are herbivores who are supposed to eat grasses and be allowed to forage. Similarly, pigs are omnivores and are supposed to munch on some bugs and grubs, not government-subsidized corn and soy in feed bundles. When animals are pasture-raised and graze on grass and grubs, their meat has more omega-3 fats and fewer omega-6 fats, approximating a 1:1 ratio. In addition, it has more healthy vitamins and minerals. Meat from ruminants like cows and sheep also contains an anti-inflammatory polyunsaturated fat called conjugated linoleic acid (CLA), which has been associated with decreased obesity, cancer, and cardiovascular disease.[18]

I'm generally okay with 3 ounces of organic, grass-fed, pasture-raised red meat about once or twice weekly.

> "Remember, *what they eat,* **you eat.** And none of us needs those dangerous compounds in our body."

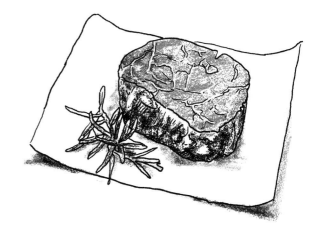

---

[18] L. J. den Hartigh, "Conjugated linoleic acid effects on cancer, obesity, and atherosclerosis: a review of pre-clinical and human trials with current perspectives," *Nutrients* 11, no. 2 (2019): 370.

PROCESSED MEAT

I want you to avoid highly processed meats, meaning the ones that don't look like the sources from which they came. Examples would be sausage, hot dogs, deli meats, cured meats, corned beef, beef jerky, and bacon that has been treated with preservatives like nitrates and nitrites and is full of additives, fillers, preservatives, gluten, and sometimes high-fructose corn syrup.

Nitrites are added to meats to preserve their pink color and provide the salty flavor consumers want. Without nitrites, the meat would turn brown quickly and look less appetizing. The problem is that when these nitrites are exposed to temperatures over 266°F, they turn into nitrosamines, which are carcinogenic. My kids and husband happen to love bacon, so it's a treat in our house on a weekend or when hosting friends. I recommend buying uncured meats when you do decide on this indulgence to avoid preservatives and other unappetizing chemicals. Steer clear of products with the words *nitrate, nitrite,* or *celery salt* (which can have hidden nitrites) on the ingredient list. And cook bacon low and slow to prevent the formation of nitrosamines as well as other toxic carcinogenic chemicals like PAHs (polycyclic aromatic hydrocarbons) and HCAs (heterocyclic amines).

A connection has been made between processed meats and increased risk of cancer, but the effect is small and convoluted. The World Health Organization (WHO) reviewed over 800 studies and issued a headlining report linking processed meats to a 20 percent increased risk of colorectal cancer.[19] The headlines many of us saw following the publication of that report didn't qualify the increase by talking about the natural statistical occurrence of colorectal cancer, which is about a 5 percent lifetime risk. So, if eating bacon every day raises the risk of colorectal cancer by 20 percent, then the lifetime risk for someone of average health goes from 5 to 6 percent. The only problem is that we generally don't eat bacon in isolation, and the people eating bacon every day are not at average risk. Unlike my children, most people don't eat one or two slices of responsibly sourced, organic, grass-fed, uncured bacon alongside a full plate of phytonutrient-rich plants. Americans eat processed meat in the context of a bacon-egg-and-cheese sandwich or with other inflammatory foods. And that combination makes it a bit harder to tease out the real risk of cancer when it comes to processed meats.

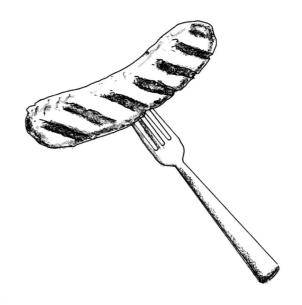

---

[19] R. L. Santarelli, F. Pierre, and D. E. Corpet, "Processed meat and colorectal cancer: a review of epidemiologic and experimental evidence," *Nutrition and Cancer* 60, no. 2 (2008): 131–44.

POULTRY & EGGS

Let's talk chicken now, since that's the poultry most of us eat. In my mind, poultry is a neutral food: it is not great for you, but it's not horrible, either. Chicken is a little lower in inflammatory saturated fats than red meat. It's also a rich source of protein, and it's tasty in a variety of ways.

It's important to buy organic, antibiotic-free, pasture-raised poultry. The free-range label is often misleading; it doesn't mean the chickens spend much time outdoors eating bugs and grubs from the ground. Just like the feed given to factory-farmed red meat animals, poultry feed is often mass-produced, genetically modified grain. The less grain and the more bugs your poultry eat, the better, as the chickens' diet influences the nutritional value of their meat in your body. Words like *natural, cage-free, hormone-free,* and *vegetarian-fed* are pretty meaningless when it comes to buying poultry, so don't be duped!

When chickens are allowed to forage for bugs and grubs on pastures, it dramatically increases the quality and amount of nutrients in their eggs. I love seeing the gorgeous, deep yellow-orange color of nutrient-rich egg yolks. Thankfully, there are a few brands available at many supermarkets that provide this level of quality, like Nellie's. If I buy a brand of pasture-raised eggs and find that the yolks are pale yellow, I generally avoid buying that brand again.

EGGS & CHOLESTEROL

Dietary cholesterol comes only from animal sources, but you don't have to be scared of eggs and cholesterol for two reasons. The first is that eating the occasional egg in the way I describe in this book is not going to dramatically impact your cholesterol. The other reason is that about 75 percent of cholesterol is made in the liver, while only 25 percent is absorbed from food. Interestingly, there are "fancy" cholesterol tests these days that use biomarkers to tell whether someone is more genetically predisposed to make cholesterol or absorb it, so we can figure out if further prioritizing plant protein would help lower high cholesterol levels. Using such a test, I found that my genetic tendency is to absorb cholesterol from my food, so one of the things I noticed after I shifted to a plant-forward diet was a nice drop in my genetically high cholesterol to a relatively normal level. Many of my aunties who have made similar choices have noticed the same decrease.

Omega-3 eggs are from chickens who are fed flax seeds, which does contribute to the omega-3 content of their eggs. Recognize, however, that one omega-3-rich egg has only about 125 milligrams of omega-3 compared to the hundreds to thousands of milligrams in cold-water fish.

One whole egg has 6 grams of protein, so it's not the most efficient source of protein but a nice one to include in your diet. If you love eggs, I recommend eating fewer than seven whole pasture-raised eggs in a week. Do not throw out the yolks. Not only do whole eggs taste better, but you want the yolk's many antioxidants, vitamins, and minerals on your plate. Let go of the egg-white-only mindset.

GREEN TEA

Green tea might be the most anti-inflammatory food or drink on the planet. It contains antioxidant polyphenols like flavonoids and catechins, notably EGCG (epigallocatechin gallate), along with detoxifying compounds and cancer-fighting phytonutrients. Green tea scavenges and stabilizes free radicals, which can help prevent cellular damage and aid in cellular repair. Catechins have been shown to positively affect cardiovascular disease, including high blood pressure, the immune system, and overall inflammation.

One of my favorite studies demonstrating the cardioprotective effect of green tea looked at the carotid arteries of women who consumed three cups of green tea compared to those who drank less or none at all. Whether the green tea was caffeinated or not, the women who drank three cups per day had less carotid artery intimal thickness and plaque formation, which correlates to a lower risk of stroke.[20]

There's also evidence to suggest that green tea's catechins are helpful for burning fat, which may aid in weight management, but some studies have participants drinking green tea extract equivalent to seven cups per day. This kind of consumption doesn't sound balanced or in alignment with one's *Wellness Intuition*. That said, a modest amount of green tea could work well for weight management and cholesterol control. One small randomized, double-blind, placebo-controlled study followed 102 women with central obesity for twelve weeks and gave the treatment group a daily dose of 850 milligrams of green tea extract, which is equivalent to about 4 cups of green tea.[21] They found that those women lost a little over two pounds over the course of the study, most likely related to decreased ghrelin and increased adiponectin levels, in addition to decreased total cholesterol and LDL plasma levels. Ghrelin is the "hungry hormone" that increases appetite, and adiponectin is a hormone that plays a crucial role in protecting against insulin resistance, diabetes, and atherosclerosis. So perhaps a higher amount of green tea each day could be a strategy for decreasing hunger as well as metabolic risk.

---

[20] S. Debette, D. Courbon, N. Leone, et al., "Tea consumption is inversely associated with carotid plaques in women," *Arteriosclerosis, Thrombosis, and Vascular Biology* 28 (2008): 353–9.

[21] I.-J. Chen, C.-Y. Liu, J.-P. Chiu, and C.-H. Hsu, "Therapeutic effect of high-dose green tea extract on weight reduction: a randomized, double-blind, placebo-controlled clinical trial," *Clinical Nutrition* 35, no. 3 (2016): 592–9.

MATCHA

Matcha is all the rage these days. It comes from the same plant as regular green tea, but farmers grow matcha by covering their tea plants several weeks before harvest to shield them from direct sunlight, which boosts chlorophyll production (giving matcha its gorgeous green glow) and increases the anti-anxiety amino acid L-theanine content. L-theanine is one of my favorite adaptogenic supplements for improving energy and decreasing anxiety. The harvested leaves of matcha are then ground into a fine powder and packaged for sale.

To enjoy matcha traditionally, mix a teaspoon into 8 ounces of hot water to make a frothy tea. If you're fancy, you can use a bamboo whisk. If you're not, then just stir well with a spoon. You can also find matcha in tea bags, which is much easier. I also love matcha collagen, which blends in the power of collagen proteins, making anti-inflammatory living a little easier.

Since matcha is the whole tea leaf, it has many more antioxidants and more caffeine than traditional green tea. One teaspoon of matcha has about 70 milligrams of caffeine compared with 15 to 30 milligrams in green tea or 60 to 100 milligrams in a cup of coffee. I recommend consuming matcha (and caffeinated green tea in general) before noon to avoid it compromising your ability to fall asleep at night.

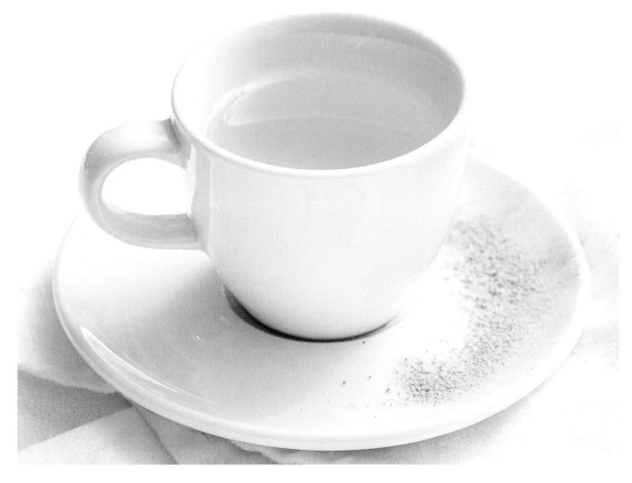

HELPING YOUR PALATE
TO LIKE GREEN TEA

My husband and I drink at least two cups of green tea every day, usually throughout the morning after our first cup of coffee. I hated the taste of green tea the first time I tried it as a college student at my future in-laws' house. I distinctly remember politely taking a sip and then letting it cool on the table while pretending to look engaged in conversation, hoping they wouldn't notice that I didn't drink the Japanese crown jewel.

Many of my patients decline my suggestion to drink green tea because of its distinctive taste, so I have developed a few helpful suggestions over the years based on my own journey. First, buy a good brand and steep it for only thirty seconds to a few minutes. If left to steep too long, the astringent tannin flavor becomes pronounced, making the tea bitter. I also recommend easing into green tea with blends of other delightful ingredients like lemongrass, ginger, or toasted rice. But watch out for teas with added ingredients like citric acid, "natural flavors," sugar, or stevia.

While I love hot beverages at breakfast, green tea can be a nice pick-me-up in the early afternoon with a square of extra-dark chocolate. The tea warms your palate just enough that the chocolate will pleasantly melt. And, unlike the caffeine jolt of coffee, the smoother release of caffeine in green tea—especially when combined with the fat of extra-dark chocolate—leads to a gentle increase in productivity. If you don't want the caffeine in tea, you can easily make your tea decaffeinated by discarding the water after steeping for a minute and then allowing it to steep for another few minutes in a fresh cup of hot water. Caffeine is the first component to be steeped out of tea, followed by catechins a few minutes later and tannins several minutes after that.

I love the ritual of a cup of tea. It causes me to slow down my mind and savor the moment, which can be a nice reminder amidst the flood of activity in a day. Tea can be an important part of your *Wellness Intuition* not just when it comes to food, but also to your mental well-being.

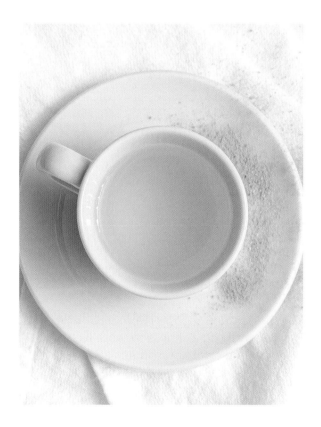

DETOXIFYING HERBS & SPICES

It's impossible to detail all the gorgeous herbs and spices that exist. In fact, I could write a whole book just on them!

Over time I have come to cook with more spices than I ever did before. Some of this is due to cooking more adventurously, but a lot of it has to do with cooking more plant-forward recipes. Plant-rich cooking inherently uses more herbs and spices than animal-based dishes because meat has an intrinsic salty, umami flavor that speaks for itself. While I certainly appreciate the sweetness of broccoli and brown rice, the bitterness of Swiss chard, and the saltiness of celery, many vegetables are blank canvases and do so well with some extra-virgin olive oil and a few well-chosen herbs and spices. Herbs and spices add layers of flavor to food that make them worth more than their weight in gold.

Herbs and spices not only taste amazing, but they confer tremendous anti-inflammatory benefits to our bodies and have been used medicinally for centuries. I'll review a few examples of the phytonutrient compounds that await you as you expand your own herb drawer and spice cabinet:

- **Cinnamon** is a sweet spice that brings unparalleled richness to food. It's loaded with powerful antioxidants such as polyphenols that aid in cardiovascular protection by decreasing LDL and stabilizing blood sugar by increasing sensitivity to insulin. Cinnamon is warming to the body and increases circulation, which may contribute to its cardiovascular effects. Additionally, cinnamon is antimicrobial and may help prevent fungal and bacterial infections. See my note on page 203 about buying true Ceylon cinnamon.

- **Cloves** are a sweet aromatic spice that provides protection from environmental toxins, blood sugar ups and downs, and cancer. Its compound eugenol is a potent antioxidant that reduces free radicals and the inflammatory response in the body, which may be helpful for conditions like arthritis as well as protective of the digestive tract and liver.

- **Coriander and cilantro** (the leaves of the coriander plant) are a natural way to detoxify the body from heavy metals and reduce oxidative stress on cells. These herbs can also help keep blood sugar more even-keeled! Coriander and cilantro are a delicious part of many dishes from Mexican, South American, Indian, and other Asian cuisines.

- **Garlic** is a zesty allium that is anti-inflammatory, antibacterial, antiviral (boosting virus-fighting T cells), immune-boosting, and cardioprotective and releases antiplatelet enzymes to prevent coronary artery blockages within minutes after being crushed or chopped. The less you cook garlic, the better it is for you. Treat yourself and buy peeled garlic cloves to make it easier to use.

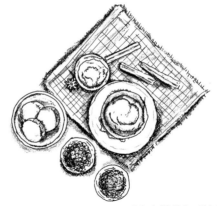

- **Ginger** is a spicy-sweet root that's excellent for digestion because it acts as a prokinetic agent, meaning it keeps things moving through your system. This makes it helpful for digestive ailments like slow digestive transit (including gastroparesis), nausea, reflux, and constipation. It's also an antioxidant powerhouse and a potent anti-inflammatory that acts similarly to COX-2 inhibitors nonsteroidal anti-inflammatory drugs (NSAIDs) like ibuprofen and naproxen.

- **Parsley** brightens flavors as a mild bitter green that marries well with many other spices, which is probably why it's used so often across multiple cuisines from Italian to Greek to Middle Eastern traditions. Parsley has antioxidant and antitumor properties and promotes good breath. It's also a helpful de-bloater because of its diuretic properties and can be helpful in managing blood pressure. You have to try my Crispy Parsley recipe on page 282. It's my favorite way to enjoy this herb.

- **Turmeric** has a cheery bright yellow color (and will stain your clothes–be careful!) and provides a bit of earthy grounding to dishes. It works similarly in the body to ginger as an NSAID. Turmeric is used medicinally for multiple inflammatory conditions, like osteoarthritis, inflammatory bowel disease, allergies and asthma, and cardiovascular disease. The trick to getting total body absorption of turmeric is to combine it with piperine, the active alkaloid in black pepper. Ever notice that most recipes with turmeric also have black pepper? Other cultures have known of this culinary power combo for centuries. I use turmeric in multiple recipes in this book because it's one of the best spices for your health. I typically use turmeric powder for cooking, but it also comes in root form similar to ginger if you'd like a fresh, vibrant flavor. It can also be taken in supplement form if it's hard for you to get into your diet on the regular.

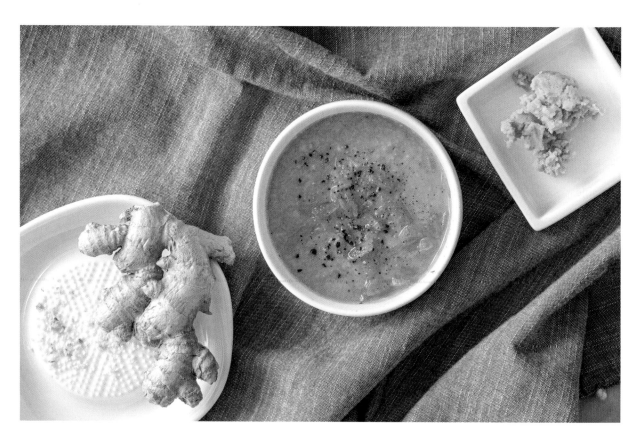

EXTRA-DARK CHOCOLATE

I'm sure you can tell from the recipes in this book that I have a love affair with dark chocolate. What's not to love? It's delicious, nutritious, and oh-so-satisfying.

Extra-dark chocolate is generally at least 85 percent cacao (cacao being the pure form of chocolate that closely resembles its raw, natural state) and is rich in saturated fat, a key component in our diet used for building cell membranes and other important lipid functions. The saturated fat in dark chocolate, however, is made mostly of stearic ("stee-air-ic") acid. Stearic acid, unlike the saturated fatty acids found in animal proteins, is anti-inflammatory and doesn't appear to raise LDL the way other saturated fats do. The antioxidants and flavanols in chocolate may also prevent LDL oxidation, which makes them less sticky in our arteries and may be meaningful to the prevention of heart attack and stroke. And an ounce of chocolate can reduce blood pressure levels a few notches, which may be a dual effect of the antioxidants and flavanols combined with magnesium.

Speaking of magnesium, a 100-gram bar of dark chocolate has 200 to 300 milligrams of magnesium, which is more than half of the recommended daily value, but I don't recommend eating that much at one time. It's been hypothesized that women crave chocolate because we tend to be a little magnesium deficient, so cravings for the dark stuff could be Nature's way of getting us what we need.

The lower the cacao percentage, the less potent these anti-inflammatory flavanols are and the more chocolate you have to eat to get the same level of benefit. For instance, if we compare raw cacao powder (which is 100 percent cacao) to dark chocolate to milk chocolate, we can see that in order to get 200 milligrams of flavanols, we'd have to ingest most of our calories for the day.[22]

200mg of Flavanols

1¾ tablespoons unsweetened, non-alkali-treated cocoa powder	20 calories
1 tablespoon raw cacao powder	65 calories
2 ounces dark chocolate	320 calories
10½ ounces milk chocolate	1,580 calories

[22] K. B. Miller, W. J. Hurst, N. Flannigan, et al., "Survey of commercially available chocolate- and cocoa-containing products in the United States. 2. Comparison of flavan-3-ol content with nonfat cocoa solids, total polyphenols, and percent cacao," *Journal of Agricultural and Food Chemistry* 57, no. 19 (2009): 9169–80; B. Liebman, "Behind the headlines: the science may surprise you," *Nutrition Action Healthletter* January/February 2015.

I find extra-dark chocolate incredibly satiating. It's a little sweet, but not too sweet. It satisfies the need for a little something in the middle of the afternoon, but once you eat a piece or two (or three!), you can be done with it and move on with your day, in contrast to other sugar hits that leave your body searching for more. The high percentage of saturated fat in extra-dark chocolate turns on brain chemicals signaling satiety.

So, ultimately, extra-dark chocolate is a superfood and one I recommend you build into your daily habit. I eat some almost every day and keep it in my bag when traveling since it's the perfect snack.

If you find extra-dark chocolate too bitter, ease into it. Rome was not built in a day, and you don't have to love extra-dark chocolate the first time you try it. If you're eating milk chocolate like it's your job, switch to semi-sweet chocolate and then work your way into extra-dark over the course of a few months.

I hear patients talk about extra-dark chocolate not melting in their mouths like creamy milk chocolate. The relative chalkiness can be a turnoff. First, try warming your palate with a warm liquid like green tea. If that doesn't help the chocolate pleasantly melt, try a different brand; some brands of dark chocolate are super smooth while others can be gritty. Steer clear of emulsifiers like lecithins and alkali-processed chocolate if you can. This may be another example of a food you have to try several times with different brands to get the hang of it. I encourage you to persevere!

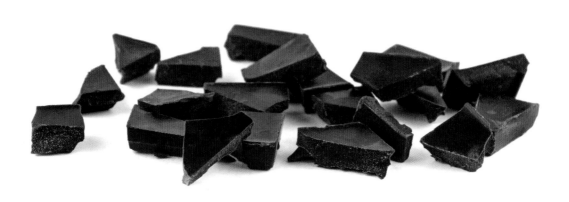

COFFEE & ALCOHOL

Coffee and alcohol are two wonderful drinks on opposite ends of the energy spectrum. When used in the right amount at the right time, they can be a healthy part of everyday living. But recognize that they are drugs—coffee is a stimulant and alcohol is a depressant—so you need to proceed with care. As noted below, they are amazing and helpful to our health up to a point, but thereafter they can have disastrous effects.

Both coffee and alcohol can be vehicles for sugar and processed additives in the form of creamers and mixers. I encourage you to keep these to a minimum and eliminate them if they contain noncaloric sugar substitutes. Coffee and alcohol can be consumed with less-than-optimal foods as well. There's a reason coffee and donuts go hand-in-hand in exactly the same way that drinking beer makes people crave potato chips. I encourage you to be careful.

COFFEE

Don't feel guilty about a little caffeine from coffee (or green tea, for that matter). Research shows there may be benefits to consuming modest amounts of caffeine, especially when it comes to preventing cognitive decline, but positive associations exist in connection to all-cause mortality, cardiovascular mortality and disease, incidence of cancer, and other neurological, metabolic, and liver conditions.[23] Each cup of coffee or shot of espresso ranges from 60 to 100 milligrams of caffeine, depending on how it's brewed. *Most* people can have one or two cups of coffee (or less than 200 milligrams of caffeine) per day, but listen to your *Wellness Intuition* if you're sensitive to the activating effects or acidity of coffee. I recommend consuming most of your coffee before noon. Caffeine can stick around in your system for up to twelve hours, depending on your individual metabolism, and may interfere with sleep. I also advise pregnant women to limit caffeinated beverages.

Coffee is inherently bitter, and many people don't like the taste unless it's masked by sugar, sugar substitutes, or creamers of various types. If you don't like your coffee black—which I encourage you to work up to over the course of time—then use real substances in your coffee and keep them to a minimum. Use real cream or half-and-half, or try coconut cream or a smoother plant milk like oat milk or one made from higher-fat nuts like macadamia or pine nuts. Use real sugar or maple syrup if you need sweetness, but don't use stevia, monk fruit, or sucralose (Splenda). If your morning brew is looking like a glorified milkshake or keeping you full for a substantial amount of time, then you might want to rethink your cup of joe.

---

[23] R. Poole, O. J. Kennedy, P. Roderick, et al., "Coffee consumption and health: umbrella review of meta-analyses of multiple health outcomes," *BMJ (Clinical research ed.)* 359 (2017): j5024.

ALCOHOL

Here's a subject that won't win me friends, since I tend to think we overconsume alcohol as a society.

Alcohol is delicious and contributes to feeling relaxed. And light to moderate consumption is positively correlated to better cardiovascular health, including lower rates of heart attack, heart failure, ischemic stroke, and diabetes along with lower risk of dementia and osteoporosis.[24] Alcohol, especially red wine, is known to positively influence the cardioprotective, happy cholesterol HDL. In fact, the highest HDL level I've ever seen of 144 was in a hospitalized patient with alcohol withdrawal who drank upwards of a bottle of vodka per day. (Unfortunately, even when he was sober, his walk was permanently crooked and he could not maintain his balance because his years of alcohol abuse had destroyed his cerebellum, the part of the brain that coordinates motor movements.)

We know that the positive effects are quickly negated by disastrous effects to almost every organ system in the body when alcohol is regularly consumed in excess or in the form of binge drinking (consuming several drinks in a relatively short time). One of the most significant immediate effects of alcohol for both habitual and binge drinkers is that it affects the integrity of the gastrointestinal tract and damages the gut microbiome balance, as well as interferes with the immune response by damaging T cells, macrophages, and neutrophils from protecting the natural barriers in the gut and airway.[25] We also know that alcohol severely inhibits our ability to enter the deep, restorative sleep that our bodies need to repair themselves during the night.

So where's the happy medium?

As my favorite cardiologist colleague says, "Ladies, it's one drink a day and you can't save it up." I like this idea because it emphasizes that the upper limit of acceptable alcohol use is one drink per day for women and two drinks per day for men. Unfortunately, our bodies are not adept at detoxing more alcohol than that. That means you can't have three drinks on Thursday even if you didn't drink Monday through Wednesday.

While one or two drinks daily is a good start, I recommend being even more prudent with alcohol. When I look at all the evidence and factor in the socioeconomic impacts of alcohol, *most* people might enjoy a drink up to three or four nights per week, but only if it brings you joy. There's no reason to start drinking alcohol if you don't enjoy it. And if you've struggled with substance abuse or you're sensitive to the depressing effects of alcohol, then abstaining will be better for you.

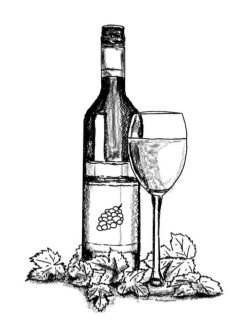

---

[24] J. B. Standridge, R. G. Zylstra, and S. M. Adams, "Alcohol consumption: an overview of benefits and risks," *Southern Medical Journal* 97, no. 7 (2004): 664–72.

[25] D. Sarkar, M. K. Jung, and H. J. Wang, "Alcohol and the immune system," *Alcohol Research: Current Reviews* 37, no. 2 (2015): 153–5.

PROCESSED FOODS & SUGAR

News flash: sugar is bad for you…but it's so delicious!

Treat sugar like the treat that it is and enjoy it sparingly. Remember, a treat is no longer a treat if you have it all the time.

Most of us are hip to the overt sources of sugar in our diets, like candy and desserts. But we need to be detectives and watch for sugar masquerading as healthy food. A good example is processed whole-grain products like most breakfast cereals and whole-grain breads. These are not real foods and should be limited in the diet.

It's a good practice to sweeten foods ourselves, as food companies almost always add more sugar than we would. Sweetened yogurt is one of my pet peeves; a common brand of light strawberry yogurt packs 4¾ teaspoons of sugar in just 6 ounces. Buy plain yogurt and sweeten it yourself with fruit or a little honey if you find it too sour. Better yet, buy coconut yogurt, which is naturally sweet and needs no doctoring.

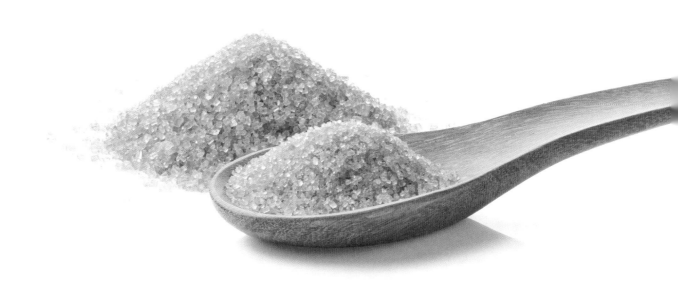

SUGAR IS SUGAR

Many patients ask me about which types of sweeteners are the most healthy. To be fair, sugar is sugar, no matter where it comes from. That said, maple syrup and honey may be superior to table sugar or agave due to their natural state and lower fructose content. Grade A dark maple syrup and locally sourced honey also carry the benefit of multiple anti-inflammatory antioxidants and immune system modulation along with a richness of flavor that surpasses that of regular sugar.[26]

Okay to Have in Small Amounts	Use Very Sparingly	Eliminate Completely
Raw coconut sugar, blackstrap molasses, honey, maple syrup, agave, dried fruits	Barley malt, beet/date/grape sugar, brown rice syrup, cane sugar, caramel, carob syrup, dextran, dextrose, diastase, diastatic malt, ethyl maltol, evaporated cane juice, fructose, fruit juice concentrate, galactose, glucose, lactose, malt syrup, maltodextrose, maltose, monk fruit, muscovado sugar, panocha, rice syrup, sorghum syrup, stevia, sucrose, treacle	High-fructose corn syrup, artificial nonnutritive sweeteners like acesulfame potassium, aspartame, saccharin, and sucralose

[26] S. Samarghandian, T. Farkhondeh, and F. Samini, "Honey and health: a review of recent clinical research," *Pharmacognosy Research* 9, no. 2 (2017): 121–7.

NONCALORIC SWEETENERS: THERE'S NO SUCH THING AS A FREE LUNCH

Sweeteners—whether caloric or noncaloric—have consequences in the body. I always tell patients, "There's no such thing as a free lunch." And nowhere is that more clear to me than in the form of noncaloric sweeteners.

Always choose nutritive sweeteners (those with calories) over nonnutritive ones (those without calories, usually in the form of artificial sweeteners). The jury is out for me on stevia and monk fruit, which are natural but processed nonnutritive sweeteners, because I'm unsure of the downstream effects they have on the body. A study published in *Nature* suggests that nonnutritive sweeteners disrupt the probiotic-rich microbiome, which independently increases the risk of metabolic diseases like diabetes and obesity.[27] Avoiding metabolic disease is often *why* we turn to noncaloric sweeteners in the first place.

What we know for sure is that sweetness in the diet begets more cravings for sweet foods due to the impact of the happy neurotransmitter dopamine, which is part of our brain's reward circuit. When we eat or drink sugar, dopamine is released, and that makes us feel amazing; the problem is that we have to continue to consume sugar to get the same effect, and we experience a bit of "pain" right after the initial dopamine hit, which makes us want more and more. Turning off cravings for sugar is akin to detoxing from illicit drugs because the effect of dopamine is so powerful. You're not making up the unpleasant sensations in your body that you feel during the first few days of taking a break from sugar.

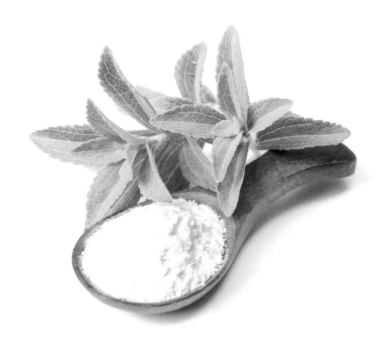

[27] J. Suez, T. Korem, D. Zeevi, et al., "Artificial sweeteners induce glucose intolerance by altering the gut microbiota," *Nature* 514 (2014): 181–6.

AVOID SWEETENED BEVERAGES

I recommend avoiding sweetened beverages like soda, juice, sweet tea, coffee drinks, and sports drinks like the plague. Sweetened beverages aren't good for us at all; they are just vehicles for disastrous consequences, including obesity and metabolic syndrome.

Many beverages, including soda, are made with high-fructose corn syrup (HFCS), an ultra-processed derivative of corn that is preferentially metabolized by the liver. Over time, the liver becomes taxed and begins to get inflamed, leading to elevated liver enzymes and eventually the deposition of fat into the once-functional tissue. This condition is called non-alcoholic fatty liver disease (NAFLD) because the liver appears similar to the way it looks when taxed with alcohol. Eventually, NAFLD causes a decline in liver function, leading to a whole host of other problems.

All sweetened beverages are bad for us, even if they don't have HFCS in them. Choosing a drink made with regular cane sugar over one made with high-fructose corn syrup is like the difference between a D- and an F on your report card. They're both terrible and will likely get you grounded.

Juices and sports drinks are especially tricky because they are marketed as healthy choices for active kids. You want your whole family to get vitamins and minerals from real fiber-rich fruit and vegetables and get electrolytes from a little pinch of salt in your water (or try Dr. Katie Life Water on page 306).

A NOTE ON PROCESSED FOODS

I've spent a bit of time talking about the landmines of processed foods, but I include them in the tip of the food pyramid (refer to page 99) to show you how few of your daily or weekly calories should be spent on ultra-processed foods. Sometimes, however, your heart wants what it wants. And maybe that's some chips or a cookie. If it's a one-off or a departure from your regular assortment of healthy food, don't worry about it. In fact, I sincerely want you to enjoy the indulgence. Savor it, and take some time to appreciate whatever it was about that food that had you at hello. Understanding your *Wellness Intuition* necessitates some wiggle room...but follow a processed food indulgence with a plant-forward, fiber-rich meal to keep yourself on track.

The bottom line on sugar and processed foods: choose natural sources of sugar very carefully and work to limit or eliminate the rest.

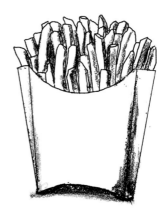

FIND BALANCE
ON YOUR PLATE

Start by making vegetables at least half of your plate at each meal, including breakfast.

If you're not used to eating vegetables at breakfast, it can seem strange at first. Very few Americans naturally desire vegetables for breakfast. It takes some rethinking about how to put your meal together, but I promise, it will become second nature to you and to your family. The first time I served my then-four-year-old boys vegetables at breakfast, they looked at me like I had two heads. I shrugged and said, "Yeah, guys. This is what we're doing now." They balked a little bit and pushed their vegetables around their plates, but eventually they ate them. One day I didn't have any left-over roasted vegetables to serve them (imagine the horror!), so I didn't put any vegetables on their breakfast plates. Both boys suddenly disappeared, and I found them around the corner in the living room high-fiving each other.

If you just can't fathom vegetables at breakfast, then I'll give you a pass for that one meal.

Here's a guide to finding balance on your plate that might be helpful:

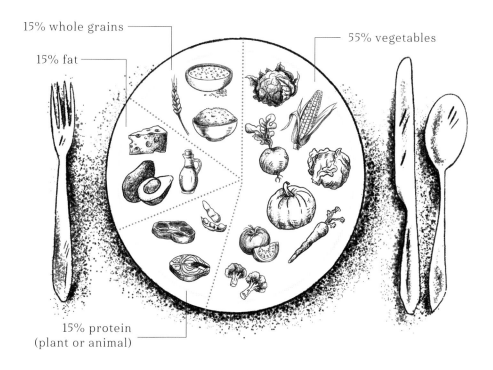

15% whole grains

15% fat

55% vegetables

15% protein
(plant or animal)

Note that my chart is in terms of *real estate, not percentage of calories.* (This becomes important because, as you know, fat is more calorically dense than vegetables, meaning that 100 calories of broccoli looks drastically different from 100 calories of almonds.)

If you start with at least half of your plate real estate in vegetables, then you're going to find better balance in your digestion and in your diet.

FOLLOW THE 80/20 RULE

I seem a little strict, right? Well, that's where the 20 percent comes in. No one needs to be perfect. Just like in other parts of life, if you do well 80 percent of the time, then you don't need to feel guilty about the remaining 20 percent. This girl loves sweet desserts, crusty bread, savory cheeses, robust wines, salty french fries, and juicy burgers, so I make allowances for indulgences like those and plan for them.

I think about indiscretions in our diets as being like little paper cuts. One or two paper cuts hurt but don't bother us too much, and we can generally move on with our days, maybe noticing some inconvenient stinging or sensitivity. But if we were constantly getting paper cuts, the damage to our poor fingers would compound over time, and we'd become really uncomfortable.

Imagine this same idea in your body, specifically in the gut, and be on the lookout for when a tiny paper cut becomes a bit more pronounced in the form of headaches, fatigue, skin irritation, indigestion, or just not feeling well. That's when you come back to your *Wellness Intuition* and lean into what makes you feel great.

A NOTE ON FOOD SENSITIVITIES & ALLERGIES

Not everyone is made to eat every food. Lots of people have food sensitivities. They just don't know it because they aren't paying attention.

Food sensitivities can cause inflammation in the body just like allergies do. The difference is that true food allergies can be fatal, as in the case of anaphylaxis due to a peanut or shellfish allergy. If a person who has a sensitivity to peanuts accidentally eats a peanut, their immune system will respond in a way that's similar to the inflammation from a bee sting discussed in Chapter 1. The difference between an uncomfortable bee sting and generalized anaphylaxis is that the inflammation in anaphylaxis is so profound that it overcomes the body's ability to rebound. Anaphylaxis can include many signs, but it generally involves profound swelling especially in the respiratory tract, making it difficult to breathe, accompanied by a massive dilation of blood vessels leading to severe hypotension. It can be life-threatening if not aggressively treated.

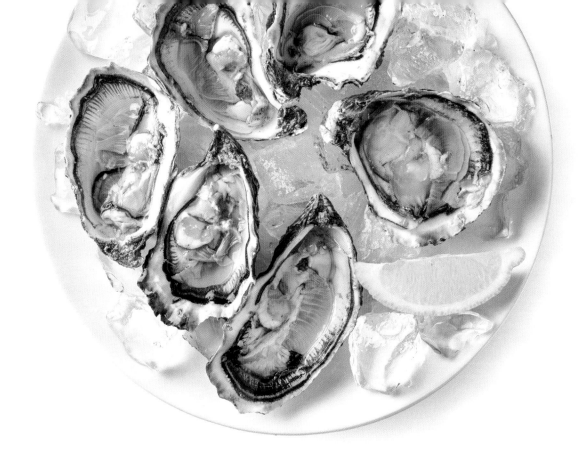

FOOD SENSITIVITIES & YOUR *WELLNESS INTUITION*

True food allergies can be measured more easily than food sensitivities. Your allergist can do a skin prick test or test for immunoglobulin E (IgE) antibodies in your blood. IgE is the natural antibody protein that the immune system makes when responding to an allergen. The more IgE your body produces in response to an allergen, the more profound your reaction when you come into contact with that food.

Unfortunately, it's not as easy to measure food sensitivities via immunoglobulins. Newer tests exist that evaluate for immunoglobulin G (IgG) and A (IgA) antibodies, but these tests are not as reliable as the IgE test and are sometimes influenced by the last time you ate that particular food. For example, if you do a food sensitivity test and you have high IgG antibodies to walnuts, but you eat one-quarter cup of walnuts every day on your oatmeal or salad, then it's hard to tease out whether it's a true sensitivity. Likewise, if a food sensitivity test says you have very little IgG antibodies to crab, but you never eat crab, it's tough to know whether it's a true negative. I still use these tests in my practice because they can be useful for some patients, but I recognize their shortcomings and guide patients through the maze of food elimination and reintroduction in a methodical way.

A better way to discern food sensitivities is to tap into your *Wellness Intuition* and simply pay attention to what happens in your body when you eat a particular food. Do you become bloated or develop a faint rash whenever you eat sesame seeds? Do you get a loose stool every time you eat raw cauliflower, but cooked cauliflower seems to be fine? Most food sensitivities seem to show up in the gastrointestinal tract as bloating or stool changes, but I find a strong correlation with the skin along with vague symptoms like fatigue, brain fog, joint pain, depressed moods, sinus congestion, and headaches.

One of the best examples I have of this food sensitivity phenomenon involved my patient Serena, a young and vibrant mom who happened to have type 1 diabetes. She went to her endocrinologist and said she was having profound fatigue after breakfast, to the point where she wanted to take a nap. The doctor reviewed her blood sugar control and found that Serena was covering her blood sugar at breakfast appropriately with insulin. Serena started keeping a detailed food journal and would write down every time she felt fatigued after breakfast. She quickly saw the pattern of having fatigue only after weekday breakfasts of chia seed pudding with vanilla, raspberries, and almond butter. She ate chia seeds, raspberries, and almond butter on their own

or with other foods on many other occasions, so she smartly deduced that she might have been reacting to vanilla extract. Sure enough, once she removed the vanilla from her morning pudding, she soared through the day like normal. Now she knows that if she eats something that has vanilla extract in it, she may feel tired afterward.

Thankfully, most food sensitivities are not life-threatening, but they can severely compromise your quality of life and lead to festering inflammation in the body. Leaving even small amounts of inflammation unchecked is a recipe for feeling poorly and taxes your system too much.

If you're curious about whether you have food sensitivities, start by tuning into your *Wellness Intuition*. Pay attention to the way you feel after you eat. If you decide that a food elimination is in order, I recommend starting with the foods people are commonly sensitive to: gluten, dairy, nuts, soy, shellfish, beef, pork, caffeine, alcohol, citrus, and nightshades such as tomatoes, bell peppers, potatoes, and eggplant. This list is the backbone of the plant-forward *Dr. Katie Detox*, which I detail for you in Chapter 12.

HEALING THE BODY

What I've discovered in my personal and professional life is that once we quell the inflammation from food sensitivities with thoughtful elimination and simultaneously heal the gut lining, we can often go about enjoying small amounts of foods on our sensitivity list without much issue. My patient Serena who is sensitive to vanilla extract is able to tolerate small amounts of it in roasted or baked foods without much of an issue. She just doesn't put vanilla in her chia pudding anymore.

So, if I recommend a food in *Dr. Katie's Anti-Inflammatory Diet* that doesn't agree with you, you should avoid it for now but then work with your Integrative healthcare provider to heal that food sensitivity so that you can regularly enjoy a robust array of plant-rich, anti-inflammatory foods.

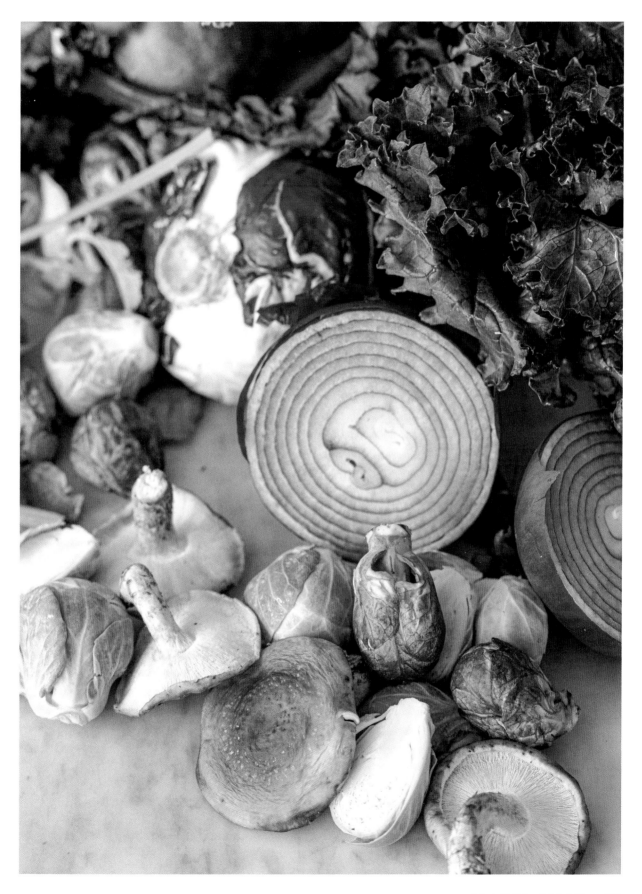

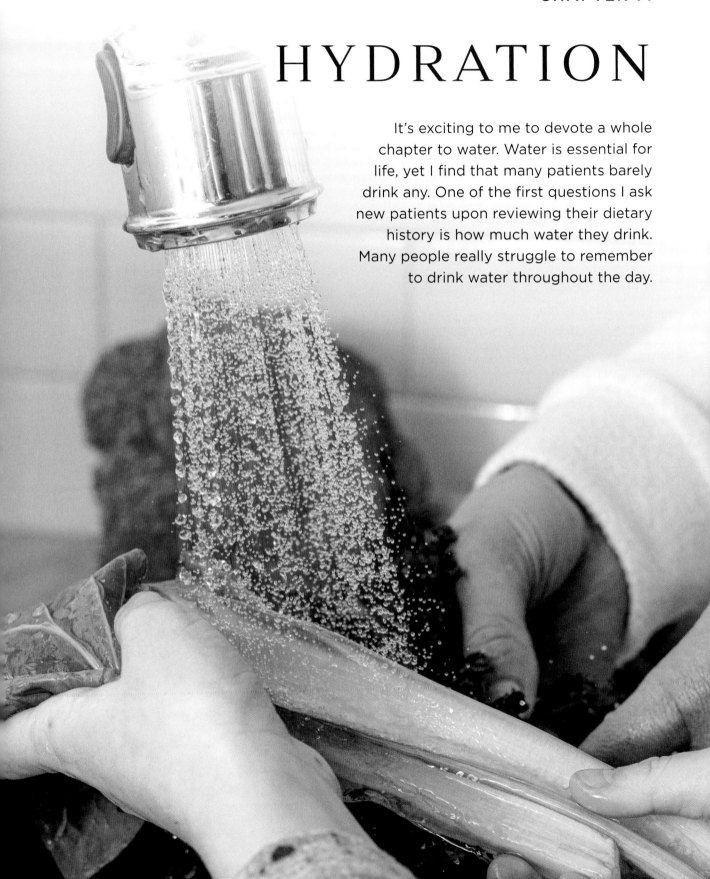

CHAPTER 7

HYDRATION

It's exciting to me to devote a whole chapter to water. Water is essential for life, yet I find that many patients barely drink any. One of the first questions I ask new patients upon reviewing their dietary history is how much water they drink. Many people really struggle to remember to drink water throughout the day.

WHY HYDRATE

It's important to stay well hydrated for so many reasons. First of all, our bodies are mostly water, and we depend on a well-hydrated system for optimal function. Our water intake influences regulation of body temperature, joint lubrication, infection prevention, nutrient delivery to cells, ease of digestion, sleep and wake cycles, cognition, and mood. Proper water intake also influences the skin, helping it to stay supple and lessening the likelihood of wrinkles. (If nothing else makes you drink water, vanity should!)

Another reason to stay well hydrated is that it helps to regulate the body's hunger and satiety hormones. Sometimes our bodies misconstrue hunger for thirst, making us think we're hungry when in fact we're just thirsty.

The next time you're hungry, especially if it's been only an hour or two since you last ate, have a large glass of water and do a small chore. See if the hunger sensation passes. If it does, you were likely dehydrated.

HOW MUCH WATER DO YOU NEED?

Everyone's water needs are different, but most people need to drink 2 or more liters of water per day. Experts recommend at least half of the ideal body weight in ounces. Newer guidelines are up to 1 ounce of water per pound of body weight! For example, if your ideal body weight is 140 pounds, then you should be drinking 70 to 140 ounces per day, which equates to more than 2 liters (64 ounces).

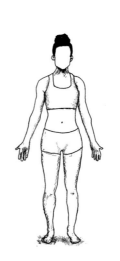

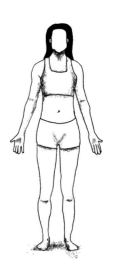

140 lbs. = 70–140 oz. of water

180 lbs. = 90–180 oz. of water.

A good judge of your hydration status is the color of your urine, which should be clear and should barely turn the toilet water yellow, similar to the color of fancy champagne. If it's darker than that (and you haven't just taken a vitamin supplement), then you should consider drinking more water.

I love water, and I drink it constantly, but too much of a good thing is not a good thing. It is definitely possible to drink too much water. Because water is hypotonic (meaning it has less solute in it compared to our blood volume), drinking too much water can dilute your natural body electrolytes like sodium, potassium, and chloride. In excess, this can be dangerous. This is why I promote adding some Dr. Katie Life Water (page 306) to your routine. Adding lemon and salt to your water balances the electrolytes to make it a little closer to isotonic. It's actually impossible to drink a truly isotonic liquid with as much solute as your blood volume because it would be so salty you couldn't stand it!

DRINK WATER BETWEEN MEALS & BEFORE DINNER

I advocate for drinking most of your daily water between meals to allow for proper digestion. Drinking lots of water while eating does two not-so-great things:

- First, it dilutes your natural digestive juices, which start in the saliva and continue into the stomach and small intestine. You want your body's digestive response to be as robust as possible to aid in the absorption of energy, vitamins, minerals, and other anti-inflammatory compounds.

- Second, drinking lots of water with meals suggests that you may not be chewing your food enough before swallowing. The natural action of chewing food releases saliva and salivary enzymes to begin the digestion process, and—along with fifty pairs of muscles and a lot of nerves—creates a moist food bolus that can be easily swallowed and moved into the stomach for further processing.

I personally limit my liquids at mealtime to less than one cup and restart drinking more earnestly about sixty minutes after eating until about twenty minutes prior to the next meal.

I also recommend that you drink the majority of your water before the late afternoon so that you don't awaken unnecessarily at night to urinate. I encourage patients to get their first liter of water in before noon.

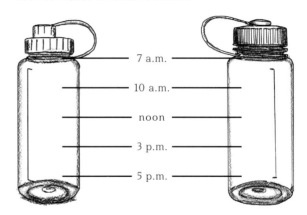

Recommended window for drinking most of your daily water

BOTTLED WATER

I don't love buying bottled water unless I have to due to the concern I have with storing water in plastic bottles and the environmental impact of single-use bottles polluting our planet. And unless you have a degree in water bottle decoding, the labels are really confusing to boot. Did you know that bottled water is often just tap water with a fancy label? If you must buy bottled water, read carefully and choose spring water, which comes from a natural source.

The better choice is a large reusable water bottle that's made of an inert substance like stainless steel or glass. If you buy a bottle that's about 1 liter (32 ounces), then you can easily keep track of your water intake over the course of the day. Plus, you'll look cool carrying it around. It brings a smile to my face to see young people posing on Instagram with their rainbow-colored fleet of Hydro Flasks. Reusable water bottles are all the rage right now and a trend I suggest you embrace.

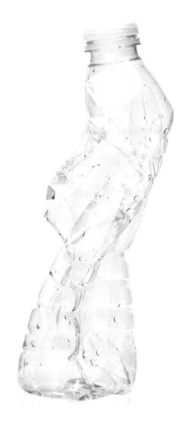

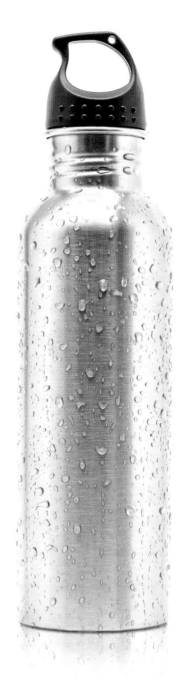

SELTZER & SPARKLING WATER

What about seltzer and sparkling water? Do those drinks count toward your total water intake? Absolutely. But with a caveat.

I recommend limiting fizzy water if you have a tendency toward acid reflux, gas, bloating, or other digestive woes. Otherwise, feel comfortable having up to a liter of bubbly water per day. I personally limit my fizzy water intake to about 16 ounces per day to avoid digestive issues. Interestingly, you may enjoy sparkling water more than seltzer, since sparkling water is naturally less carbonated and often paired with natural minerals.

If you're buying bubbly water, buy plain bubbles and add any flavoring yourself to avoid strange chemical additives. Adding a splash of pomegranate juice, a few cucumber slices, or a squeeze of citrus is a great way to make bubbly water more festive and can be a great alternative to alcohol.

As noted in Chapter 6, sweetened beverages, including fruit juice, should be avoided.

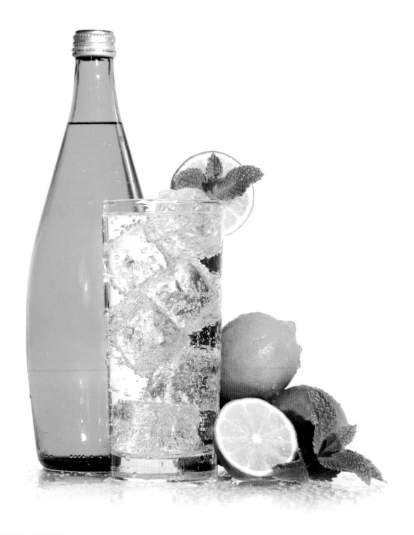

CLEAN WATER

Access to clean drinking water is a national and global problem that affects people regardless of socioeconomic status, though it disproportionately affects those living in impoverished or rural areas. Almost everything we do to advance our world has a negative impact on clean water supplies, including industrial and agricultural practices as well as household chores like laundry and showering. I grew up drinking water from a well, so while it was free of some problems, over the years our supply was fraught with other issues, including the main well drying up. Imagine waking up one morning with brown sludge dripping from the faucet into the kitchen sink. I love the idea my grandparents had on the Wehri Farm to build a cistern, which collected rainwater for washing clothes and land irrigation, but given other mounting environmental concerns, like air pollution, a cistern is not a tenable solution for most people.

One solution to having clean water at home, regardless of having city or well water, is a reverse-osmosis system at the tap, which puts water for cooking and drinking through three stages of filtration. The first filtration is usually a carbon filter, which reduces disinfection by-products and volatile organic compounds. The subsequent filtrations remove chemical contaminants like nitrates, perchlorates, arsenic, lead, toxic fluorinated chemicals, and hexavalent chromium, which none of us want in our water. But alas, no system is perfect. It's not wise to install a whole-house system for several reasons. It not only removes chlorine, which can be a problem for bacteria growth in water pipes, but also removes essential minerals like magnesium, calcium, and iron. The reverse-osmosis process also wastes a lot of water, about three times as much as it treats; that's why a tap system only in the kitchen might be the most economical and practical for your household.

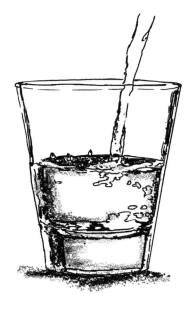

> "Almost *everything we do to advance* our world has a **negative impact** on clean water supplies."

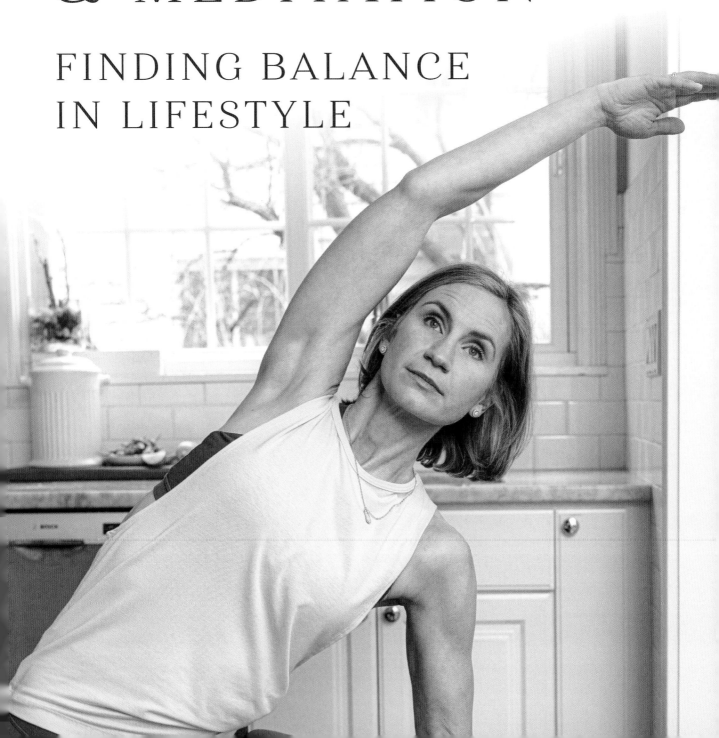

CHAPTER 8

MOVEMENT, REST & MEDITATION

FINDING BALANCE IN LIFESTYLE

I've spent most of this book talking about food, but we all know that truly feeling well is not just about eating nutrient-dense food. If it were just about food, there would be no need for fitness centers or personal trainers. We'd have no need for beds because we wouldn't be sleeping. And we'd have empty churches, synagogues, yoga studios, and therapist offices because no one would need emotional or spiritual guidance.

As someone grounded in holistic body, mind, and spiritual wellness, I feel it's important to talk about taking care of more than just the nutritional aspect of health. How we move our physical bodies, how we find space for rest (both in the form of sleep and in simply taking a hot second to sit down), and how we attend to the Spiritual Self are vital pieces of wellness. And within each of these areas, we're all on a quest to find balance.

Balance is not a destination. It's not a place you magically find. And balance certainly doesn't mean all things in your health are equal. In fact, for some people, finding better balance could be heavily weighted toward food and then evenly split among the other pillars of movement, rest, and attunement to the Spiritual Self. Or, like Nikki, one of my Dr. Katie Detoxers, discovered, you could be way out of balance because the majority of your energy is going toward movement and physical fitness. Upon reflection, Nikki realized that she needed to reroute some energy to well-rounded nutrition (which for her included increasing dietary fat) and nightly rest. How do you assess your balance? This is where your *Wellness Intuition* comes in and you listen to what your body has to share.

We may recognize good balance only retrospectively. I don't often find myself saying, "Wow, I'm in balance!" It more so happens when I've been listening to my body for a period of time, and when I reflect that I feel well, I realize it's because I have been attending to my health in the right way.

My favorite quote about balance goes something like this: "You can have it all, just expect it to be a mess." And it's true. If we gun for everything all at once, we end up with chaos. I think it's better to evolve into a more optimal state of health over time, making only the changes we need in that moment or on that day, adjusting in real time to the demands of our obligations or even our moods. If I've learned one thing, it's that the body does not like drastic changes. Slow and steady wins the race.

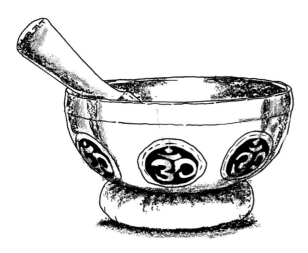

THE STRESS RESPONSE

One of the primary reasons to think about the four pillars of nutrition, exercise, sleep, and spirituality is that it brings balance to the body. And when our bodies are in a general state of balance, we are able to withstand stressors to the system.

We are all keenly aware of stress and its effects on our bodies. We generally don't feel good when we are really stressed. Our digestion may be off, we may be "tired but wired" (meaning we're fatigued but aren't actually tired and can't seem to sleep), or we may be cranky and crabby and generally unpleasant to be around. We may feel like the world is spinning around us in a hopeless tornado, or we may feel so incapacitated that we are stuck in the mud.

ADRENALINE & CORTISOL: FIGHT, FLIGHT, OR FREEZE

When we encounter a perceived threat, the hypothalamus in our brain sets off an alarm system that signals hormones in the pituitary gland to stimulate our adrenal glands to release adrenaline (in the form of epinephrine and norepinephrine) and cortisol. Adrenaline increases the heart rate and blood pressure and mobilizes skeletal muscle, while cortisol increases blood sugar, modulates the immune system, and turns off nonessential functions like digestion, reproduction, and growth so that we have the energy to fight or flee from the perceived threat. Except sometimes we don't fight or flee. Instead, we freeze. That's the feeling of being so overwhelmed that we wind up in bed under the covers, watching Netflix on a laptop and downing a pint of Ben & Jerry's.

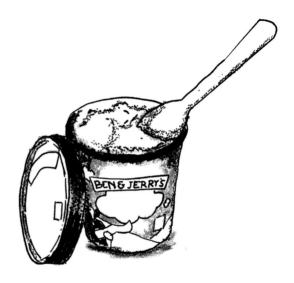

OXYTOCIN:
TEND & BEFRIEND

In addition to the fight, flight, or freeze response, we can react to stress with a "tend and befriend" response, mediated by a separate hormonal symphony that involves the hypothalamus stimulating the pituitary gland to produce oxytocin. Oxytocin is called the "love hormone" because it's intricately tied to our innate recognition of deep friendship, trust, romantic and sexual attachment, and mother-infant bonding. It's behind the warm, fuzzy fluttering you feel in your heart when you're connecting with another human or a pet.

In stressful situations, women are wired to the "tend and befriend" response, which is why many of us want to nurture something or call someone when we're stressed. This response is adaptive and positive because it suppresses adrenaline and cortisol, as long as we aren't nurturing a whole pint of Ben & Jerry's. Oxytocin release furthers the case for the importance of social interaction and community involvement throughout our lifetime.

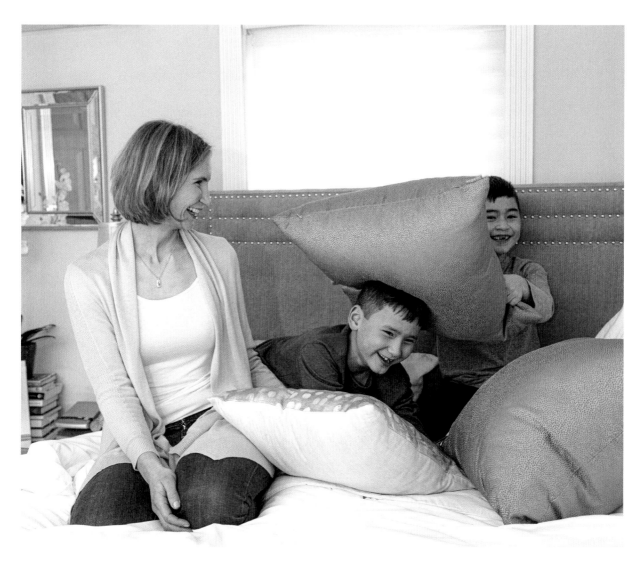

THE STOPLIGHT OF STRESSORS

Regardless of how you experience stress, you can think about the levels of stress as a stoplight. The severity of the perceived threat determines how much of your body's stress response system must be activated in order to rise to the occasion.

- **Green light stressors** are the little stressors we feel on a daily basis, and not all of them are bad. These minor stressors keep us on time for appointments, allow us to meet deadlines at work, and remind us to quickly pull our hand away from a hot pan on the stove. They keep us on our toes, last for a relatively short time, and resolve on their own. Most importantly, they cause only a brief release of adrenaline and cortisol because we can cope with them.

- **Yellow light stressors** are moderate stressors that last for longer periods, like those we experience when a family member has been hospitalized or has a longer-term illness, we go through a job change or divorce, or we start medical school and realize we're in over our heads. These stressors require care to bring them to resolution. They cause a sustained release of adrenaline and cortisol and generally make us feel yucky unless we use sophisticated coping tools.

- **Red light stressors** cause us to go into crisis mode. We can tolerate these stressors only briefly because they require so much cortisol and adrenaline that our bodies literally cannot keep up. An example would be seeing a young child run out into the street and springing into action to snatch them out of the way of an oncoming car. You know this feeling of extreme stress—your heart is pounding, and you're sweaty and nauseated and possibly feeling faint after coming down from the extreme scare. Basically, you feel terrible.

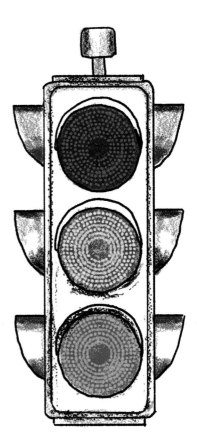

The problem with our modern way of life is that we keep piling more stressors onto our plates, so our bodies interpret even minor daily hassles as bigger threats than they really are. We forget how to cope with green light stressors, and we feel like we're constantly under attack. In medicine, this is known as sympathetic overdrive because the sympathetic nervous system continues to overreact to even the smallest stressors.

This constant need to keep your guard up disrupts your ability to live a full, healthy life. Have you ever noticed what happens when you go on vacation? When I went to Italy on a yoga retreat with my husband a few years ago, I was astounded by how well I slept despite the time change. I also noticed that my digestion worked perfectly, despite eating more gluten and dairy than I ever would at home, and I felt more like my real self than I had in months. Vacation affords us a break from reality, a chance to dial down the stress response. And dialing down the stress response removes the constant paper cuts of daily life, making it easier to find flow.

When I think about managing stress, at the heart of it is a focus on lifestyle, because how we live each day matters so much to the Self feeling at home in its own skin. If you are persistently in a state of stress, your body has no choice but to respond with the saber-toothed tiger "cortisol bath" of the red-light response. Your number one stress management tool is not popping a Xanax or having a glass of wine at night; it's mitigating the stress response with your lifestyle choices.

LIFESTYLE MATTERS

We find so many ways to take the pleasures of life and compact them into tiny bites, all in the name of efficiency. If we don't have time to cook, we can find a sodium-laden frozen meal that our bodies barely recognize as real food. If we don't have time to exercise, we can sweat bullets with an eight-minute high-intensity interval training workout and rev up our stress response rather than soothe our souls. If we don't have time to rest, we convince ourselves that we can survive on five hours of sleep or overcaffeinate. We use our smartphones while we're supposed to be resting on an acupuncture table so that we don't "waste time."

As discussed in Chapter 1, the backbone of Integrative Medicine is lifestyle, which I divide into four categories: eating, moving, sleeping, and tending to our spiritual needs. How we take care of our physical, emotional, mental, and spiritual Self is the fertile ground into which the "seeds" of everything else we do are sown. Making choices that are in line with our individual *Wellness Intuition* and balance our personal needs for food, exercise, sleep, and spirituality can fertilize the soil and change our lives.

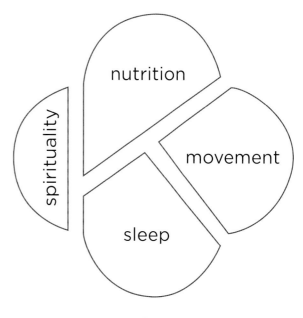

MOVEMENT

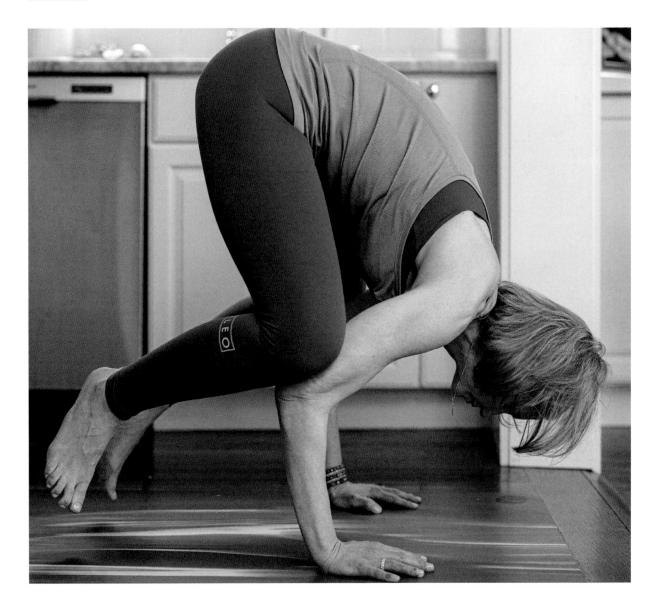

I am a big believer in exercise being a key to stress management. Exercise is my favorite feel-good pill. I realized this personally while in college, finding that the days I prioritized movement were the days I was more productive and felt happier (and noticed that exercise made my monthly menstrual cramps almost disappear). Now I recognize that exercise is my number one tool for regulating my mood, so I prioritize space in my life every day for some kind of physical movement.

There are so many resources available for you to discover forms of physical movement that feel authentic and sustainable in your life. My goal with this section is to show you how exercise fits into your overall wellness and hit a few key pointers, not to be an exhaustive list of the options. I encourage you to seek out what feels good to you in keeping with your *Wellness Intuition*.

Exercise has been directly connected to reducing risk of high blood pressure and cardiovascular disease, insulin resistance and diabetes, osteoporosis, cancer, dementia, Alzheimer's, and loss of muscle mass (sarcopenia), as well as a direct decrease in bodywide inflammation.[1] These are all excellent motivators, but I tell patients the number one reason to exercise is the production of feel-good hormones called endorphins. Multiple studies show that moderate exercise like walking is just as effective as using SSRIs (selective serotonin reuptake inhibitors) for the treatment of depression and anxiety.[2] And you don't have to do a lot of exercise to get the job done: walking as little as three times per week is meaningful enough to make an impact on mental health.

There's also extensive research to show that exercise influences our sleep and regulates our circadian rhythms. One of the best ways to get your motor started in the morning (regardless of how you slept) is to get exposure to sunlight outdoors in combination with a little movement, otherwise known as a morning walk. I advocate waking at the same time every day, so follow your 6 a.m. wakeup with a twenty-minute walk.

LITTLE BY LITTLE THROUGHOUT THE DAY, & STANDING HELPS

Exercise doesn't have to happen all at once. If you find yourself with five minutes to take the stairs before work or ten minutes to take a walk after lunch, seize the opportunity; it all adds up. Your goal is about 150 minutes per week of gentle aerobic exercise, but the more active you are, the better.

I'm sure you've heard the phrase "sitting is the new smoking." American desk workers can sit for up to fifteen or more hours per day, and recent evidence from epidemiological and experimental studies makes a persuasive case that too much sitting should be considered a standalone component of calculating future risk of diabetes and cardiovascular disease.[3] Did you know you burn an additional 50 calories every hour just by standing? I joke with patients who comment on my standing desk that if I stand for three hours during the day, I can earn a glass of wine at night.

When it comes to dedicated exercise, do the best you can. If you only have time for a twelve-minute walk before work, try to make up the time on other days when you have more flexibility. Instead of beating yourself up for slacking off, acknowledge that you did the best you could and enjoy those minutes as "me time." In fact, I encourage you to think about the time you reserve in your schedule for exercise as a deposit in your bank account of energy so that you can live fully and give back to others.

[1] D. Furman, J. Campisi, E. Verdin, et al., "Chronic inflammation in the etiology of disease across the life span," *Nature Medicine* 25 (2019): 1822–32.

[2] J. A. Blumenthal, M. A. Babyak, K. A. Moore, et al., "Effects of exercise training on older patients with major depression," *Archives of Internal Medicine* 159, no. 19 (1999): 2349–56; G. Stathopoulou, M. B. Powers, A. C. Berry, et al., "Exercise interventions for mental health: a quantitative and qualitative review," *Clinical Psychology: Science and Practice* 13, no. 2 (2006): 179–93.

[3] D. W. Dunstan, B. Howard, G. N. Healy, and N. Owen, "Too much sitting—a health hazard," *Diabetes Research and Clinical Practice* 97, no. 3 (2012): 368–76.

GENTLE, JOYFUL MOVEMENT

I want to emphasize that *gentle* exercise is the way to go. I find that some of my patients exercise way too intensely, fueling hormonal imbalance, sparking appetite, and actually increasing stress hormones like cortisol and adrenaline. Your goal is a level of 6 to 7 out of 10 on the exertion scale that makes you just a little breathless, so that if you were having a conversation, you wouldn't be able to speak sentence after sentence nonchalantly. If you feel like someone should mop you up off the floor after you complete your high-intensity interval training or you have significant fatigue several hours after exercise, then you may be working out too hard.

I encourage you to exercise with family or friends, even if they live far away. One of my favorite things to do is a walk-and-talk by phone. Walking and talking is a beautiful, healthy way to catch up with those who are important to us and sure beats a Zoom happy hour where we're sitting and drinking alcohol in front of a screen.

BALANCE, STRENGTH & MUSCLE MAINTENANCE

It's also important to work on balance and strength, especially if you're at risk for osteoporosis. (Those who are most at risk of osteoporosis are generally postmenopausal Caucasian or Asian women who have thin body frames, an endocrine disorder like thyroid disease or menstrual irregularities, a smoking history, poor nutritional habits, or a family history of osteoporosis.) While having weak bones can cause a fall, most osteoporotic fractures happen because people are not as strong or stable as they could be and find themselves in unsafe conditions like slippery showers or icy sidewalks. Do yourself a huge favor and start your muscle building as soon as possible.

Our independence as we age is directly related to our ability to retain muscular strength and function. When I'm doing squats, I'm not thinking about how great my butt is going to look in my swimsuit this summer; I'm thinking about how, when I'm ninety-plus years old, I'm still going to be able to squat on my own toilet and care for myself, just like my grandmother.

Aim to do at least two sessions per week of an activity that builds strength. I like light weights and lots of repetitions, like in a barre or Pilates workout, or using body weight in the form of planks or squats. If you want to multitask in your movement endeavors, I recommend yoga because it involves building both strength and balance and recenters the spirit.

"Do yourself a huge favor and **start your muscle building** as soon as possible."

REST

What if I told you I had a magic pill that would decrease your inflammation and susceptibility to infections; regulate your hunger and satiety hormone signals; decrease your risk of heart disease, diabetes, and cancer; make you more pleasant and less irritable; and improve your cognitive and physical stamina? You'd probably say, "Yes! I'll take it!"

That's what sleep does for you. Sleep makes almost everything better. It's the time our bodies use to heal, detoxify, and recharge our systems. Taking time for adequate rest is one of the best things you can do for your body.

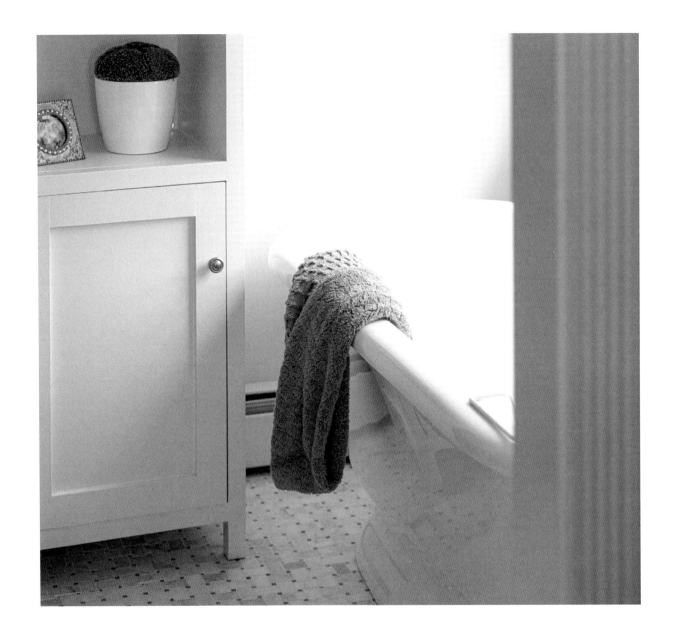

SETTING THE STAGE FOR SLEEP

Anyone who has struggled with sleep knows that you can't *make* yourself fall asleep. Sleep is passive—it's something that happens to you, something you relinquish yourself to. This idea of letting go and relinquishing yourself to rest is important, especially for those of us who are go-go-go throughout the day. I find that most of my patients with sleep issues are not insufficiently sleepy but excessively awake, victims to that "tired but wired" feeling I talked about earlier in relation to how stress manifests in the body. It's virtually impossible to fire on all cylinders from the time you wake up in the morning until the moment your head hits the pillow.

Most people won't just magically fall asleep at night unless they're exhausted or they're one of those enviable people who never experience sleep issues. The mind and body need a wind-down period, an opportunity to settle and ground yourself after a full day of learning and experiences. I recommend giving yourself at least forty-five minutes to come down from the day. This wind-down period needs to be device-free to avoid blue-light stimulation (which excites rather than relaxes the brain) and could include any number of relaxing activities, including a warm bath with magnesium salts, a cup of chamomile tea, a non-stimulating book, restorative yoga, prayer, or meditation.

University of Rochester neurosurgery professor Maiken Nedergaard says our brains are like dishwashers because they clean up toxins while we sleep.[4] Our brains have only two functional states—awake and partying, or asleep and cleaning up. Dr. Nedergaard simply says, "You can either entertain the guests or clean up the house, but you really can't do both at the same time." I like this idea. It's only by relinquishing to rest that we are able to do the good work of cleaning up.

YOUR SLEEP RHYTHM

How much sleep do you need? This is an individual answer based on your homeostatic sleep drive and circadian rhythm.

Your *homeostatic sleep drive* is the amount of sleep you naturally need to feel rested. Most adults need seven to nine hours per night, but there are a few who truly need only five hours and some who need a whopping twelve hours to feel rested. The best way to know your homeostatic sleep drive is to remember back to your younger years (when fewer people have sleep issues) and think about how much sleep you needed to feel great. There's your answer.

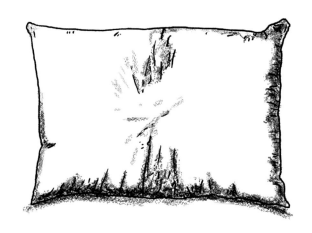

---

[4] J. Hamilton, "Brains sweep themselves clean of toxins during sleep," All Things Considered, October 17, 2013, https://www.npr.org/sections/health-shots/2013/10/18/236211811/brains-sweep-themselves-clean-of-toxins-during-sleep.

A CONSISTENT WAKE TIME

I have found that having a consistent wake time is one of the keys to protecting sleep architecture. Over the course of the day, our brains build up the neurochemical adenosine, which basically suppresses nerve cell activity and causes a feeling of drowsiness. After about sixteen hours, the amount of adenosine reaches a critical level, and we start to feel sleepy.

Of course, you can disrupt this adenosine buildup by drinking caffeine. In fact, that's how caffeine works—it competitively binds to adenosine receptors so you temporarily feel less tired. Once the caffeine is metabolized (which happens at different rates for different people), adenosine is able to continue binding to its receptors, and you start to feel sleepy again.

The best way to feel tired at a predictable time at night is to have a consistent wake time and get exposure to morning sunlight. Morning sunlight along with a consistent wake time helps your body settle into your natural circadian rhythm, helping you to feel tired at night and fall asleep more easily from the predictable nerve cell relaxation influenced by accumulated adenosine.[5]

It's important not to shortchange your sleep on either end. I think this point is especially important for teens and young adults who are likely to stay up late studying or hanging out with friends, though almost all of us engage in some amount of "social jetlag" on the weekends when we stay up later than usual and try to sleep in the following morning. In the first part of the night, the brain is pruning connections, deciding what it wants to keep of the new information you experienced during the day. In the latter half of the night, the brain is strengthening and storing those memories so that you can call upon them later. If you stay up late watching TV, you miss out on the pruning. If you wake up early to catch a morning flight, you miss out on the storing. One of the best things we can encourage the young people in our lives to do is to get the amount of sleep they need to feel rested.

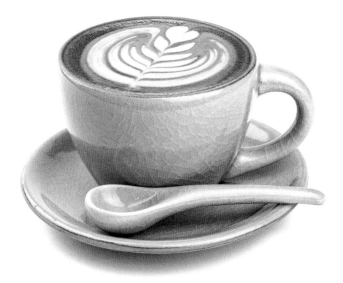

---

[5] D. Furman, J. Campisi, E. Verdin, et al., "Chronic inflammation in the etiology of disease across the life span," *Nature Medicine* 25, no. 12 (2019): 1822–32.

THE OLDER WE GET, THE LESS WE SLEEP

Sleep habits change as we age, and my elder patients often have unrealistic expectations that they will sleep the same number of hours and through the night like most teenagers do.

When we're older, our sleep pattern can become more like that of a baby or small child, where we sleep a few hours and then are up for a little while, and then fall asleep again. These interruptions are normal, but of course they are annoying and can be troublesome if getting back to sleep is difficult due to a busy mind. As I say to patients, it's not the thing that wakes us up that keeps us awake. For example, if you awaken at night to urinate or because of a perimenopausal night sweat, once you finish peeing or the hot flash is over, you should theoretically be able to fall right back asleep. But that's not the way it happens for so many of us. Generally, we are kept awake by our wandering mind focusing on everything from the mundane events of the day we just lived or tomorrow's to-do list, or perhaps to more anxiety-provoking thoughts and worries about how tired we might be tomorrow because of our present sleep difficulties.

While it's impossible to prevent yourself from waking, you can lessen your chance of waking by avoiding daytime naps. If you must nap during the day, I recommend limiting naptime to twenty minutes or less to protect your ability to fall asleep at night.

REST IS IMPORTANT, TOO

Sleep isn't the only kind of rest our bodies need. Rest can simply be finding moments to slow down and allow your brain to pause, and it can happen multiple times during the day.

It's physically easier to rest while sitting in a chair or lying on a couch, but you can even rest while standing up. Resting allows your brain to let go of everything that it's toggling while coming back to the breath, a word that's soothing, like a mantra, or a moment of gratitude for making it to this point in the day. Give yourself some space in the day to rest.

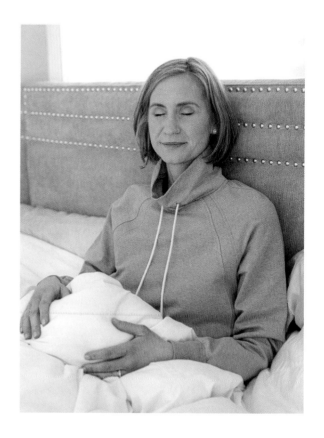

"**Resting** *allows your brain* to let go of everything..."

MEDITATION & THE SPIRITUAL SELF

All of us have an innate need to connect to our Spiritual Self. This is the "real" you, the Self that lies deep in your belly and guides your thoughts and actions. It's the Self you show to true friends and close family. In Chinese Medicine, this is where the flow of Qi (pronounced "chee"), our vital life energy, originates. This true Self is tightly woven into the fabric of your *Wellness Intuition*, governing what feels right for your body. Your true Self is nourished by people and activities that bring you joy and taxed by irritating people or situations.

You can think of your Spiritual Self as a bank account. Deposits are made with meditation, gentle exercise, nutritious food, restorative sleep, deep passions, and time spent in community with those you cherish. Withdrawals are made by everything else–doing laundry, handling mundane work tasks, arguing with your partner, disciplining your kids, paying bills–the list goes on and on. Attending to your Spiritual Self is about finding more deposits than withdrawals.

MIND-BODY MEDICINE & THE AUTONOMIC NERVOUS SYSTEM

One of the best ways to attend to the Self is with mind-body medicine, which includes everything from movement-based forms of meditation like yoga and tai chi to religious forms of meditation like prayer and Bible study to mindfulness meditation. It doesn't matter how you connect to that deeper part of yourself; it only matters that you do.

From a science perspective, research shows that mind-body medicine affects our autonomic nervous system. This background part of our nervous system is always in motion, like our heart beating and our digestive function. Western medicine divides it into two parts: the sympathetic and parasympathetic nervous systems. But recognize that this concept of duality exists in ancient systems of medicine as well, except it is described in a much more beautiful and holistic way. For example, in Chinese Medicine, we call this understanding *yin* and *yang*. In Ayurveda, a similar duality is described in terms of *soma* and *agni*, or *ojas* and *tejas*.

Our sympathetic nervous system is our "fight, flight, or freeze" response. You know this overactivation as the sweaty palms, heart racing, stomach churning feeling you get right before a big presentation or the quick-as-a-dime reflex you have to jump out of the way of an approaching car. I'm sure you've also experienced a hypoactive stress response, where you literally freeze, paralyzed by the cortisol bath of your nervous system.

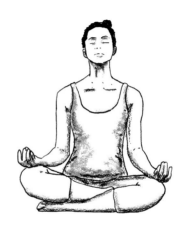

In contrast, our parasympathetic nervous system is our "rest and digest" response. This part of the nervous system is mediated by the vagus nerve and allows us to relax, sleep, digest our food, and have sex. It's the yin to the yang of the overactivated nervous system.

As discussed earlier in this chapter, most of us don't have a healthy balance between our fight, flight, or freeze response and our rest and digest response. Many of us spend much of our time in sympathetic overdrive as if we were running from saber-tooth tigers. Our bodies interpret this stimulus as a signal to produce stress hormones like cortisol and adrenaline. Chronic cortisol elevation can lead to worsening insomnia, weight gain, and other downstream hormonal disturbances.

One way to increase our parasympathetic response is by engaging in mind-body modalities. Robust systematic reviews including multiple trials and thousands of participants show that spending time doing activities like yoga and meditation has incredible positive effects on the body due to the decrease in stress hormones during the relaxation response.[6]

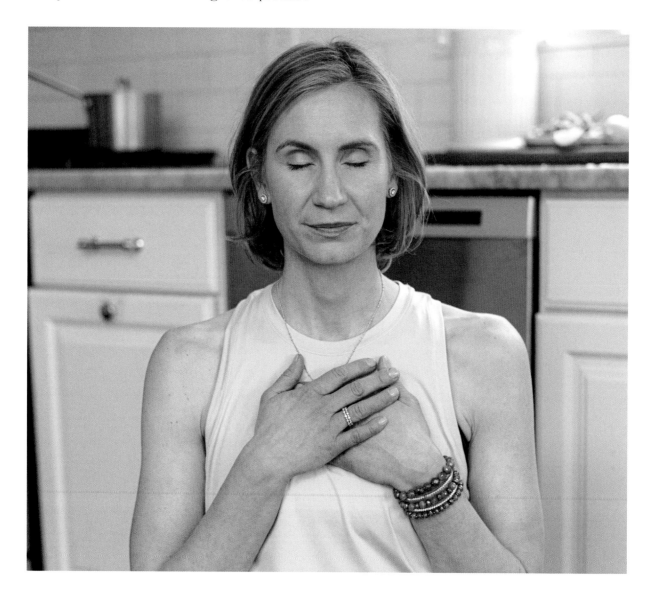

[6] M. Goyal, S. Singh, E. M. Sibinga, et al., "Meditation programs for psychological stress and well-being: a systematic review and meta-analysis," *JAMA Internal Medicine* 174, no. 3 (2014): 357–68.

YOU CAN CHANGE YOUR BRAIN

Our brains have the beautiful capacity to remodel themselves over time, called *neuroplasticity*. This ability means that practicing relaxation techniques helps us relax more and more over time.

Neuroscientists like to say "neurons that wire together fire together." You know this in your own life as the ability to quickly learn lyrics to a catchy, upbeat song after hearing it on the radio a few times a day for a week. The same is true with relaxation techniques. The brain-body connection is strong, and attending to a mind-body practice can change your brain and body to react more calmly over time. It's important to engage in regular practice. Just like you don't go to the gym one time to do biceps curls and expect completely toned muscles, the relaxation response requires gentle attention each day to allow you a better and better response. Sometimes it's hard to be patient, but you've chosen to read this book because you value a nonpharmaceutical approach.

I imagine mind-body modalities along a spectrum. At one end are the more pure forms of meditation like mindfulness, where you focus on the breath and allow thoughts to come and go without attachment or judgment. At the other end are purely religious forms, like praying or attending a service. Scattered across the middle are the blended types of meditation, like guided meditations that gently relax the body or use imagery to help people find their happy place. Another broad type of mind-body medicine is movement-based meditations like tai chi, qi gong, and yoga. Whatever type you choose to do is perfectly fine–I just want you to do it. Make some space in your life for amazing things to happen.

HOW TO START PAYING ATTENTION TO YOUR SPIRITUAL SELF (OR GIVE MEDITATION THE GOOD OLD COLLEGE TRY)

Starting a meditation practice can feel overwhelming, so I teach my patients some simple breathing exercises along with what I call "Meditation for the Busy Person." My advice is to begin with a guided muscle relaxation that takes five to ten minutes each day. Many free meditations exist–I have some on my website, www.DrKatie.com–so I encourage you to try a few different kinds to see what kind appeals to you.

I advise all patients to give meditation "the good old college try." You need to do it almost daily for two or three weeks before making up your mind about its effect on your life. I encourage you to choose any form of meditation that feels good to you. Try your hand at various breathing exercises, progressive muscle relaxation, guided imagery, or even a movement-based meditation. At the same time, start to tune into your *Wellness Intuition*. Look at all areas of your life–your sleep, concentration, energy, and irritability–and determine if you're a little better off than before. But cut yourself some slack and know that it could take longer to get into a mindful state that requires constant grace to welcome back the busy brain.

I started meditating when my children were about five months old and we were sleep training. Since I was no longer utterly exhausted, if my boys woke me up, I found I was having trouble reinitiating sleep. I began with a relaxing form of breathwork called the 4-7-8 breath and added in some gentle muscle relaxation. Over the course of several months, I trained my monkey mind to calm itself so that I could fall back asleep. Although my sleep meditation techniques are generally effective, they don't work every time, but using them is certainly better than the alternative of lying awake worrying about being tired tomorrow.

I've also had times in my life when a religious meditation felt more appropriate. When pregnant with my boys, I felt a deep need to thank God and wanted to honor that gratitude by attending church. If prayer or religious services speak to you, then attend to your Spiritual Self with those modalities.

These days, I find myself doing more yoga, but yoga didn't come easily to me at first. I tried yoga classes for a whole year before I understood the concept of savasana. Savasana is the pose generally taken at the end of a yoga class where you lie flat on your mat and soak in all the goodness of your practice. At first, I thought savasana was a waste of time and only suitable for making a to-do list for the rest of the day, but now it's my favorite pose. I love knowing that my only purpose in those minutes is to lie on my mat and relax. That's bliss!

I've found that doing yoga three times a week is my personal sweet spot, but I encourage everyone to make space for it at least once a week. While focusing on my breath and movements during yoga, I can more easily let go of my busy brain and connect to my Spiritual Self, and I feel nourished. I have my most positive body image while doing yoga because I realize how strong and beautiful I inherently am. But yoga is not for everyone. The great thing about mind-body modalities is there are so many different ones to try.

MINDFULNESS & THE DEFAULT MODE NETWORK

Remember how I suggested that not all rest comes in the form of sleep? Mindfulness meditation is active rest where you pay attention to your thoughts and feelings and accept them without judgment, without believing there's a right or wrong way to think or feel. It can be enjoyed at any time of the day, in any position, while doing almost anything. During mindfulness, you let go of ruminating over the past or worrying about the future by staying in the present moment. Mindfulness has been studied extensively, and the outcomes show benefits to a multitude of conditions, from acute and chronic pain management to mental health of expectant mothers.[7]

Why should we practice mindfulness or meditation in general? Because it gets us out of the nonhelpful daydreaming brain called the Default Mode Network (DMN). The DMN is the background story, the scenarios that the brain makes up while it's not actively engaged. It's the unhelpful rumination about the past and worry about the future that we all find ourselves doing constantly. It's estimated that we spend *at least half* of our waking moments in our heads, not engaged in the present moment, spinning stories about our reality that may or may not be true.

---

[7] A. Shires, L. Sharpe, J. Davies, and T. Newton-John, "The efficacy of mindfulness-based interventions in acute pain: a systematic review and meta-analysis," *PAIN* 161, no. 8 (2020): 1698–707; Z. Shi and A. MacBeth, "The effectiveness of mindfulness-based interventions on maternal perinatal mental health outcomes: a systematic review," *Mindfulness* 8, no. 4 (2017): 823–47.

And studies show that the more time we spend in the wandering brain, the less happy we are.[8] Mindfulness meditation has been associated with reducing activity in the DMN.[9] It's a way to short-circuit the brain into experiencing more joy.

You can certainly practice mindfulness while in a stationary position. It would be ideal to have a few short breaks during your day when you could sit down, close your eyes, and come back to your breath, allowing the many thoughts that enter your mind to remain unjudged and float away on a balloon or cloud, knowing that you can come back to them later.

You can extend mindfulness into all parts of your day with a little awareness. When was the last time you put on your shoes and truly focused on how your foot slides into the shoe and how you tie the laces? Or chopped vegetables in preparation for dinner and focused on the act of chopping? Um, never.

If you're like me, while you put on your shoes, you have a trillion thoughts about everything you need to accomplish after you walk out the door, along with a healthy dose of worry about how to get it all done combined with rumination about how a past project didn't go so well because of *x*, *y*, or *z*.

But what if you slowed down and really did one thing at a time? That's a way to find mindfulness in tiny nuggets throughout your day that doesn't require a sit-down practice. It's impossible to say what effect this could have on your physical, mental, emotional, and spiritual health, but I would bet my life on it being positive.

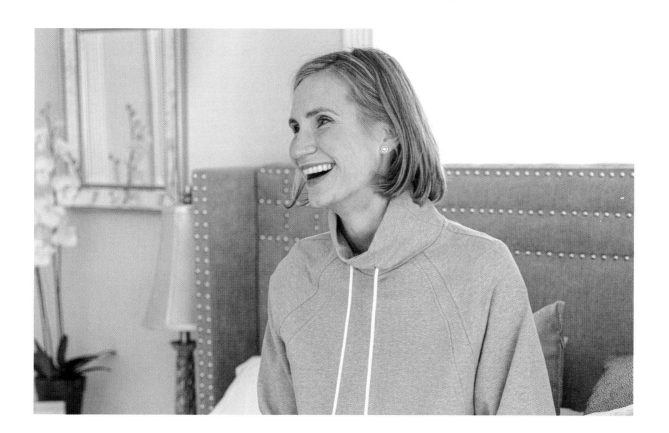

[8] H. Zhou, X. Chen, Y. Shen, et al., "Rumination and the default mode network: Meta-analysis of brain imaging studies and implications for depression," *NeuroImage* 206, no. 1 (2020): 116287.

[9] K. A. Garrison, T. A. Zeffiro, D. Scheinost, et al., "Meditation leads to reduced default mode network activity beyond an active task," *Cognitive, Affective & Behavioral Neuroscience* 15, no. 3 (2015): 712–20.

Above all else, when it comes to nourishing your Spiritual Self, the most important part is to do things that bring you joy.

Joy is not the same as happiness. Happiness is an intense emotion that is brought on by external triggers and tends to be rather fleeting. We feel like we're on the top of the world, but that feeling isn't sustained because we feel it due to circumstantial and temporary situations that are outside of ourselves.

Joy is different. Joy is an internally cultivated feeling of contentment that's relatively consistent, despite what's happening around you. It comes when you make peace with yourself and have a strong connection to your Spiritual Self, an enduring feeling that persists despite frustration and challenges. Joy is a choice to fuel yourself with satisfying relationships, make space in your life to take care of yourself, recognize gratitude, forgiveness, generosity, and acceptance, and belly laugh from time to time.

My hope is that you'll nourish your Spiritual Self by discovering your internal joy.

MEANINGFUL CHANGE

There are many entries into living a full, authentic life, and this chapter was a quick primer on how to build fertile soil with meaningful lifestyle choices in addition to eating a nutrient-dense, plant-forward, anti-inflammatory diet. Obviously, none of these interventions is a silver bullet. Understand, however, that the tiny changes you make to move your body more joyfully, prioritize rest, and connect to the real You is a pathway to bringing about meaningful change.

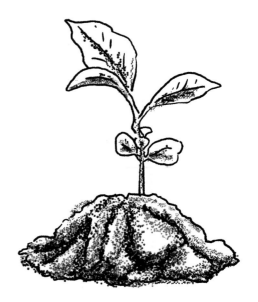

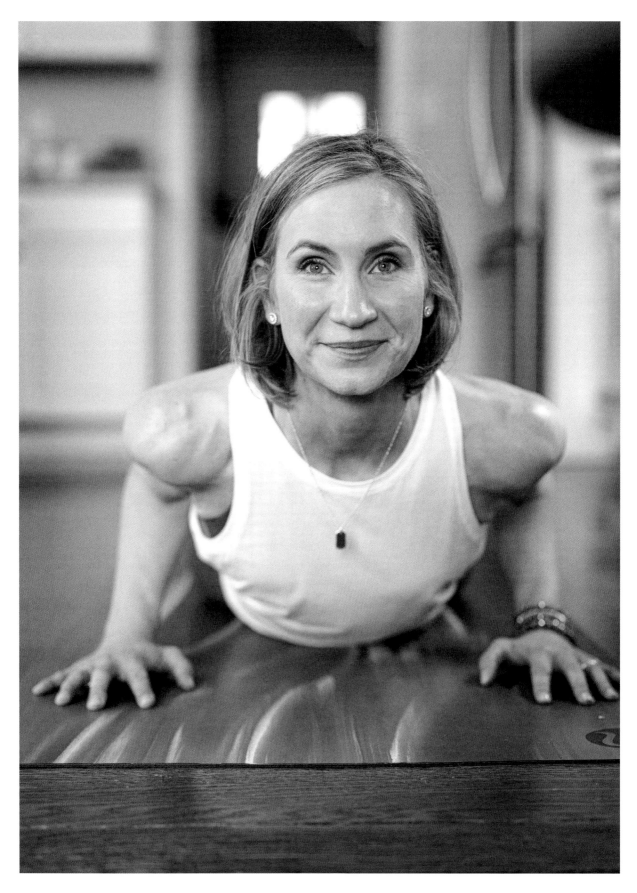

CHAPTER 9

ESSENTIAL SUPPLEMENTS FOR A PLANT-FORWARD LIFE

One of my favorite things to tell my patients is that we can't supplement our way to good health. Supplements are, after all, supplemental. Nature has a way of creating wholesome beauty for our plates that we couldn't possibly replicate in pill or powder form. That said, there are a few high-yield vitamin and supplement pearls that you can include as part of your daily regimen to ensure you're getting what you need if you're following a plant-forward lifestyle.

I could write a whole book about vitamins, minerals, and supplements. There's so much to say! All vitamins and minerals are important. You need iodine and selenium for thyroid health. You need calcium to build bones and keep your heart beating rhythmically. You need iron to make hemoglobin so that your red blood cells can efficiently carry oxygen to your tissues and organs. This chapter is not meant to suggest that these essential nutrients are not good in supplement form, because they may be—*for you.* It's so important to tap into your *Wellness Intuition* and evaluate your daily choices in order to figure out which vitamins and supplements may work in your life. In general, if you follow the advice I give in this book, you're likely to pick up these crucial nutrients from food and may not need to supplement. As we all know, food-based nutrition is the best possible source for fueling our bodies, but talking to your personal physician is always a good move before making changes.

So let's talk supplements!

MAGNESIUM

Magnesium might be my favorite supplement. I just love how versatile it is. Magnesium is helpful for a variety of conditions, including sleep problems, headaches, menstrual cramps, restless legs, muscle achiness and cramps, constipation, and general anxiety or stress. Magnesium allows the nervous system to relax, which is quite helpful right before sleep, and many women tend to be a bit magnesium deficient relative to men.

Why does supplemental magnesium solve so many different problems? It's because magnesium is so universally useful in the body. In fact, it's a cofactor involved in the activation of over 300 enzymes and required to make adenosine triphosphate (ATP), the body's main energy source. We need magnesium for the health and function of virtually every tissue and organ, from the brain to the heart to the bones to our endocrine glands for hormone production.

Magnesium is available in the diet in the form of leafy greens (another reason to eat kale!), nuts, seeds, chocolate, avocados, legumes, and tofu.

Supplementing with magnesium can be tricky, as the type of magnesium salt a supplement contains can change its effects on the body, specifically in the digestive system.

If you tend toward constipation, then a bit of magnesium citrate or oxide can be helpful; otherwise, choose magnesium glycinate or another chelated magnesium. Doses of approximately 400 milligrams at night are standard, but I've seen higher dosing as long as serum RBC magnesium level is normal. Magnesium and omega-3 fatty acids are two of the few supplements safe for pregnant and lactating women. You can also consider massaging magnesium oil or cream into your skin or bathing in magnesium salts (like Epsom salts) for alternative forms of absorption.

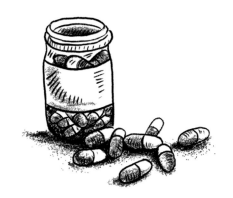

OMEGA-3 FATTY ACIDS

Omega-3 fats are another essential nutrient that's hard to get in the diet unless you're eating a regular amount of cold-water fatty fish like wild salmon, black cod, halibut, herring, sardines, tuna, and mackerel. You can also find omega-3 fatty acids in plant sources like flax seeds, chia seeds, and walnuts, but the conversion rate of alpha linolenic acid (ALA) to the usable EPA (eicosapentaenoic acid) and DHA (docosahexaenoic acid) is poor and not as bioavailable.

We see a positive effect in the body with just a modest amount of omega-3 fats in the diet. Just one or two 3½-ounce servings of wild fatty cold-water fish is enough to have a positive impact and is generally equivalent to taking a daily fish oil supplement. If you're not eating 3½ ounces of fatty cold-water fish at least once weekly, I recommend supplementation. As you may remember from Chapter 6, my lovely patient Diane had some major neurological symptoms from being omega-3 deficient because this compound is critical to the body's optimal function.

Unfortunately, the typical American diet leads to an imbalance of anti-inflammatory omega-3 and inflammatory omega-6 fats due to our unhealthy consumption of processed foods and oils like vegetable, corn, and soybean oil. But Diane's story suggests that even a healthy eater can struggle with omega-3 consumption, especially if one is following a plant-forward or completely vegan lifestyle.

Like vitamin D_3, omega-3 supplements should be taken with a meal that contains fat. I recommend taking them with dinner. I find that omega-3 supplements help me sleep better, and evidence shows that omega-3 supplementation may improve sleep, especially in children.[1] And when kids sleep better, adults sleep better, too. I also recommend omega-3 supplementation to pregnant and nursing women who cannot make cold-water fish a regular part of their diet because these fats are crucial for baby brain development.

I generally recommend that adults get 1,000 to 1,200 milligrams of a combination of EPA and DHA per day. Children need less omega-3 fats than adults because they are physically smaller.

Unfortunately, fish oil supplements don't taste very good when chewed and can give us a little "fish burp" reflux even if we swallow the whole gel capsule. Taking fish oil with a meal or storing the bottle in the freezer can alleviate this problem. I've bargained with my boys to eat wild fish twice weekly in exchange for not making them chew omega-3 supplements. Maybe you can convince your youngsters to do the same!

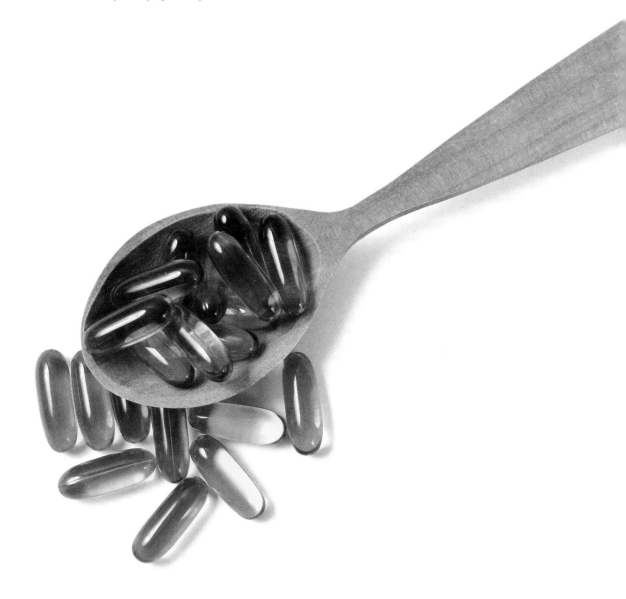

[1] P. Montgomery, J. R. Burton, R. P. Sewell, et al., "Fatty acids and sleep in UK children: subjective and pilot objective sleep results from the DOLAB study—a randomized controlled trial," *Journal of Sleep Research* 23, no. 4 (2014): 364–88.

VITAMIN B$_{12}$

You need vitamin B$_{12}$ in your diet to support your nervous system and make efficient red blood cells, and only a few plant foods naturally have B$_{12}$ in them, like seaweed, mushrooms, and nutritional yeast. Animals naturally make B$_{12}$ in their gut by way of the anaerobic bacteria that make up their microbiome, so if we eat animal protein, we naturally get some vitamin B$_{12}$. But absorption of B$_{12}$ is a complicated process based on age, robust stomach acid, medication use, and damage to the gut's integrity from disease or prior surgery, so it's not as simple as eating some animal protein.[2]

Not everyone needs to supplement with vitamin B$_{12}$. It's best to talk with your doctor and have your level tested so that you know how much to take. The lab reference range for B$_{12}$ is huge, usually from about 250 to 900 pg/ml. You want to have a level somewhere in the upper middle of that range.

Most vitamin B$_{12}$ supplements are whopper doses, so you can pretty easily oversupplement if you're not careful. The best way to take a B$_{12}$ supplement is under the tongue, usually in the form of a sublingual lozenge, so that it bypasses metabolism by the liver and gets straight into the bloodstream. Vitamin B$_{12}$ is also available by intramuscular injection, but studies show that sublingual dosing is effective, too, and it's a whole lot more comfortable. I find vitamin B$_{12}$ energizing, so I recommend taking it earlier in the day. If you're not deficient and just trying to improve your B$_{12}$ level, taking 1,000 mcg a few times per week can work wonders.

Due to genetic variations, some of us benefit from taking a special kind of B vitamin supplement. If you read your vitamin label, you'll see that both B$_{12}$ and its cousin folate can be *methylated*. Genetic variations like the MTHFR mutation that lead to methylation problems are getting a lot of press these days due to our expanding knowledge that inability to methylate properly can prevent absorption of B$_{12}$ and folate. Vitamins B$_{12}$ and folate are critical for the production of energy in the mitochondria; they are also linked to anxiety and depression because they are crucial to the building blocks of serotonin and other neurotransmitters.[3] Of late, you can easily get sophisticated tests done with your Integrative Medicine doctor to show a variety of genetic variations called single nucleotide polymorphisms (SNPs). An MTHFR mutation is just one of the many SNPs you could test for. Another option is to have your Integrative doctor order a homocysteine level. Homocysteine—an inflammatory marker—builds up in the body when the body doesn't have enough of its methylated vitamin cofactors.

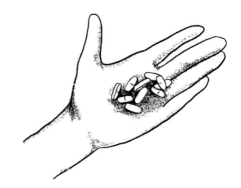

[2] R. Obeid, S. G. Heil, M. Verhoeven, et al., "Vitamin B$_{12}$ intake from animal foods, biomarkers, and health aspects," *Frontiers in Nutrition* 6 (2019): 93.

[3] O. P. Almeida, L. Flicker, N. T. Lautenschlager, et al., "Contribution of the MTHFR gene to the causal pathway for depression, anxiety and cognitive impairment in later life," *Neurobiology of Aging* 26, no. 2 (2005): 251–7.

VITAMIN D

Vitamin D is so hard to get in the diet that almost everyone needs to supplement, even if you eat animal products (which is where vitamin D is almost exclusively found). I see lower-than-recommended vitamin D levels in almost every patient who is not taking a vitamin D supplement. Poor vitamin D levels are associated with all kinds of health issues, including heart disease, cognitive impairment, asthma, cancer, insulin resistance and blood sugar control, and the bone-softening condition called rickets.

Vitamin D levels are almost universally a problem because the best way to get vitamin D is to step outside, and most of us do not spend as much time outdoors soaking up the sun as we should. As discussed in Chapter 2, vitamin D is naturally created in our bodies when we expose ourselves to sunlight, and the best way to increase vitamin D levels is to expose a good amount of skin to the sun for at least twenty minutes every day. This is virtually impossible for most of us to do in the cooler months unless we want to freeze to the bone.

It's important to get vitamin D in our bodies because it is crucial to the absorption of other important nutrients, like calcium, iron, magnesium, phosphorus, and zinc, through the gut. Vitamin D is not really a vitamin but a prohormone, which is a precursor to the synthesis of other hormones.

Vitamin D is found naturally in foods like the oily fish mackerel, sardines, herring, and salmon, as well as egg yolks, red meat, liver, and porcini mushrooms. It's also added to a lot of foods, like milk (hence the reason your low-fat milk carton says "vitamin A & D fortified") to help the general public get more of this essential nutrient.

My advice is to ask your doctor to check your vitamin D25-OH level first so that you know what your level is. (Vitamin D25-OH is the standard test we use, but other vitamin D tests exist that are useful in other areas of medicine.) This level will help you decide how much to take on a daily basis. The consensus on vitamin D25-OH levels varies; I like to see my patients with D25-OH levels between 40 and 70 ng/ml, though 30 ng/ml is technically the cutoff for deficiency. Recognize that these numbers are subject to change over time, but this is the most accurate way to view vitamin D25-OH levels in my opinion given the current knowledge.

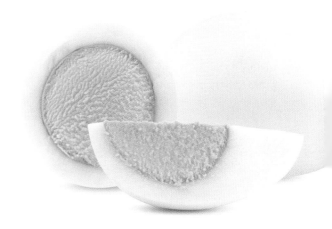

"**Vitamin D** is *crucial to the absorption* of other important nutrients, like calcium, iron, magnesium, phosphorus, and zinc, through the gut."

Vitamin D25-OH Levels

<30 ng/mL	Deficient
30–40 ng/mL	Insufficient
40–70 ng/mL	Optimal
>70 ng/mL	By recommendation of your doctor for specific conditions

I recommend that you take a vitamin D_3 supplement throughout the year. Unless you're deficient (in which case you'd need more), most people do well with about 1,000 IU per day. D_3 is available over the counter and is more bio-available than D2, which means you get more bang for your buck in terms of absorption and usability in the body. (Interestingly, vitamin D2 is prescription vitamin D and is the way doctors generally replete low vitamin D25-OH levels in patients.) Vitamin D_3 is a fat-soluble vitamin, so it needs to be taken alongside a meal with fat in it. Since you're hip to eating fat at every meal, it shouldn't matter too much what meal you take your vitamin D_3 with. You can support your vitamin D supplementation with exposure to sunshine and eating cold-water fish like salmon once or twice a week.

You may see vitamin D in combination supplements with calcium and vitamin K_2 (usually as menaquinone-7, or MK-7). Vitamin D ensures that calcium is absorbed in the gut, and K_2 ensures that calcium is easily integrated into the bone matrix.[4] Calcium cannot be utilized effectively without D_3 and K_2. Vitamin K_2 additionally prevents the progression of arterial calcification and supports proper blood clotting. A combination of calcium, D_3, and K_2 may work for you, so it's an option to discuss with your Integrative doctor. Vitamin K_2 is naturally made by the intestinal microbiome, which gives us another reason to eat a fiber-rich diet so that we can keep our probiotics happy.

Note: If you have active cancer, inflammatory bowel disease, hyperparathyroidism, or granulomatous disease like sarcoidosis, you may not be able to supplement with vitamin D_3 due to risk of high calcium levels. As with every recommendation in this book, it's important to tailor your vitamin D_3 intake to your individual constitution.

---

[4] A. J. van Ballegooijen, S. Pilz, A. Tomaschitz, et al., "The synergistic interplay between vitamins D and K for bone and cardiovascular health: a narrative review," *International Journal of Endocrinology* 2017: 7454376.

ABSORPTION
OF SUPPLEMENTS

As you know, supplements are just the icing on the cake of what you should mostly be able to accomplish with mindful dietary choices. If you need to supplement, please do. But be aware of your levels so that you can keep track of whether you are actually absorbing what you're taking. If your levels don't improve with supplementation, then taking more could be useful. Even better, have a conversation with your doctor about how to enhance your absorption. You could have an underlying problem with your digestion and absorption that needs to be addressed.

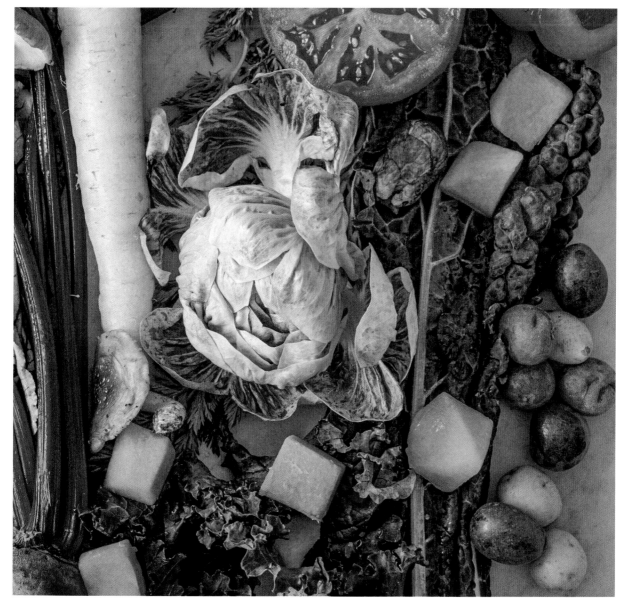

CHAPTER 10

DR. KATIE'S LIFE KITCHEN

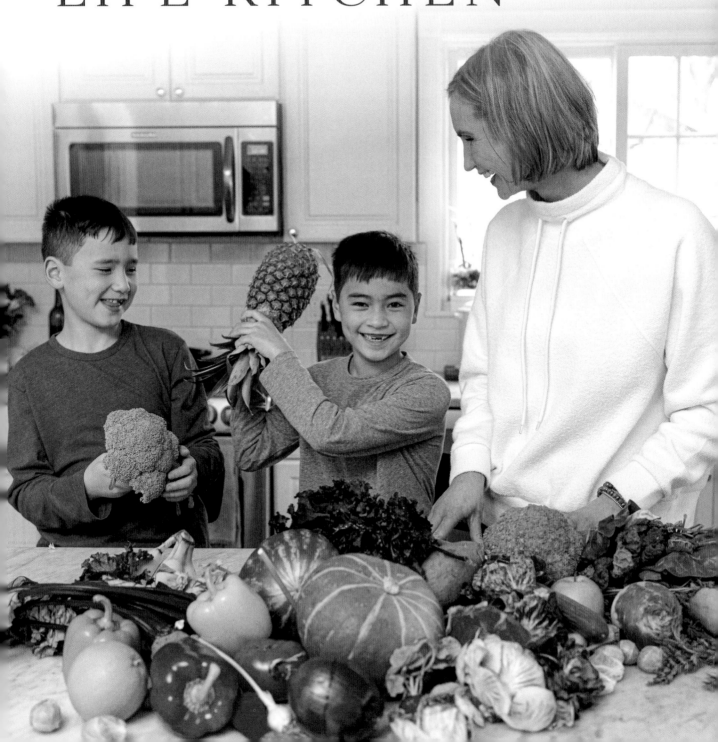

This chapter dives into what I call "Dr. Katie's Life Kitchen." Why "Life Kitchen"? Because I incorporate all of life into the way that I cook. At its best, cooking should be joyful and fun, inspirational and delicious. But it's also important that it's practical. It doesn't feel good to walk away from an afternoon in the kitchen with nothing more than a measly platter of green beans, no matter how many steps or spices went into making them. I want to see results from my efforts, so I choose and design recipes to make sure of that.

Interestingly, the Sanskrit word *Hridayam*—which translates to "that which nourishes and heals the heart" and "the heart of your home"—is also used to describe the kitchen. As you can tell from this book, I think the expression of full health and healing starts with the way we take care of our bodies, which is centered around nourishing food.

I'll start with some life hacks for managing kitchen basics, then talk about stocking your refrigerator and pantry and useful tools for plant-forward cooking. I'll also address concerns about digestion and food aversions.

COOKING AT HOME

Cooking at home is vital to a healthy lifestyle because it gives you control over the ingredients you use and, ultimately, how you fuel your body.

I recognize that home cooking is not the most convenient, so I recommend batch cooking (accompanied by leftovers!) and allowing yourself some grace along the way. After all, we aren't born great cooks. I personally discovered my skill—and my passion—for cooking in my mid-thirties as I began to experiment more and get more comfortable. I also have some hacks for adapting your existing repertoire of favorites. Let's start by exploring a few core concepts of *Dr. Katie's Life Kitchen*.

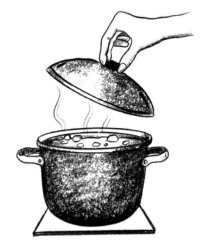

INGREDIENT CONTROL

The number one reason to create food in your own kitchen is ingredient control. Ingredient control is simply the idea that when you're in charge of what goes into your food, you tend to make better decisions than someone would make for you. I always say there's a reason the salad or soup from your favorite corner spot tastes different or better than the one you create at home. It's because they're adding things to your food that you don't normally add–namely extra salt, fat, or sugar. Not-so-great ingredient control can also occur in our own kitchens when we're cooking for someone not in our immediate family and we want our dish to taste *extra* delicious. If you're like me, you're tempted to throw in an extra smidgen of salt or an extra tablespoon of maple syrup to ensure your guests really like your cooking. Believe me, most food preparation businesses are doing the same thing, but we're not just talking about an extra pat of butter.

WEEKEND BATCH COOKING

I do most of my cooking on the weekends because that's when I have the most time. It's hard for me to come home after a big day and spend an hour in the kitchen, though I recognize that for others such time might be stress-relieving and energetically pleasing. My husband and I generally cook enough on the weekends that we have enough leftovers to get us to midweek. I also enlist my wonderful nanny, Angie, to roast multiple trays of vegetables and prepare several cups of whole grains for us while she's here during the week so that we can always piece together a healthy hodgepodge of fiber, fat, and protein if my Sunday soup doesn't last as long as I thought it would.

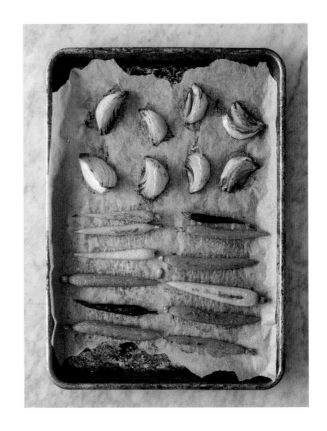

PRACTICE, PRACTICE, PRACTICE

I wish I could offer a big shortcut around the elbow grease needed to cook, but it doesn't exist. What I can offer you are some small shortcuts in the form of batch cooking meals that serve more than two people and make for good leftovers, along with some tricks and tools that will enhance your efficiency.

But do you know what enhances your efficiency the most? Practice. So roll up your sleeves and practice cooking. Practice is how I became a good cook, a good doctor, and a good mom. Thankfully, we have the rest of our lives to continue practicing.

"Do you know what enhances your efficiency the most? **Practice.** *So roll up your sleeves and* **practice cooking.** *Practice is how I became a good cook, a good doctor, and a good mom. Thankfully, we have the rest of our lives to continue practicing."*

DR. KATIE'S HACKS FOR MAKING RECIPES HEALTHIER & MORE PLANT-FORWARD

If you're cooking from someone else's recipes or you want to adjust some of your family favorites, a few simple Dr. Katie hacks can make almost any recipe a bit healthier and more plant-forward. Try the following:

- Multiply the vegetables in the recipe by two or three times and incorporate more staple vegetables like carrots, celery, and onions (which you are likely to have on hand).

- Choose a leaner cut of organic animal protein when possible (for example, sirloin steak instead of rib-eye or pork loin instead of pork chop).

- If the recipe calls for a heavy dressing or sauce, decrease the fat by one-third.

- Decrease all sugar by one-third to one-half (or more), including natural sweeteners like maple syrup or honey.

- Substitute plain full-fat Greek yogurt or coconut yogurt for sour cream and plain kefir for buttermilk.

- Cook or garnish with nutritional yeast instead of a sprinkle of cheese.

- Double the garlic and increase the herbs and spices to taste.

- If you are sautéing vegetables and the pan starts to look a little dry, add 1 to 3 teaspoons of water or broth before adding more cooking fat.

STOCKING YOUR KITCHEN FOR PLANT-FORWARD COOKING

The biggest obstacle to eating nourishing food is a poorly stocked kitchen. You need to stock your kitchen with ingredients, but you also need a few well-placed tools. Let's talk about the food first.

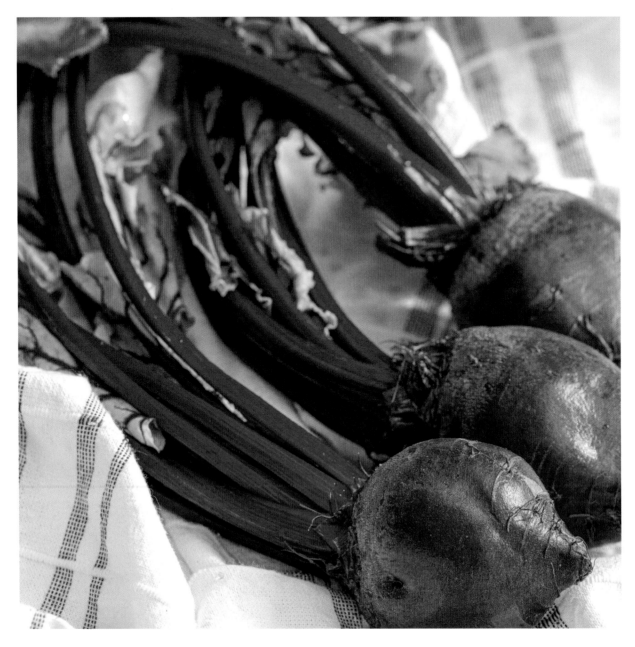

BUYING ORGANIC

If you can afford it, organic food generally tastes better and is better for you because it decreases your exposure to pesticides. And avoiding pesticides is always a good move. Many of the chemicals used to kill off harmful pests and prevent bothersome weeds are potentially harmful substances that disrupt the body's normal functions and may lead to conditions like infertility, neurological compromise, cancer, and respiratory problems.

It's hard to grow plants without the use of pesticides. I would know. I've been trying my hand at an organic vegetable garden for several summers, and each year I get frustrated with some bug or animal that decides to munch on my prized possessions.

But eating organic is expensive, which can make it prohibitive for many people. The question my patients always ask is whether eating organic is really worth it. The answer is that it depends.

USE THE DIRTY DOZEN & THE CLEAN FIFTEEN

The Environmental Working Group (EWG) is a tremendous resource with free information that will allow you to do a deeper dive into the world of organic food if you'd like. The EWG puts out a list every year called the Dirty Dozen, which are the twelve most pesticide-laden vegetables and fruits. If budget is a big concern, then I recommend you prioritize buying these organically. The EWG also publishes the Clean Fifteen, which is a list of the conventionally grown vegetables and fruits you can buy with the least pesticide residue. These lists will get you started in the world of buying organic.

At my house, the general rule is that we buy organic if we eat the peel, and we buy conventional if we don't eat the peel. Thus, we almost always buy organic apples and strawberries, but we don't always buy organic bananas or avocados.

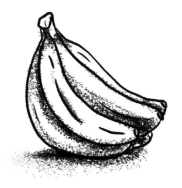

EAT THE PEEL

I love eating the peels of my produce when possible. This saves me tremendous time in the kitchen and increases the fiber content of my food.

I started experimenting with not peeling vegetables and fruits a few years ago when a patient told me she ate kiwi with the peel on in an effort to increase her fiber intake after she was diagnosed with celiac disease and could no longer eat the gluten-containing whole grains to which her smooth digestion was accustomed. I was bewildered at the thought of eating a whole kiwi, skin and all. Didn't the peel taste fuzzy in her mouth? She said she got used to it after a few times and now kind of liked it. So I tried it. She was right—the first few times it was a bit strange, but then I got used to it. Now I almost never peel kiwis because it saves me time and gives me added dietary fiber.

I generally recommend keeping the peel on most produce if you can. The only things I peel before eating these days are fruits like oranges and mangoes and hard exterior shells like those found on butternut or spaghetti squash. The smaller squashes generally have more delicate skin that softens right up when roasted. I never peel eggplants, carrots, potatoes, or other root vegetables.

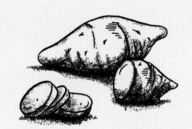

ALWAYS BUY ORGANIC WHOLE SOY & ANIMAL PRODUCTS

I recommend two groups of food that should be prioritized as organic if possible: whole soy and animal products. You'll notice in my recipes that I don't specify organic except in these two circumstances.

When buying whole soy products like tofu, tempeh, edamame, and soy milk, always buy organic. You don't want genetically modified organisms (GMOs) in your body. You also want to avoid GMO soy because it may be less nutrient-dense and contain more herbicide residue than organic soy.

Organic, grass-fed, pasture-raised, antibiotic-free animal products are worth the extra cost. After all, we eat what they've eaten, and it makes no sense to buy organic spinach and then skimp on the animal protein. You want to stay away from less-expensive meats from factory-farmed animals because they generally eat mass-produced, genetically modified grains treated with pesticides and are given hormones and antibiotics, all in an effort to fatten them up quickly and inexpensively. We don't want those dangerous compounds in our bodies.

FRESH OR FROZEN?

Frozen vegetables and fruits are totally fine in my book. They make life easy because they are available at all times of the year, keep for months, and are sometimes less expensive than fresh. And, to boot, they are more nutritious than their nonfrozen counterparts because they are flash frozen right after picking, thus locking in their gorgeous phytonutrients, vitamins, and minerals, which prevents them from degrading over time on a store shelf.

Shockingly, fresh produce is sometimes months old by the time it makes it to the produce aisle. For example, apples can remain "fresh" for up to ten months in a temperature-controlled facility with the help of the gaseous compound 1-methylcyclopropene, which blocks ethylene gas and thus prevents ripening.[1] Ever notice that apples picked fresh off the tree taste so much better than the ones in the store? Buying fresh produce straight from a farmer is an even better way to know that it's just left the earth.

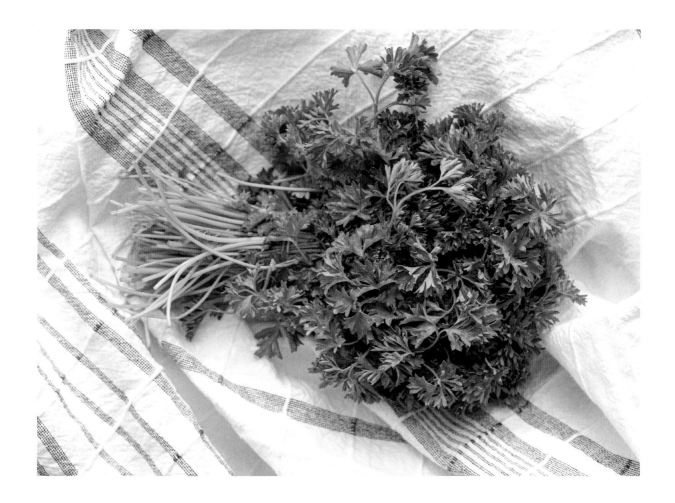

---

[1] A. Dubin and C. Serico, "That apple you just bought might be a year old—but does it matter?" *TODAY*, October 13, 2014, https://www.today.com/food/apple-you-just-bought-might-be-year-old-does-it-2D80207170.

DR. KATIE'S KITCHEN PHARMACY: STAPLES FOR PLANT-FORWARD COOKING

As plant-forward cooking becomes more mainstream, ingredients like quinoa and ground flax seeds are becoming easier to find. Many of the ingredients in my recipes will be familiar to you if you've already been exploring what cooking with more plants looks like.

I'll review some of the most important pearls for your refrigerator and pantry shelves. Many of these foods are covered in other parts of the book as well, especially in Chapter 5 and in the recipe notes. Here we go!

ARROWROOT FLOUR

Throw out your cornstarch and pick up this thickening agent made from a root vegetable. The next time you want to thicken a sauce, whisk in 1 to 3 teaspoons of arrowroot.

AVOCADOS

This humble fruit is a superfood for sure. It's rich in anti-inflammatory monounsaturated fatty acids and provides a clean creaminess to any dish, from breakfast to dessert. I buy avocados at different levels of firmness so that I have about one ripe avocado every two days. You know an avocado is ready to be used when its flesh yields slightly to the gentle pressure of your thumb.

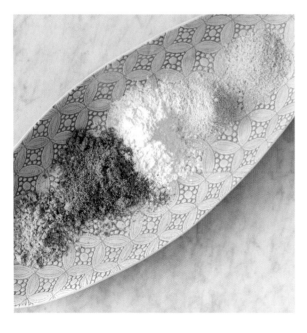

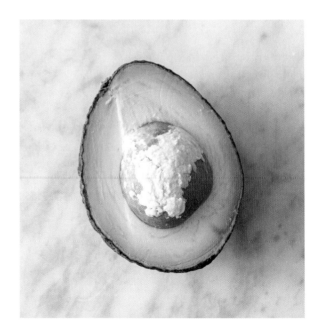

BEANS & LEGUMES

The heart of plant-forward protein is beans and legumes. While it might be less expensive to buy dried beans and cook them yourself, I definitely push the easy button when it comes to canned beans and prioritize spending more on a brand that's pressure-cooked with kombu to ease digestion. If I'm short on time and need a quick protein for a salad, I often just sauté rinsed canned beans in olive oil with some simple spices until they're golden brown. It's a family favorite and takes about five minutes. If I have time, I'll sprout dried beans and lentils on my countertop before using them in recipes. (See page 220 for more on sprouting.)

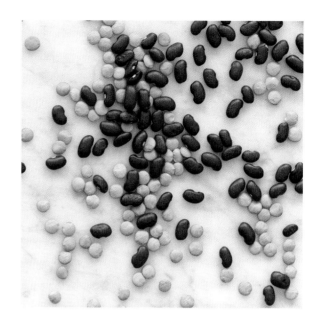

BREAD & CRACKERS

Bread is not evil. In fact, it's delicious and can even be nutritious, as is the case with my Whole-Grain Nut & Seed Bread (page 294). If you want something less dense and more like traditional bread, head to a local sourdough bakery. Instead of yeast, sourdough uses the magic of microbial fermentation to make the bread rise. This fermentation naturally breaks down some of the gluten, making it easier to digest for many people who are sensitive to wheat and gluten. Truly fresh bread is good for only a few days, so slice off what you think you may want and then freeze the rest in a zip-top bag. If you're buying a more robust bread made with heavier flour or nuts and seeds, choose the heaviest loaf.

Seed crackers are one of my favorite snacks to pair with hummus, nut butter, or salsa and work well as a crunchy side to a salad or soup. You can create your own crackers with my Whole-Grain Nut & Seed Bread or buy them. Just make sure all of the ingredients in store-bought crackers are words you recognize as real food.

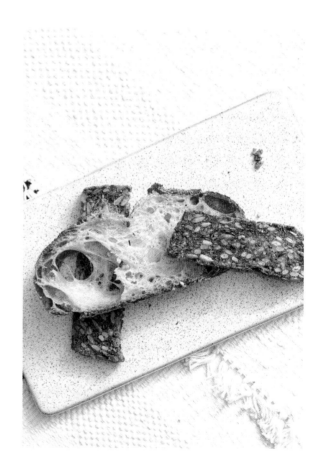

BROTH

I recommend keeping bone broth in the freezer or pantry. I generally prefer bone broth to traditional stock because of its superior flavor and nutrient density. I love to cook whole grains in this nourishing tonic; it gives whatever you put it in a deeper flavor and increases satiety due to its protein and mineral content. Bone broth is also known to support digestion and repair the intestinal wall if it's inflamed. You can make your own bone broth by putting leftover organic chicken, beef, or pork bones in a pressure cooker with water and a little apple cider vinegar. If you are vegan, you can substitute vegetable stock for bone broth in any of my recipes.

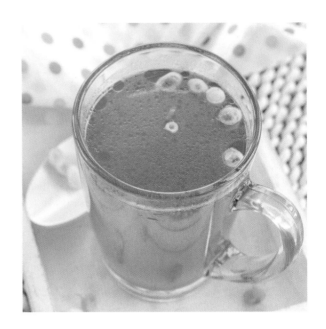

CHOCOLATE, CACAO NIBS & COCOA

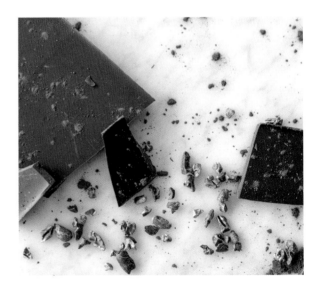

- **Chocolate:** Dark chocolate is my favorite food in the whole world. The antioxidants and flavanols in chocolate are a delicious dream of cardiovascular benefit and combine with anti-inflammatory saturated fatty acids to make for a satiating sweet. The higher the percentage of cacao, the more benefit you get without a sugar rush. My recipes call for specific percentages of dark chocolate to guide you. If you're new to the world of dark chocolate, start with a lower percentage and work your way up over time. Try to find brands without alkaloids or lecithins, which are generally added to improve flavor and texture.

- **Cacao nibs:** These little crunchy joys are small pieces of cocoa bean with a deep bitter chocolate flavor. They are low in sugar and high in fat, making them a satiating addition to a smoothie (like my Recovery Smoothie on page 248), trail mix, or dessert. Just be careful about eating them too late in the day; I find them pretty energizing.

- **Cacao powder:** I recommend choosing cacao powder over cocoa powder. Traditional Dutch-processed cocoa has a less acidic flavor profile that some people prefer, but the alkaline wash results in fewer phytonutrients.

COCONUT

I didn't like coconut as a kid, but now it's one of my favorite flavors. Its high saturated fatty acid and medium-chain triglyceride content makes it a win for keeping you satiated. I love coconut in all forms, from canned coconut milk to shredded or flaked coconut to coconut yogurt and coconut oil. The most important thing is to buy full-fat, unsweetened coconut products for two reasons: first, they taste better, and second, coconut is inherently sweet.

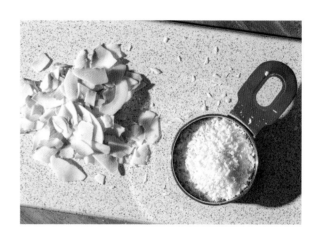

- **Canned coconut milk:** Full-fat unsweetened canned coconut milk without additives like guar gum is a great alternative to full-fat dairy, and leftover milk can be frozen in ice-cube trays or used in smoothies, sauces, soups, or desserts.

- **Canned coconut cream:** Full-fat unsweetened canned coconut cream is the thickest part of canned coconut milk. It generally comes in smaller cans, which are useful when you want more concentrated fat and flavor or to dollop on desserts or fruit—or you can make your own by following my Coconut Whipped Cream recipe (page 334).

- **Shredded coconut:** I prefer unsweetened shredded coconut to coconut flakes for the recipes in this book, but I keep both types in my kitchen. Coconut flakes are yummy for a snack or when you want some texture, but I find shredded coconut works better in granola, baking, and cooking.

- **Coconut yogurt:** Full-fat unsweetened coconut yogurt is one of my favorite foods. It's versatile, from being a creamy base for dairy-free dips to an alternative to sour cream in recipes to being a dessert topped with fresh berries. My favorite way to enjoy it is topped with granola and chopped Black Mission figs in the morning. Coconut yogurt naturally separates, so I store mine upside down in the fridge until first use to encourage mixing. (I store my nut butters upside down too for the same reason.) If you have leftover yogurt that is too watery, add a tablespoon of chia seeds and refrigerate overnight to make a thicker, fiber-rich yogurt for the following day.

- **Coconut oil:** When buying coconut oil, I recommend organic, cold-pressed, virgin oil. Unrefined coconut oil has a lower smoke point than refined, so if you notice that your pan is smoking, throw the oil away and start over. And if you spill some, just use it as a natural moisturizer for your hands. (You can channel your inner Dr. Katie at the same time by closing your eyes and picturing a tropical beach while finding a mindful moment.) Coconut oil is white and hard at cooler temperatures and clear and liquidy at higher temperatures, and you'll notice it changes over the seasons. If it's too hard to scoop out, you can warm the jar gently in a hot water bath in your sink.

- **Coconut butter:** There's a reason coconut butter is called coconut manna: it's truly heavenly. I find a few teaspoons of coconut butter with some green tea before a morning strength workout to be just the right amount of nutrition to power me through my planks. Coconut butter is simply dried coconut that's been blended into a paste, and it's the perfect blend of protein, fat, and fiber. Store it next to your coconut oil and use it in smoothies, stir it into hot beverages, add it to soups or stews for sweetness, top oatmeal with it, or spread it on toast.

COLLAGEN & PROTEIN POWDER

The jury was out for me on collagen until recently, but now I incorporate it into my diet a few times per week. Collagen is the most abundant protein in our bodies and the "glue" that holds the body together. It's found in blood vessels, bones, muscles, skin, tendons, and the digestive tract, giving us strength and flexibility. Collagen comes from both land and sea animals, including beef, chicken, fish, and eggshells. You'll find collagen in a generally tasteless powdered or liquid form that can easily be added to smoothies or other beverages.

I don't regularly use protein powders, but many of my patients do, so my recommendations are to use a plant-based protein like pea and make sure that it doesn't have sweeteners added to it. Protein powder should not be sweet (after all, it's ground-up protein), so be suspicious if you have one that tastes great when mixed with water or milk. You can see from the Recovery Smoothie on page 248 that I also like to use silken tofu for protein in a smoothie.

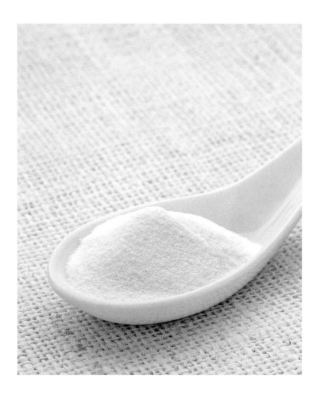

FISH SAUCE

Fish sauce, a staple in Southeast Asian cuisine, is made from fish or krill that have been coated in salt and fermented. It provides a grounding umami flavor to dishes and is used in small quantities. It has a distinct smell, so I generally don't put my nose too close to the bottle when I'm adding it to my Thai Coconut Curry Noodle Soup (page 266).

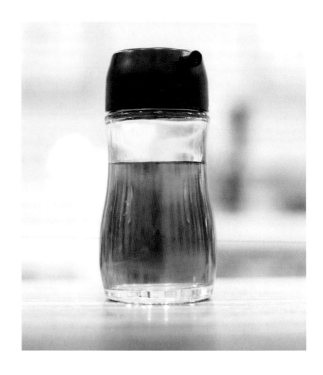

FLOUR & OTHER BAKING STAPLES

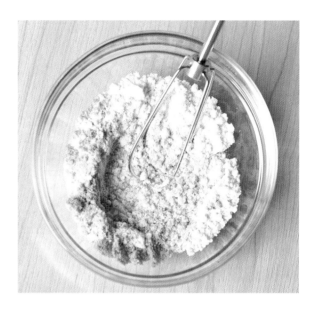

- **Flour:** I primarily use oat flour and almond meal in my gluten-free baking, mostly because they're both easy to make on the spot in a food processor because my kitchen is always stocked with rolled oats and almonds. Almond meal is particularly amazing because it is so rich in fat and protein (not to mention calcium, magnesium, and potassium) that it anchors your appetite with less volume. If you're buying almond flour, opt for unblanched natural almond flour or almond meal, which is the whole almond ground up, giving it a brown color and a coarser grind. Blanched almond flour has the fiber-rich skins removed, making it more refined and light yellow in color. I use small quantities of regular all-purpose flour, but if I want a gluten-free option, I use gluten-free 1:1 flour. I store fragile nut flours such as almond flour in the refrigerator or freezer for freshness.

- **Baking powder:** Look for a brand that's free of aluminum.

- **Chickpea crumbs:** These are a great gluten-free breadcrumb option for making homemade veggie burgers (like the Mushroom Burgers on page 276) or as a crunchy breading for roasted vegetables.

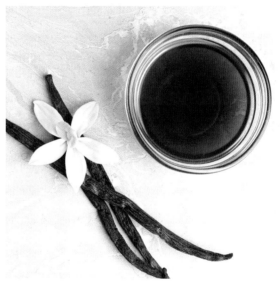

- **Vanilla extract:** I would love to cook more with whole vanilla beans because they taste so much better, but this beautiful substitute works wonders. Buy pure vanilla extract and check the label to avoid artificial flavorings.

GARLIC & ONIONS

Alliums are true workhorses in the kitchen and are part of most savory recipes for good reason. They are like fertilizer for your microbiome because they are rich in the indigestible prebiotic starches that our probiotics like to munch on.

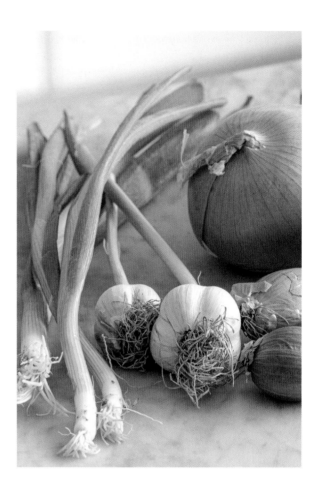

- **Garlic:** This zesty allium is anti-inflammatory, antibacterial, antiviral, immune-boosting, and cardioprotective. Within minutes of being crushed or chopped, garlic releases antiplatelet enzymes to prevent coronary artery blockages. The less you cook garlic, the better it is for you. Treat yourself and buy peeled garlic cloves to make it easier to use in the kitchen. Store peeled garlic in the refrigerator and garlic bulbs in a dark ventilated place.

- **Onions:** These nutrient-dense alliums are high in fiber, fight heart disease and cancer, and get their astringent taste from sulfur-containing compounds and flavonoids. Onions are also a source of quercetin, known for reducing bodywide inflammation, so take off only the outermost layer of onion skin before chopping. I generally use yellow onions, shallots, and green onions (also called scallions), but sometimes I like red onions or sweet Vidalia onions for color or flavor. Onions with edible green tops (like scallions, chives, and leeks) should be kept in the refrigerator, while those with papery skins should be stored in a dark ventilated place. Soaking raw chopped or sliced onion in water before using mellows out its biting flavor.

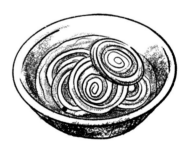

HERBS & SPICES

On a plant-forward diet, you need more flavor in your food. One of the biggest transitions I made from my Midwestern meat and potatoes diet to the way I eat now was the incorporation of more herbs and spices.

Herbs and spices not only provide a punch of flavor, but most are anti-inflammatory powerhouses due to their phytonutrient profiles. They enhance digestion and elimination, provide cardiovascular protection, police rogue cancer cells, keep blood sugar stable, fight bacteria and viruses, detoxify environmental toxins and heavy metals, and are inherently good sources of essential minerals.

- **Herbs:** Many home chefs skip the step of adding fresh herbs to their dishes, but a sprinkle of parsley or cilantro is a great move. Not only are herbs visually pleasing, they provide a bright, fresh taste. Use heartier herbs like oregano, rosemary, sage, and thyme to add depth to cooked dishes and leafy-looking herbs like basil, cilantro, dill, mint, and parsley closer to the end of cooking and as a garnish. I keep a variety of leafy herbs in the refrigerator crisper drawer at almost all times to make it easy. (I've tried to grow herbs on my deck, but no matter what organic measures I use, the squirrels and chipmunks feast on them before I have the chance.) And, sure, store-bought herbs go bad in about a week, but you deserve it. I'm a fan of dried herbs in cooking when I don't have access to fresh, with the equivalent being about 1 tablespoon of fresh herb to 1 teaspoon dried.

- **Spices:** Stock a convenient spot in your kitchen with little glass jars of spices. Gone are the days of spices sitting for years. You'll find that once you get into spices, you'll run through them quite fast, which is great because they lose their potency over time. Some of the spices used in my recipes include allspice, black pepper, cardamom, cinnamon, cloves, cumin,

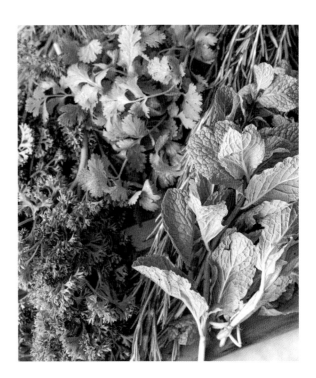

fennel seeds, ginger, nutmeg, paprika, and turmeric, but I also have bay leaves, cayenne, chile powder, and red pepper flakes. I buy my spices already ground, but you can use a mortar and pestle if you want the freshest, zestiest taste.

- **A note on ginger and cinnamon:** In my recipes, I specify whether I want you to use ginger powder or grated fresh ginger. I prefer Ceylon cinnamon because it's sweeter and lower in the compound coumarin (found in larger amounts in the more common cassia cinnamon), so if you're using cassia cinnamon, you may want to decrease the quantity a little since it's a bit spicier.

If a particular herb or spice does not appeal to you, consider substituting a different herb that looks similar, like using flat-leaf parsley or basil instead of cilantro.

For more health specifics on herbs and spices, check out pages 139 and 140, where I discuss especially powerful anti-inflammatory herbs and spices.

KOMBUCHA

Kombucha is a fizzy, tangy drink made from fermented tea combined with fruit juice and spices. The good little probiotics in kombucha support your own microbiota, and it can be a healthy addition to your diet along with other fermented foods like yogurt, kefir, kimchi, sauerkraut, miso, and natto. The first time I had kombucha, it was way too strong for me. I was not prepared for the sour flavor characteristic of all fermented foods. If the flavor is too strong for you, too, I have found diluting kombucha with a bit of sparkling water helpful. I recommend keeping kombucha to about 4 to 8 ounces at a time to avoid digestive issues and to buy kombucha with less than 5 to 8 grams of sugar per 8-ounce serving to avoid a sugar bomb.

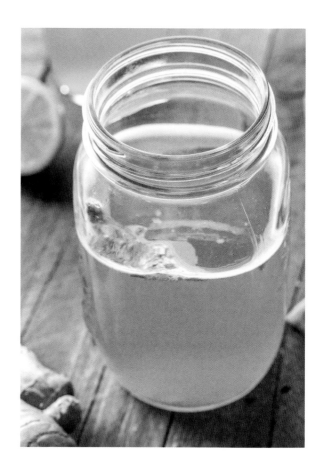

One of my all-time favorite baking secrets is using kombucha when I need extra moisture and the recipe already has enough fat from oil or butter. Kombucha adds a lightness due to its effervescence and works in everything from muffins to waffles to my Ginger Mandarin Almond Torte (page 332). It also makes a nice substitution for a liquid in a recipe if you don't happen to have something like juice or plant milk on hand.

LEMONS & OTHER CITRUS

It's a near emergency at my house if we don't have lemons. I use lemons daily in my Dr. Katie Life Water (page 306), and I find them so helpful for adding brightness to dishes that need a flavor lift. The zest of lemons and other citrus like limes and oranges can transform your baking, as in my Ginger Mandarin Almond Torte (page 332). Lemons enhance digestion and help to eliminate toxins, so starting your day with a glass of warm or cool lemon water may be the best early-morning move you could make, especially before a cup of coffee.

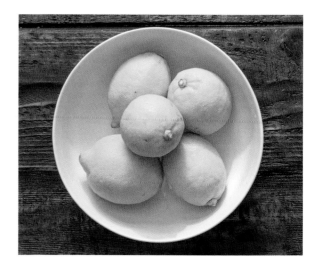

I buy lemons that have smooth, dull skin with smaller "pores" that are not rock hard because I find they have more juice and are easier to squeeze. When cutting lemons into wedges, I lop off the ends and then slice them into six wedges, cutting off the white pith in the center and removing the seeds. I store extra wedges in a glass container in the refrigerator for future use.

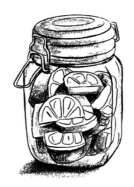

MACA

Maca is a beautiful Peruvian cruciferous root vegetable with a malt taste, sold in powdered form. It's known in herbal medicine for being a vitality-enhancing adaptogen. Adaptogens are plants and herbs that help us adapt to stress. Maca is naturally uplifting, so don't use it if your mood and energy are already very positive or if you're feeling anxious. As with all adaptogens, I recommend you consult your Integrative Medicine doctor about maca before trying it in my Maca Cacao Hot Chocolate recipe (page 310). I store maca powder in the pantry.

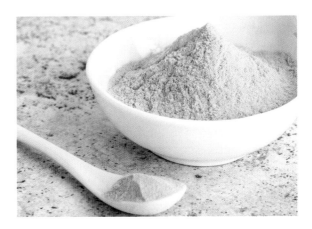

MISO

Miso is a paste made from fermented soybeans or chickpeas. It's naturally rich in beneficial bacteria that support digestive health and provides a salty umami richness to cooking. I generally buy white miso because of its versatility and mild flavor, but you can take it up a notch with yellow and red miso.

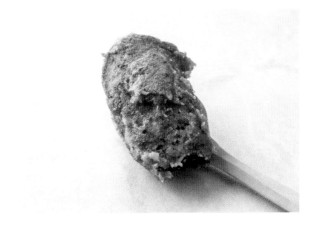

MUSHROOMS

Mushrooms have an earthy sweetness and add a satisfying meaty texture to plant-forward dishes. Mushrooms are one of the few sources of vitamin D in our diets. They are also packed with B vitamins and phytonutrients that boost immunity and are anti-cancer. I mostly use shiitake mushrooms at home, but my family loves all varieties. Mushrooms should be cooked before eating because cooking destroys potentially harmful substances. Plus, cooked mushrooms taste better and allow for better phytonutrient absorption. Store mushrooms in the refrigerator in a resealable plastic bag and thoroughly wash and dry whole mushrooms before cooking them.

For more health specifics on mushrooms, check out page 127, where I discuss them as part of my anti-inflammatory diet.

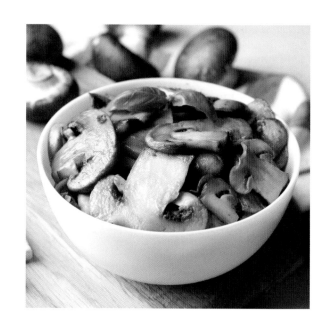

NUTRITIONAL YEAST

Nutritional yeast is an inactive form of yeast used for seasoning. It's a good source of B vitamins and protein and confers a savory, umami-rich flavor that's similar to cheese. You can sprinkle nutritional yeast on everything from salads to roasted vegetables to whole grains. It is available at most grocery stores in flake and powdered form. I prefer flakes because I like the texture, but the powdered form may be easier to stir into dressings or sauces. I keep a bottle of nutritional yeast on my counter next to the salt and pepper to encourage its use.

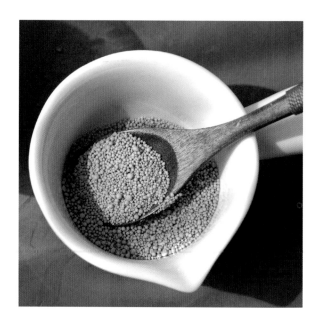

NUTS & SEEDS

I adore nuts and nut butters because they taste great and have the perfect blend of digestive fiber, muscle-supportive protein, and heart-healthy fat along with essential bone-building minerals. I keep a stock of raw almonds, Brazil nuts, cashews, hazelnuts, peanuts, pecans, pistachios, and walnuts in the pantry at all times. I recommend buying raw nuts in bulk and either eating them raw or toasting them on the stovetop or in the oven yourself, since food companies tend to both salt *and* toast nuts, and you don't want that extra salt in your diet on the regular.

Soaking raw nuts in water for ten minutes before eating softens them and enhances digestion for many people. If you want to make a cashew cream sauce like my Lemony Basil Cashew Cream (page 300), soak cashews in boiling water for thirty minutes or in room-temperature water for at least two hours before blending.

I also keep a steady supply of raw seeds in the kitchen. Seeds confer similar benefits to nuts, mainly being the ideal blend of fiber, protein, and fat. I store delicate seeds like hemp and flax in the refrigerator and sturdier seeds like chia, pumpkin, sesame, and sunflower in the pantry. I buy hulled seeds in bulk and then store smaller amounts in pretty glass containers for everyday use. Like nuts, I suggest you toast your own seeds when desired and soak raw seeds before eating if they cause you digestive strife.

Flax seeds are particularly useful in a plant-forward diet. Flax seeds in ground form are the best way to absorb the nutrition of this fiber-rich omega-3 fat. I use whole seeds when I want texture, like in my Whole-Grain Nut & Seed Bread (page 294). You can purchase pre-ground flax seeds at your grocery store, or you can buy whole seeds and grind them yourself with a dedicated coffee grinder.

"Flax eggs" are especially convenient in plant-forward baking as a replacement for eggs. The best method is to mix 1 tablespoon of ground flax seeds with 3 tablespoons of

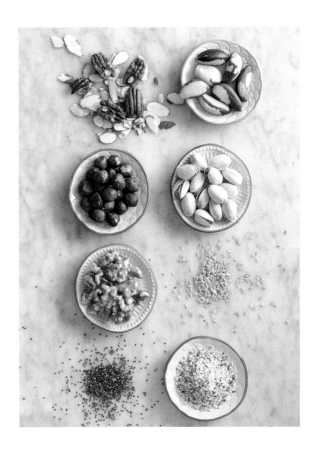

warm water and allow the mixture to thicken for about ten minutes before using. This yields one flax egg.

I keep several types of nut and seed butters available for daily use on everything from morning pancakes to seed bread, rotating through them to encourage phytonutrient variety. I like texture in my nut butters, so I buy crunchy varieties with the exception of tahini and cashew butter, which are super creamy and smooth. Be wary of nut and seed butters that have any ingredient other than nuts or seeds, especially added oils like palm oil or added sugars. I store nut and seed butters upside down to encourage mixing of the nut and seed oils, as separation occurs naturally when the butter sits for a bit. I like tahini (a savory sesame seed butter) made from both black and white sesame seeds and am a huge fan of tahini that comes in a squeeze bottle because it makes a tahini drizzle so easy.

OILS

Extra-virgin olive oil (EVOO) gets the most use in my kitchen because of its flavor and top-notch health benefits from anti-inflammatory monounsaturated fats. Extra-virgin means it's the oil that came from the first cold-pressing of the ripe olive fruit. I love it with everything from roasted vegetables to salad dressing to light sautéing. It's important to store EVOO in a darker-colored bottle. I buy it in larger jars and decant it into a wine-sized bottle with a pour spout for ease in the kitchen. And I keep a fancier, more expensive EVOO for dressings and raw uses, while I use a more economically priced EVOO for cooking and baking.

When I need an oil for higher-heat cooking or something with a more neutral flavor, I use avocado oil. I also love the deep flavor of toasted sesame oil, but I tend to add it at the end of cooking to Asian-influenced dishes. And who can beat the taste of coconut oil, especially when you want a slightly sweeter profile, like in an Indian or Thai curry or with granola? (See page 199 for more on coconut oil.)

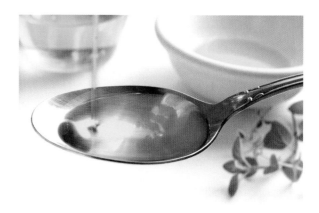

I also love the flavor of grass-fed Irish butter and clarified butter, also called ghee. Ghee provides a buttery flavor without the milk solids of unclarified butter that give some people digestive woes. Ghee also happens to be one of the few sources of the anti-inflammatory messengers short-chain fatty acids, which are the by-products of happy probiotic bacteria that munch on fiber. I store ghee at room temperature, but the refrigerator works well, too.

See my discussion on healthy fats on pages 119 to 125 for more health insights.

PLANT MILK

There are many types of nondairy milk, each with its own flavor and nutritional profile. For my recipes, you can use whichever plant milk you'd like, including almond, cashew, hemp, soy, or my personal favorites, macadamia and walnut. Just make sure it's unsweetened and unflavored. Note that coconut milk comes both in a beverage form similar to other plant milks and in canned form, which I specify when used in a recipe. Once opened, use plant milks within a week and store in the refrigerator.

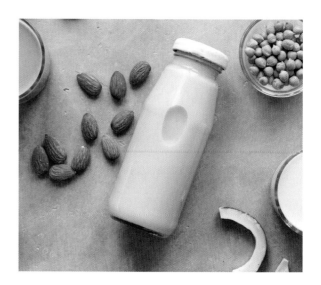

SALT & PEPPER

Sea salt makes almost everything taste better. It highlights all flavors and actually increases your ability to detect sweetness in foods, which is why it's included in every delightful dessert recipe.

I keep fine sea salt, coarse sea salt, flaky sea salt, and kosher salt in my kitchen. The workhorses for me are coarse sea salt and kosher salt, but most of my recipes call for fine sea salt because it's more commonly used and dissolves easier. I personally love the saltier bites that you occasionally get when you eat food seasoned with kosher or flaked salt, but you should use what you like.

You don't have to be afraid of salt if you're home-cooking plant-forward meals and drinking a few liters of water every day. Most of us only get into problems with salt when we're eating processed foods, which is why you wake up feeling bloated and almost hungover after eating something that you didn't make yourself. You need salt for electrolyte balance, especially if you sweat when you work out. If you want to level up, look for pink Himalayan salt or grayhued Celtic salt, which provide more essential minerals and nutrients.

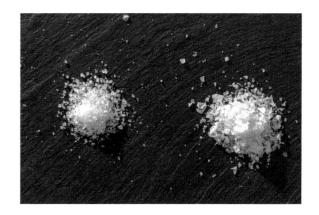

Black pepper is the yang to the yin of salt. Black pepper brings a deep richness to food and provides a specific texture that just tastes so nice on a salad or soup that's already been brought to the dinner table. It is also essential for the absorption of spices like turmeric, so make sure you pair those. I buy whole peppercorns and grind them fresh just before using. When measuring pepper for recipes, I grind my peppercorns into a small bowl and measure from there, but I encourage you to wing it with freshly ground pepper.

SEA VEGETABLES: DULSE, KOMBU & NORI

Adding iodine-rich sea vegetables like dulse, kelp, kombu, nori, and wakame to your diet is a great way to get the essential mineral iodine. You'll remember from the discussion on page 197 that kombu is helpful for the digestion of legumes. Crumbled sheets of nori taste great on a salad or soup, and little snack packs of roasted nori are a great way to introduce this food to children or dubious adults.

Using shakers of sea vegetable flakes like dulse or kelp is an easier way to incorporate iodine into your diet. I keep these shakers next to my salt and pepper grinders to encourage their use.

You can find sea vegetables in the international foods aisle of your grocery store.

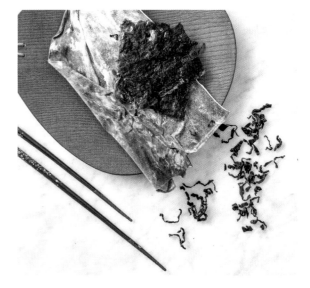

SWEETENERS

Sugar is sugar, no matter where it comes from, but there are a few sources of dietary sugar that are less processed and more mineral-rich, including blackstrap molasses, coconut aminos, coconut sugar, dried fruit, honey, and maple syrup. A little goes a long way, so take care when adding these sweeteners to recipes. I generally don't use agave; I prefer maple syrup and honey because they are lower in fructose. I also steer clear of nonnutritive (noncaloric) sweeteners like stevia, monkfruit, and artificial sweeteners. If you're used to sugary treats, it might take your taste buds a bit of time to adjust.

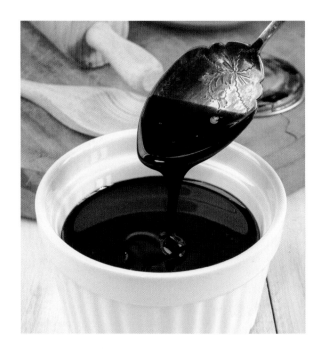

- **Blackstrap molasses:** Blackstrap molasses creates a deeply sweet, satisfying flavor and is an excellent source of plant-based iron, which is essential for all of us, but particularly for growing children and menstruating women.

- **Coconut aminos:** This caramel-colored sauce is promoted as an alternative to liquid aminos, soy sauce, and tamari, but it is so much sweeter that I think it should be considered like maple syrup or honey. Even though it's made from the fermented sap of a coconut palm combined with salt, coconut aminos don't taste much like coconut. The combination of salty and sweet is delicious with tempeh, tofu, or animal proteins or in soups or stews for a salty-sweet flavor burst. In fact, any time you're unsure of the flavoring in your cooking, you can probably add a smidge of coconut aminos and elevate the culinary experience.

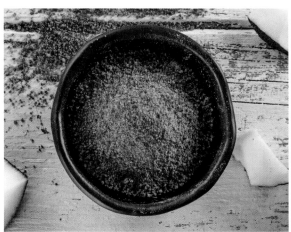

- **Coconut sugar:** Coconut sugar is less processed than traditional granulated cane sugar, so in my kitchen it has become our granulated sugar option for baking.

- **Dried fruit:** Having an assortment of dried fruit on hand is a great way to sweeten a homemade trail mix or salad. I keep prunes, Medjool dates, blueberries,

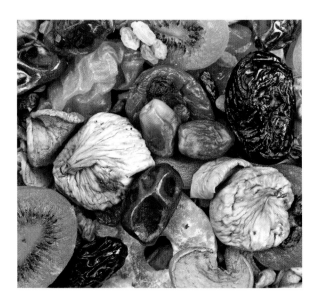

cranberries, goji berries, tart cherries, apricots, and a raisin medley stocked in my pantry. Just buy unsweetened and check that the only ingredient on the label is the fruit itself.

- **Honey:** Generally, the richer the color of honey, the more nutrients it provides. Buying local honey can be helpful for those who struggle with allergies, since exposure to local bees and pollen is like your own form of homeopathy. And a teaspoon of honey has been shown in studies to be as effective as over-the-counter cough suppressant during a respiratory illness.[2] I like raw honey, which is more solid at room temperature. If I need it to be in a liquid form, I just gently warm the vessel in a hot water bath in the kitchen sink. I like the stickiness of honey when making granola or other things that I want to bind together, like my Spiced Nut Mix (page 326).

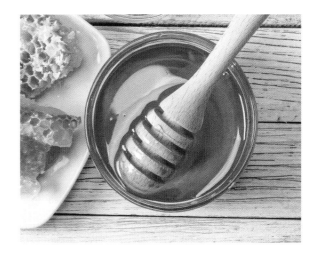

- **Maple syrup:** I like grade A dark maple syrup, which is darker in color and richer in flavor than other types. Maple syrup is lower in fructose than honey, so it's my go-to sweetener if I just want a touch of sweetness in a matcha latte or a cup of black tea with plant milk.

TAMARI, SOY SAUCE & AMINOS

These flavorful savory liquid seasonings are similar, but there are some key differences between them:

- **Tamari and soy sauce:** Both tamari and soy sauce are made by fermenting soybeans; tamari is usually gluten-free. Compared with most soy sauces, tamari is darker, less salty, and has a richer umami flavor, so I generally prefer it to soy sauce. Don't buy reduced-salt soy sauce because you'll probably end up using more to get the desired taste. From ice cream to soy sauce, I'm a big fan of buying the real deal and just consuming less.

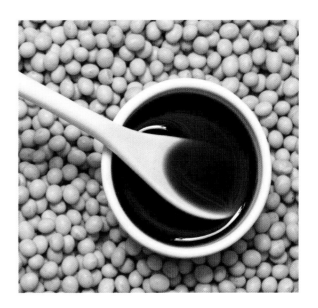

---

[2] O. Oduwole, E. E. Udoh, A. Oyo-Ita, and M. M. Meremikwu, "Honey for acute cough in children," *Cochrane Database of Systematic Reviews* 4, no. 4 (2018): CD007094.

- **Liquid aminos:** Liquid aminos looks and tastes similar to soy sauce. It's made by treating soybeans with an acidic solution to break them down into free amino acids, which gives food a savory, salty flavor. You can purchase liquid aminos in a shaker bottle or as a spray, which is a fun way to add just a hint of umami to your food.

- **Coconut aminos:** See my thoughts on this flavorful salty-sweet seasoning in the previous section.

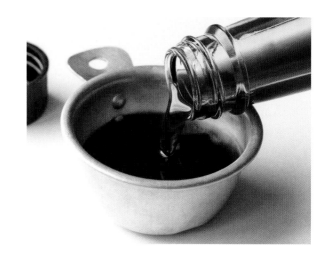

TEMPEH & TOFU

Tempeh and tofu are amazing whole soy products that pack a ton of protein. I keep a supply of organic silken tofu, extra-firm tofu, and tempeh in the refrigerator. I prefer tempeh made from soybeans to bean- or lentil-based tempeh because of the protein content, but the latter makes a great substitute if you are sensitive to soy. Make sure to buy organic soy to avoid exposure to genetically modified organisms. See my discussion of preparing plant proteins later in this chapter for more health and kitchen prep specifics.

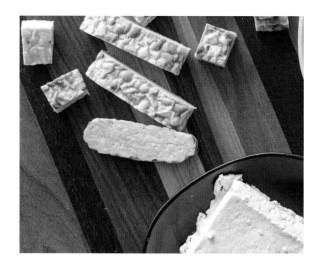

VINEGARS

I love an astringent, sour taste in my food, so I like to use vinegars in combination with sweet, salty, and earthy flavors in cooking.

- **Apple cider vinegar (ACV):** My top vinegar pick is apple cider vinegar because of its tremendous medicinal properties and potent bite, but I recognize that not everyone wants to dive in, so start with small amounts and work your way up. Buy raw, unfiltered organic

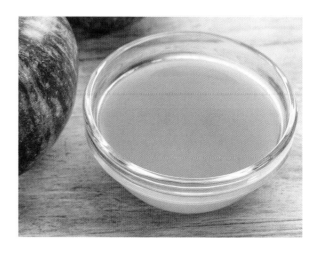

ACV, which looks a bit murky from sediment in the bottle, which is where all the proteins, enzymes, and friendly bacteria live. Just shake it up before use. For more on ACV, check out my Spiced Apple Toddy on page 314.

- **Sweet vinegars:** I love the sweetness of thick balsamic vinegar in salad dressings, rice vinegar in Asian dishes, and red wine vinegar in Greek food. Just make sure your balsamic vinegars are 100 percent balsamic vinegar and not wine vinegar with flavoring or coloring added to it. Real balsamic vinegar is expensive, but it's worth the price because a little goes a long way.

DR. KATIE'S LIFE KITCHEN FAVORITE BRANDS

These products are available on Amazon and at Whole Foods, Trader Joe's, Fresh Direct, and many specialty or independent stores.

Amino acids: Bragg

Apple cider vinegar: Bragg

Beans: Eden Organic

Bone broth: Fire & Kettle, Bonafide Provisions, FOND

Buckwheat noodles (soba): Eden Selected

Butternut squash and pumpkin, canned: Farmer's Market

Chickpea crumbs: Watusee

Chocolate, dark: Theo 85%, Alter Ego organic 85% to 100%, Evolved 100%

Coconut aminos: Bragg

Coconut butter: Artisana

Coconut milk, canned unsweetened full-fat: Native Forest Simple No Guar

Coconut oil: Nutiva

Coconut yogurt: Anita's, Cocojune, Culina

Crackers: Mary's Gone, Flackers

Fish sauce: Red Boat

Flours, meals, and baking aids: Bob's Red Mill

Kombu: Emerald Cove

Kombucha: GT's Gingerade, Health-Ade

Maple syrup: Boon Farms Grade A Dark

Miso: Miso Master

Nori: GimMe snack pack, Shirakiku snack pack, Emerald Cove sheets

Nut and oat milks: Elmhurst, MALK, Three Trees

Nut and seed butters: Trader Joe's Salted Almond Butter, Artisana, Once Again, Nuttzo Power Fuel, Crazy Richard's

Nutritional yeast: Bragg

Salt: Maldon sea salt flakes

Sea vegetables: Emerald Cove

Spices: Simply Organic, Spice Islands Organic, Frontier Organic

Tahini: Mighty Sesame Co., Kevala, Artisana Organics

Tea: Traditional Medicinals, Numi, Ito En

Tempeh: Lightlife Organic

Tofu: Nasoya Organic

Whole grains: Bob's Red Mill, Lundberg Family Farms

HOW TO WASH PRODUCE

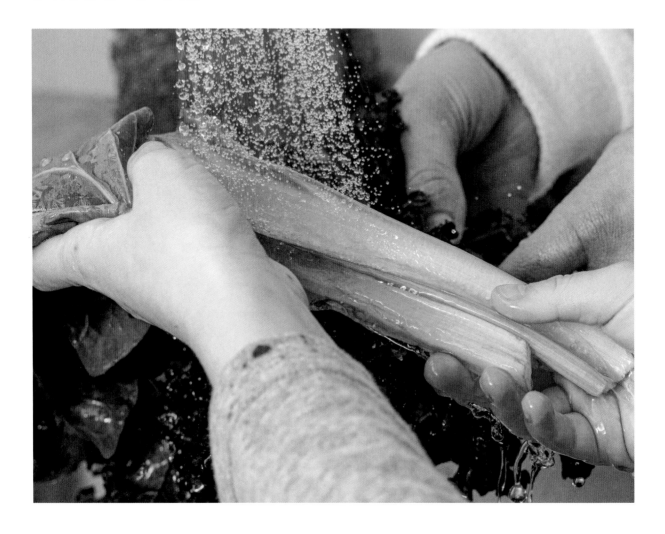

If you eat the peels, you'll want to wash your produce thoroughly, especially if you didn't buy organic. Most of us just rinse our produce under running water before we use it, but recognize that friction is your friend, meaning a little elbow grease with a vegetable brush is helpful. A vegetable brush can easily be thrown in the dishwasher to be cleaned.

If you're more serious about reducing pesticide exposure, you can use a dilute solution of apple cider vinegar, hydrogen peroxide, or baking soda to clean your produce. Some newer evidence suggests that a baking soda soak might be the best way to clean produce.[3] When washing fruits and vegetables, simply soak them in a bowl of water with a teaspoon of baking soda for at least a minute. If you have fifteen minutes, soak them longer. Then swish them around and drain.

---

[3] T. Yang, J. Doherty, B. Zhao, et al., "Effectiveness of commercial and homemade washing agents in removing pesticide residues on and in apples," *Journal of Agricultural and Food Chemistry* 65, no. 44 (2017): 9744–52.

HOW TO PREPARE VEGETABLES

There are a few different methods for preparing vegetables. You can use any method you want; just promise me you won't boil your vegetables to death, deep-fry them, or use the microwave as a cooking vehicle. (Microwaving for short periods to reheat something is okay, but you'd be surprised at how many leftovers taste just fine straight out of the fridge or left for twenty minutes to come to room temperature.)

Here are some ways to prepare vegetables:

- **Steaming:** Any vegetable can be steamed. It's best to steam only long enough so that the vegetable is still on the crisp side. You know you've gone too far when your broccoli has turned dark green and is limp. I generally follow steaming with a shock in an ice water bath to stop the cooking process and preserve the vegetable's vibrant color. This sounds more complicated than it is: after draining the hot water, just add ice cubes and cold water to the vegetables in the cooking pot until they cool down.

- **Sautéing:** Any vegetable can be sautéed in a pan with a little avocado, coconut, or extra-virgin olive oil over medium heat along with some yummy herbs and spices. If your oil starts to smoke, your heat is too high. Start over with a clean pan and fresh oil and give it a go at a lower temperature. If your pan starts to get dry, add a little water or broth to encourage concurrent steaming. This sauté-steam combo works particularly well for hearty vegetables like Brussels sprouts.

- **Roasting:** This is my favorite method for preparing vegetables because it's the easiest and tastiest. The hot, dry oven air causes the sugar in the vegetables to caramelize, which leads to a beautiful golden brown crisp on the edges and an enhancement of sweetness, all while making the vegetables soft. It's a kid-friendly, crowd-pleasing way to serve vegetables. Use my Easy Roasted Vegetables recipe on page 286, which includes a handy chart for commonly roasted vegetables. (Roasting works for fruit, too! Check out my Sheet Pan Roasted Chicken with Pears, Figs & Swiss Chard recipe on page 264.)

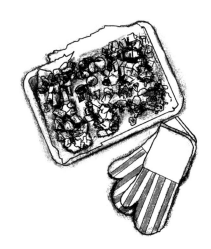

THE BASICS OF ROASTING VEGETABLES

1. **Preheat your oven to 425°F.** You need a high temperature to break down the sugars in vegetables and encourage caramelization. (The one Dr. Katie exception is when roasting mushrooms, which I personally prefer at 350°F.) Remember that convection ovens can be about 25°F hotter and cook faster than conventional ovens, so you may need to adjust the temperature and time downward if you're getting burnt vegetables.

2. **Pick a metal sheet pan with low sides.** Glass baking dishes don't conduct heat as well, and high sides will trap steam in the pan, making your vegetables mushy.

3. **Roast directly on the pan, or line your pan with unbleached parchment paper for easy cleanup.** Aluminum foil is so 1990s and leaches heavy metals into your food, so I don't recommend using it.

4. **Dry your vegetables after washing.** Wet vegetables will steam in the oven and could become rubbery.

5. **Cut your vegetables into roughly $\frac{1}{2}$- to 1-inch chunks.** Having vegetables of a uniform size will help them all to cook at the same rate. You can be super efficient and roast different vegetables on the same pan by cutting denser vegetables like winter squash, potatoes, and root vegetables into smaller pieces and less dense vegetables like broccoli and cauliflower a little bigger.

6. **Toss your vegetables in an adequate amount of avocado, coconut, or extra-virgin olive oil, sprinkle with salt and pepper (and any other herbs and spices you like), and spread them out on the baking sheet *cut side down*.** One of my patients taught me that almost every vegetable tastes great sprinkled with a little garlic powder—and she was right! Don't roast your vegetables with maple syrup, honey, or other sugars because they will burn. (You don't need to add sugar anyway. The caramelization process will take care of developing the sweetness for you.) And placing vegetables cut side down will create the golden color you're looking for.

7. **Roast for five to fifty-five minutes, turning the veggies once or twice.** They're done when they're crispy and a little brown on the outside and tender on the inside. More delicate vegetables like mushrooms and leafy greens need only a short amount of roasting time, while hardier veggies like cabbage and root vegetables may need more time in the oven.

HOW TO PREPARE WHOLE GRAINS

You'll want to prepare whole grains in bulk, creating leftovers that will make future meals easier. Most whole grains will keep in a covered container in the refrigerator for at least several days, and, refrigerating grains may increase their resistant starch content, which makes them even better fuel for your probiotic microbiome. I've laid out the most common whole grains and how much liquid to use when cooking them in my Hearty Whole Grains recipe on page 290.

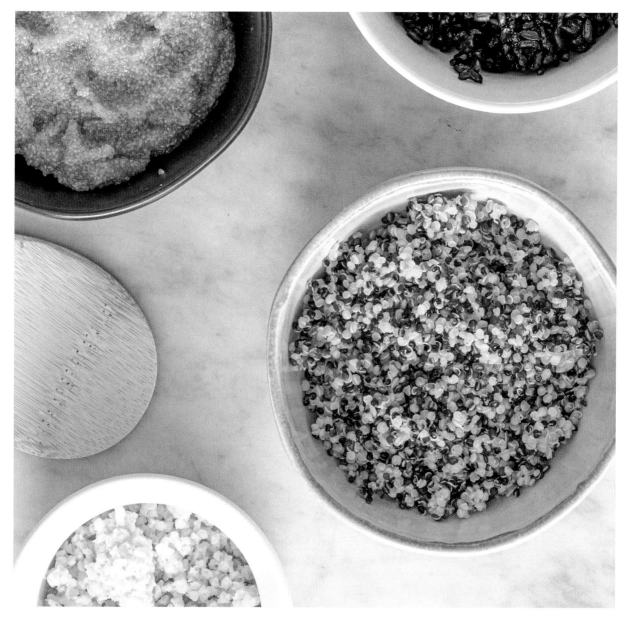

COOKING WHOLE GRAINS

I recommend rotating through the many beautiful whole grains available to ensure that you get a variety of phytonutrients in your diet. Quinoa is nutritious, but so are barley, farro, and millet.

Soaking and rinsing whole grains before cooking them removes extra starches, bitterness, and any impurities. If you skip this step, add a few extra tablespoons of liquid when cooking.

Making fluffy whole grains in a rice cooker is so much easier than the stovetop method and almost foolproof. Give yourself the gift of ease in the kitchen and invest in a rice cooker. You deserve it. My Hearty Whole Grains recipe on page 290 includes instructions for both cooking methods.

While I recognize that whole grain purists love just using water for cooking, I prefer to cook grains in nourishing bone broth along with a pinch of fine sea salt. Bathing whole grains in bone broth is a great way to add flavor and get powerful immune-boosting nutrients and protein from natural collagen, an important structural component of bones and joints, muscles and tendons, hair and nails, and blood vessels.

If I don't use bone broth, I mix in a teaspoon of extra-virgin olive oil, virgin coconut oil, or toasted sesame oil after cooking to make the whole grain taste extra yummy and provide some fat to balance out the fiber. For an extra special treat, you can cook your grains in a combination of canned unsweetened coconut milk and water, which provides both fat and a sweet flavor, like in my Almond Furikake Crusted Halibut recipe on page 268.

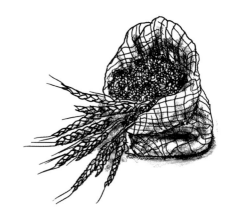

CHANGING THE GLYCEMIC LOAD

Interestingly, you can change the glycemic load of the carbohydrates in foods like whole grains, many legumes, and potatoes by letting them cool in the refrigerator overnight. (You can heat them up again before you eat them!) Cooking and cooling creates resistant starch, the kind of indigestible fiber that your good probiotics in your microbiome like to munch on and turn into anti-inflammatory short-chain fatty acids. These same resistant starches may make you feel fuller more quickly as well. In one small study, researchers found that healthy adult men ate about 90 fewer calories after consuming resistant starch compared to men who got a placebo.[4] How's that for cooking chemistry? Give it a go in your kitchen and see how you feel.

---

[4] C. L. Bodinham, G. S. Frost, and M. D. Robertson, "Acute ingestion of resistant starch reduces food intake in healthy adults," *British Journal of Nutrition* 103, no. 6 (2010): 917–22.

HOW TO PREPARE PLANT PROTEINS

One nice thing about plant proteins is that many are refrigerator- and shelf-stable for a long time, making it easy to stock your pantry with them. Having a healthy stock of options makes choosing and preparing plant proteins easier.

COOKING BEANS & LENTILS

Cooking beans and lentils from scratch has its advantages. Homemade beans and lentils tend to hold their shape better and can be seasoned along the way, which you may find more appealing. Cooking times vary based on the type of legume and whether you soak them before cooking (see the tips on the next page). Most beans cook in one to two hours, and most lentils cook in twenty to thirty minutes. When you think your legumes are done, rinse a few under cold water and taste them. If they hold their shape but are tender, then you're in business.

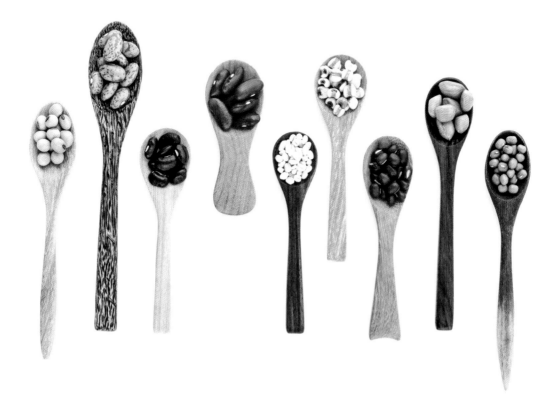

Cooking legumes from scratch has one major disadvantage: if not cooked long enough, they can cause issues with digestion. If you have digestive woes like gas or bloating that limit your desire to eat plant-based proteins, try soaking and sprouting your dried beans before cooking them (I have a post on sprouting on my website, DrKatie.com/blog, to help you), adding kombu to your cooking method, and pressure-cooking them.

- **Soaking:** Soaking dried beans and legumes in water for several hours or overnight before cooking is the most important step to easing the digestion of these plant-based proteins. Rinse them with fresh water before cooking.

- **Sprouting:** Sprouting generally breaks open the outer shell of the seed with the new sprout, which decreases a bit of the work of digestion and makes any food more nutritious and more energetically pleasing. You can easily find sprouting kits online or at your local store that use crosshatch lids to aerate the sprouting seeds.

- **Kombu:** Kombu is a Japanese sea vegetable that's a type of kelp. It contains enzymes that break down the heavy starches (called raffinose sugars) found in foods like beans. The good little probiotic bacteria in our intestines love these sugars, releasing hydrogen and carbon dioxide, which leads to bloating and gas. Kombu helps minimize this gas, thank goodness. It also contains a healthy dose of iron and iodine, two essential minerals. Add a 3- to 4-inch strip of kombu to the beans as they cook, or add the strip directly to your soup pot. After cooking, simply pull out the kombu and either chop it into fine pieces to go back into the pot or discard it. If you add it to precooked or canned beans, soak the kombu in a small amount of water for about twenty minutes, then add the seaweed and soaking water to the pot to get all of the minerals and anti-gas benefit.

- **Pressure cooking:** I drank the Instant Pot Kool-Aid a few years ago, and I haven't looked back. Gone are the days of being scared that the lid of your pressure cooker would fly off and splatter red sauce on the ceiling. The newer pressure cookers have built-in mechanisms that make them almost goof-proof. Pressure cooking helps break down the tough outer shells of beans and lentils that make them hard to digest in a brief period of hands-off time, which makes this appliance very useful. Pressure cooking also destroys lectins, a protective plant protein that can be problematic for some people.

If you're not into soaking, sprouting, or cooking dried beans, have no fear! Eden Organic brand beans are pressure-cooked before canning, so they're the ultimate shortcut. I buy canned beans by the case and store them in the basement so that they're available anytime I need them.

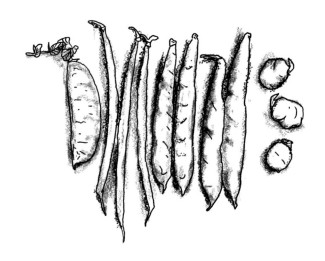

PRESSING TOFU

Pressing tofu before cooking it removes excess water and gives it a firmer, denser texture, making it easier to work with. Pressed tofu crisps and browns more easily and can be crumbled to resemble ground meat in a Bolognese or chili, for example. Pressed tofu also soaks up the flavor of the marinade or sauce in which it's cooked. Even ten minutes of pressing is worth your while, but I often press my tofu for up to twenty-four hours before use. I find thirty to sixty minutes of pressing time to be the most approachable for a busy home cook.

I'm a huge fan of my tofu press. I got it a few years ago after telling my auntie that I was wrapping my tofu in paper towels and placing a cast-iron skillet on top to remove the water. She said to me over the phone, "Katie, please.

Treat yourself to a $20 tofu press." So I bought one, and I haven't regretted it once.

Not only is a tofu press more environmentally friendly than my paper towel method, but it requires no work other than placing the block of tofu in the press and securing the pressing mechanism. If you don't have a tofu press, you can create your own by putting a block of tofu on a large rimmed plate. Simply set another plate on top, and then weight it down with a couple of heavy books for up to eight hours. You can store the pressed tofu in the refrigerator for up to three days until you're ready to use it.

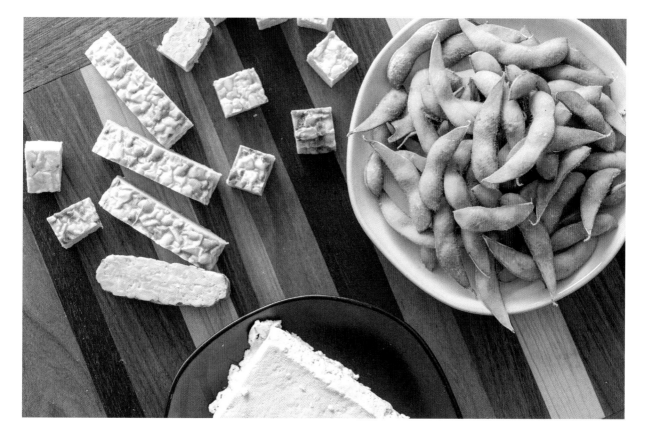

COOKING WITH TEMPEH

Tempeh is intrinsically firm, so it doesn't need to be pressed like tofu. Tempeh has an interesting flavor, like mushrooms, which I didn't care for the first few times I ate it. Now I love its flavor and texture. To make the taste milder, you can boil or steam the tempeh for ten to fifteen minutes before using it. Like tofu, tempeh tastes great with a good marinade, and the longer you marinate it, the better. I've left tempeh to marinate for up to two days, which was totally worth the flavor bomb it provided at the dinner table. If you make the Tempeh "BLT" Collard Wraps (page 272), allow your tempeh to marinate for as long as possible.

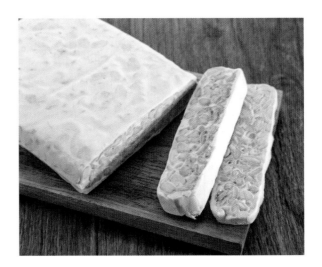

HOW TO PREPARE ANIMAL PROTEINS

Grass-fed meat and free-range poultry make their way into my diet a few times a week, mostly because they just taste good. I am diligent about buying organic animal products; if organic is not an option, then I opt for another type of protein. I rarely buy or eat farmed fish, which is loaded with toxins; I would rather eat better-quality, responsibly caught seafood, even though it costs more.

Wild fish makes an appearance in my diet at least weekly, with omega-3-rich fatty fish like wild salmon, black cod, halibut, sardines, and tuna being the stars and other fish like Arctic char, branzino, and snapper serving as a supporting cast. Living in New England, we are spoiled with oysters and wild shellfish like lobster and shrimp on occasion. You can use the organization SeafoodWatch.org to find the best options in your neck of the woods.

A proper portion of animal protein is about 3 ounces of meat and poultry or 3½ ounces of fish and seafood. Animal protein loses about 25 percent of its volume when cooked, so start with about 4 ounces for land animals and 5 ounces for seafood per person when buying animal protein at your grocery store, butcher shop, or fish market.

MARINATING

Marinating animal proteins before cooking adds moisture and changes the pH of the food, which helps reduce the production of toxic compounds if using high heat or grilling. Marinades do not have to be fancy; simple combinations of things like garlic, shallots or onions, herbs, spices, olive or sesame oil, tamari, citrus juice, salt, and pepper can make anything taste great. Interestingly, rosemary may be helpful for reducing the carcinogenic chemicals HCAs (heterocyclic amines).[5]

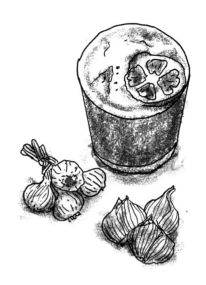

LOW & SLOW COOKING

Generally, gentle cooking methods such as baking, roasting, and stewing are better for animal proteins because they prevent the formation of PAHs (polycyclic aromatic hydrocarbons) and HCAs. As when roasting vegetables, I use unbleached parchment paper to line my pans to make for easier cleanup. The only exception is when broiling, in which case I put the animal protein directly on a well-oiled pan to prevent sticking. I generally keep broiling to just the beginning or end of cooking to help develop color.

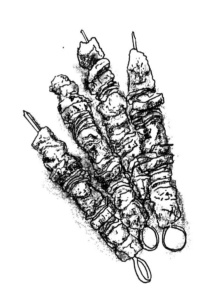

---

[5] K. Puangsombat and J. S. Smith, "Inhibition of heterocyclic amine formation in beef patties by ethanolic extracts of rosemary," *Journal of Food Science* 75, no. 2 (2010): T40–7.

GRILLING

Grilling is delicious and just so American! I mean, is there anything better than a backyard barbecue on a warm summer day with friends and family while the kids are playing nearby? But grilling on the regular is not your friend. It's important to limit meat's exposure to open flame, which can lead to the creation of HCAs and other carcinogenic compounds. If you like the taste of grilled meat or seafood, it's best to do it quickly (as in the case of hamburgers, which cook fast) to avoid charring and burning. You can also use indirect heat methods (which is more akin to baking than grilling) or to do most of the cooking in the oven at a lower temperature and finish the meats quickly on the grill for those perfect grill marks we've come to love.

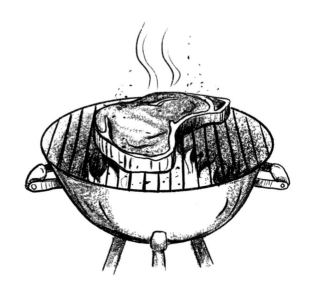

COOKING SEAFOOD

All animal protein continues to cook after it is removed from the heat, but this phenomenon is more noticeable with fish because of its thinner, flakier flesh. I recommend removing seafood to a cool surface just before it's completely opaque to prevent overdone or rubbery seafood. Nothing makes me sadder at dinnertime than a piece of overcooked fish.

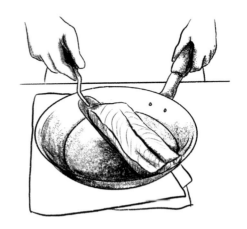

LEFTOVERS

I love leftovers. Seeing leftovers in the refrigerator is like a security blanket for me. It means I've done the work and get to reap the rewards. It removes stress from life's full plate and creates space for me to do something else with my time.

I encourage you to make larger volumes of food so that you have leftovers. There are a few things that some people don't think reheat well (though I would personally eat almost anything as a leftover), including fish. With the exception of the halibut (page 268) and salmon (page 274), everything in this cookbook can be enjoyed in leftover form. So don't make just enough Sweet Potato Pancakes (page 242) for Sunday; make enough to last you several days. Or do yourself an even bigger favor and make enough to store in the freezer.

FREEZING

While food in the refrigerator lasts only a few days, using the freezer to make the most of weekend batch cooking is a deposit in the bank of sanity. When I make a giant pot of soup, like my Creamy Roasted Broccoli Soup (page 256), or legumes, like the lentils for the Arugula & Lentil Salad (page 254), or whole grains, like my Slow Cooker Apple Pie Oatmeal (page 236), I freeze the leftovers in small containers that can be quickly defrosted in the refrigerator overnight or while I'm at work. Then, the next time I need to throw together a meal, I have precooked components to work with. If my frozen food isn't completely thawed by the time I need it, I ease it out of its glass vessel with a ten-minute warm bath in my kitchen sink.

You can freeze any of the baked goods in this book, including the Whole-Grain Nut & Seed Bread (page 294), Sweet Potato Pancakes (page 242), Morning Glory Muffins (page 244), The Chocolatiest of Cookies (page 328), and Ginger Mandarin Almond Torte (page 332). I think frozen cookies might be the best thing since sliced bread, so we freeze every type of cookie we make at my house.

"[**Freezing food**] *removes stress* from life's full plate and *creates space* for me to do something else with my time."

PACKING & TRANSPORTING

I think every recipe in this book could be transported and eaten as a leftover. I eat almost all of my lunches at work and some of my breakfasts, too, so I'm accustomed to packing tasty leftover portions in glass containers like Pyrex.

If you're making something with delicate ingredients, like the soba noodles in the Thai Coconut Curry Noodle Soup (page 266) or the arugula in the Arugula & Lentil Salad (page 254), keep the delicate ingredient separate so that it stays fresh. In the case of soba, you can add fresh soba to the otherwise complete soup when you reheat it the next day. In the case of arugula, keep the dressing in its own container and dress the greens just before eating. This will ensure that everything stays crisp or firm until you're ready to eat.

REHEATING

I generally don't recommend reheating leftovers in the microwave. You're much better off allowing a food to come to room temperature on the countertop for twenty minutes, reheating it in a 325°F to 400°F oven, or using a saucepan on the stovetop over medium heat. If you must, microwave a small quantity for a short time in a glass container covered by a paper towel. Never, ever microwave plastic. Heating plastic in the microwave can cause chemicals to leach into your food, and many of those chemicals have been identified as endocrine disruptors that have been linked to metabolic disorders and reduced fertility.

"**Never,** *ever* microwave plastic."

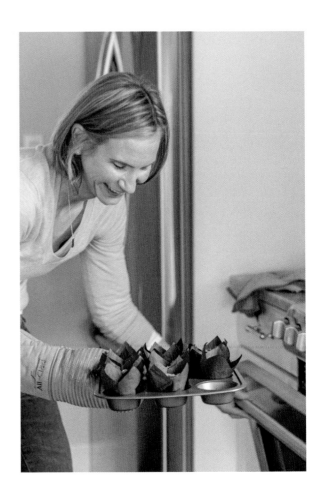

TRYING NEW FOODS

There are a ton of amazing foods out there that pack a nutritional punch, but what if you don't happen to like a particular food? Many of us have aversions to certain foods based on prior experiences (mostly from when we were children) that tarnished the way we think about them. I could recommend blueberries until I am blue in the face, but if you threw up after eating them as a kindergartner, seeing them in your oatmeal may forever trigger your gag reflex. I had an aversion to raw tomatoes on salad until I discovered their juicy sweet goodness in my mid-twenties, but as a kid I had no problem eating cooked tomatoes in sauces or soups—or in the form of ketchup, of course!

Sometimes we grow out of a food aversion by trialing the food several more times. In fact, experts think we have to try foods *up to fifteen times* before we can really reject them. That's why it's so hard to get kids to adopt new foods. It takes an obscene number of tries to help children develop a taste for a "healthy" food, and many parents just don't have the patience or the budget for so many attempts. I had to serve my two young boys salmon *eleven times* before they stopped fighting me when it appeared on their plates. Thankfully, now they eat it without much complaining...but it took a long time for that to happen.

If I talk about or use a food in a recipe that's new or strange to you, I encourage you to try it many times and in several forms before making an official decision about its place in your life. I didn't like many fermented foods like kombucha or kimchi the first time I tasted them. I diluted my kombucha with seltzer for months before I started drinking it straight. Eventually, however, my palate adjusted, and now I enjoy kombucha immensely. Give your palate space to grow and accept new foods. It's okay if something tastes a little weird at first. Sometimes we need to challenge ourselves a little to fully tap into our *Wellness Intuition.*

If you decide after several tries that a particular healthy food is not for you, I encourage you to use your food aversions to your advantage. If you don't love cucumbers, well, hey, guess what? Many other vegetables, like celery, have a similar water-filled crunch and make great substitutes.

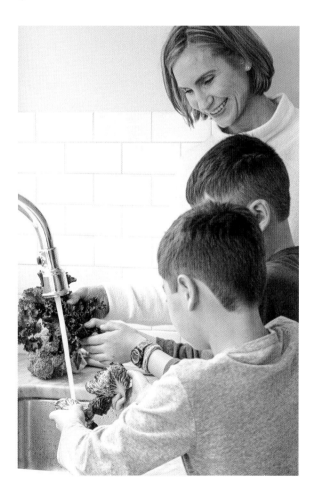

ESSENTIAL TOOLS & APPLIANCES FOR PLANT-FORWARD COOKING

There are so many tools that make things easier in the kitchen, but these are my favorites. All of these tools are available at large retail stores, specialty kitchen stores, and online.

FAVORITE TOOLS

- **Baking sheet:** You can use a 13 by 18-inch metal baking sheet with a rim (also known as a half sheet pan) for multiple purposes, from baking cookies to roasting vegetables to a cooking sheet pan dinner. I almost always line mine with unbleached parchment paper unless I'm broiling food, in which case I use a generous amount of oil to prevent sticking.

- **Cast-iron skillet:** If you don't have a cast-iron skillet that belonged to your grandmother, have no fear. Preseasoned pans are easy to find and reasonably priced. You'll want to "season" your skillet a few times per year to recreate the nonreactive hard surface that resists rust and allows used pans to be rinsed with water or wiped clean with a damp paper towel. To season cast iron, simply coat the pan with avocado oil and then place it in a 375°F oven for an hour, letting it cool in the oven. I find a 12-inch skillet to be the most versatile size.

- **Citrus press:** A citrus press makes juicing lemons a lot easier, but you can also just squeeze them with your hands. I find cutting off the ends of citrus fruit before halving makes squeezing easier.

- **Garlic press:** I'm not skilled enough with a knife to mince garlic, so I prefer to use a garlic press.

- **Ginger grater:** My ginger grater is a small dish with a rough center that makes grating roots like ginger and turmeric and radishes like daikon easier, but you could also use a Microplane or traditional grater.

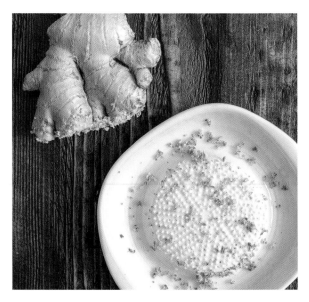

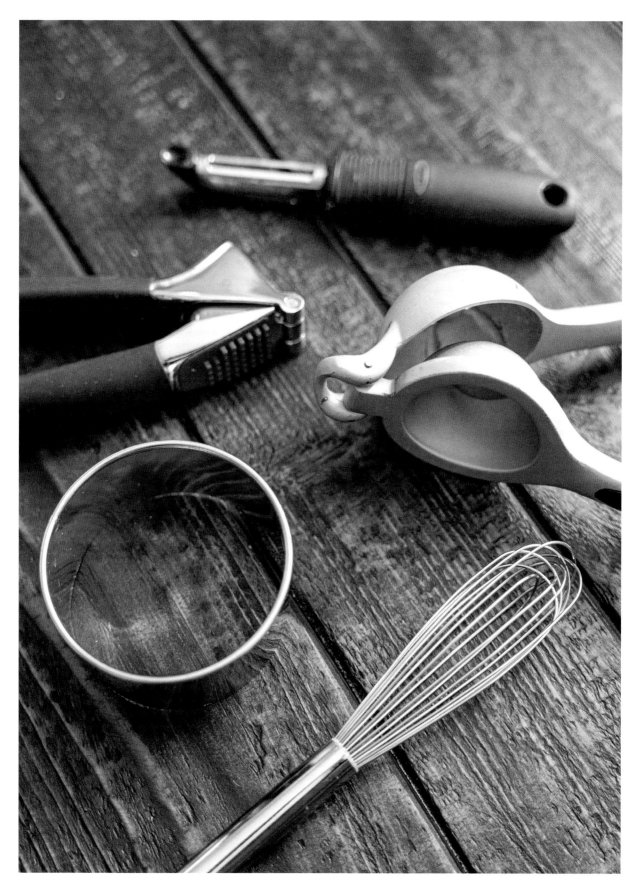

- **Glassware for storage:** I store almost all food in reheatable glass vessels, like Pyrex storage containers and mason jars. I use plastic only when I know that the vessel might be handled by a child and easily broken. Never, ever put plasticware in the microwave. If your plastic Pyrex lids begin to tear over time, you can order replacements easily.

- **Knives:** I have about fifteen different knives that I use from time to time, but the workhorses are a flat-blade chef's knife for herbs and lettuces, a thin serrated slicing knife for tomatoes and delicate produce, a paring knife for coring fruits like apples, serrated steak knives for use at the table, and a thick serrated knife for everything else, especially big, tough produce like squash and watermelon. I'm partial to the Cutco brand because their serrated knives never seem to go dull, and they offer free sharpening. Please remember to sharpen your knives regularly. You are more likely to cut yourself with a dull knife that slips than with a sharp one.

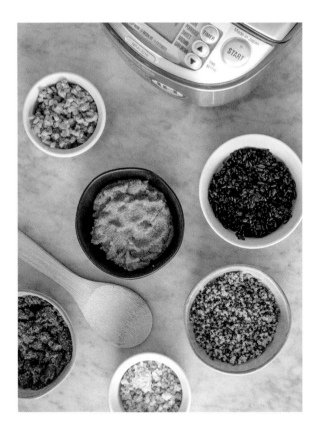

- **Mandoline:** I don't use my mandoline often, but I break it out when I want super finely sliced onions or potatoes. I bought one that uses a guide over the produce to protect the ends of my fingers, a feature I highly recommend.

- **Microplane:** I love my Microplane for zesting citrus and grating a little cheese. It also grates foods like garlic, ginger, turmeric, and daikon.

- **Parchment paper:** Parchment paper is an unsung hero because it makes cleanup so much easier. The one exception to using unbleached parchment paper is when broiling, which would cause the paper to burn; for broiling, I just place food straight on a well-oiled metal pan. I recognize that it creates waste, so I opt for unbleached parchment paper and compost it after use to make up for that negative karma.

- **Salad spinner:** My kids love to use the salad spinner, so I can often get them involved in making a salad if I offer this job to them. Not only is it fun, but it gets all the water off your lettuces and greens so that they can soak up the goodness of the dressing or the oil in which they'll be roasted or sautéed. Properly drying vegetables before roasting prevents them from getting rubbery.

- **Tofu press:** If you walk away with nothing else from this chapter, I hope you'll know that I think you deserve a tofu press. It makes preparing tofu (see page 221) so much easier and ultimately allows bland tofu to pick up the flavor of its surrounding sauces.

FAVORITE APPLIANCES

- **Blender:** I have a high-powered blender like a Vitamix, an immersion blender, and a regular blender. The Vitamix is like no other, in my opinion; the creamy texture it creates for smoothies and soups is top-notch. I use the Vitamix when I want that super-smooth texture, but use the immersion blender or regular blender when I don't mind a less smooth texture, like in my Creamy Roasted Broccoli Soup (page 256). I generally find an immersion blender easier when cooking soup and prefer a regular blender for smoothies.

- **Food processor:** A good food processor makes prepping produce so much easier. One of my favorite ways to make a finely chopped kale salad like my Kale & Quinoa Greek Salad (page 252) is to buy prewashed bagged kale pieces and throw them into the food processor. A food processor is also useful for grinding nuts, seeds, and grains into flour. You need a food processor.

- **Pressure cooker:** As I said earlier in this chapter, I drank the Instant Pot Kool-Aid and love the ease of sautéing, boiling liquids, and pressure cooking all in one pot. There are two things an Instant Pot is not as good for: cooking rice and slow cooking. This is because the heat element is at the bottom and does not encircle the whole pot, making it inconsistent and slow compared with dedicated rice cookers and slow cookers. Pressure cooking is super useful if you want to ease your digestion of plant-based proteins like beans and lentils, but it's also helpful if you have limited time and want to make a yummy soup or homemade bone broth.

- **Rice cooker:** When my Japanese then-boyfriend-now-husband bought me my first rice cooker back in medical school, I thought he was crazy, because I didn't really like rice. That's because I had grown up in a household where we didn't know such an appliance existed, so we always cooked rice on the stovetop. Friends, let me enlighten you: a rice cooker will change your life because it makes cooking tender and delicious whole grains almost foolproof. Plus, it takes one thing off your already full short-term memory list while you're cooking the rest of your meal—just set it and forget it. Check out my guide to cooking more than just rice in my Hearty Whole Grains recipe (page 290).

- **Slow cooker:** My mom is a slow-cooker genius, so I learned from the best. She taught me that using a slow cooker is a great way to feed a family of seven while actively parenting five kids. In short, it makes light work of cooking a bigger volume of food. I love a slow cooker for making everything from tender pulled pork to soups and stews to enough oatmeal for a week's worth of breakfasts. Just dump in the ingredients and you're good to go, like in my Slow Cooker Apple Pie Oatmeal recipe (page 236).

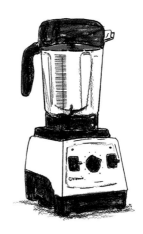

CHAPTER 11

THE RECIPES

"Appetite is the best sauce of all."

—*Anonymous*

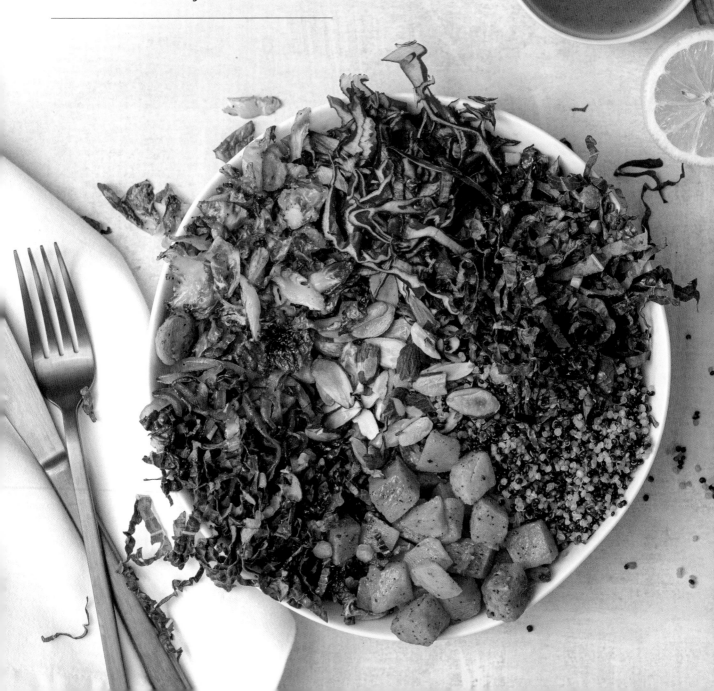

Now that we've spent the last little while shoring up your education about a plant-rich diet and well-balanced lifestyle, it's time to get to the fun part: creating in the kitchen.

My recipes are broken down into the time of day in which I think will serve you best to eat them, but recognize that they all can be eaten at any time. After all, you're not the only one who enjoys eating supper's leftovers in the morning.

Each recipe is designed to balance fiber, protein, and fat, so I recommend making it in full to ensure that you feel the effect it has on your energy and satiety, as well as the pleasure it brings your taste buds. After you eat, check in with your *Wellness Intuition* and see if you feel well. My hunch is that you will. This is no accident, but a purposeful creation from my Life Kitchen to yours.

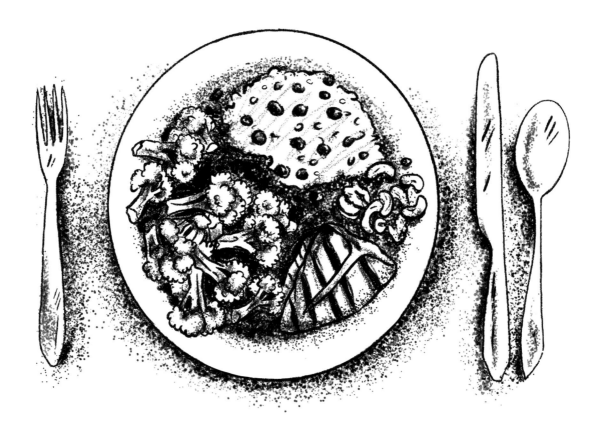

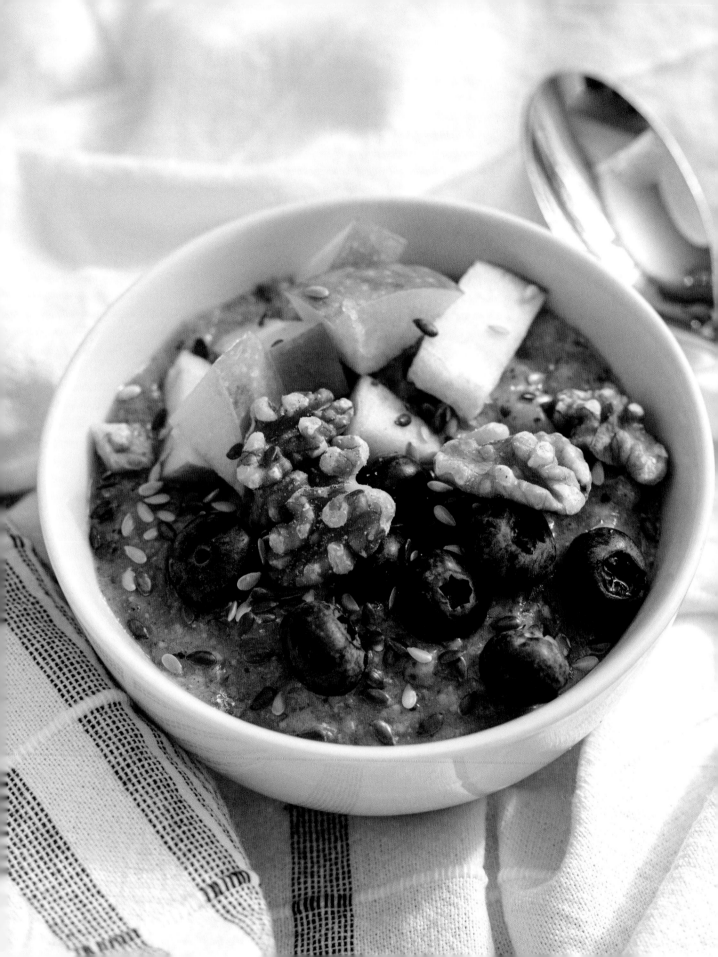

MORNING RECIPES

ENERGIZE YOUR DAY WITH A POSITIVE START

SLOW COOKER APPLE PIE OATMEAL

SERVES 6 to 8

PREP TIME: 10 minutes

COOK TIME: 2 or 4 hours

What an amazing start to the day! Steel-cut oats are a whole grain and are less processed than rolled oats (and certainly better than instant or quick-cooking breakfast porridges), making them an excellent choice for slow-burn energy. The addition of ground flax seeds and walnuts brings omega-3–rich fat to satiate, along with fiber to keep your digestion moving right along. Adding unpeeled apples gives the oatmeal a hint of sweetness and fiber-rich pectin to keep your microbiome happy. I encourage you to experiment with other delicious flavors! Note that slow cooker times are approximate and may need to be adjusted based on your own slow cooker.

1 cup steel-cut oats

¼ cup ground flax seeds

3 cups water

1 (13.5-ounce) can full-fat, unsweetened coconut milk

2 medium apples (any type), diced (do not peel)

2 teaspoons pure vanilla extract

2 teaspoons ground cinnamon

¼ teaspoon ground nutmeg

¼ teaspoon ginger powder

⅛ teaspoon ground cloves

½ teaspoon fine sea salt

Additional water or unsweetened plant milk, warmed, as needed

TOP EACH SERVING WITH:

2 tablespoons toasted walnuts, 1 tablespoon toasted flax seeds, ¼ cup Celebration Granola (page 238) or other nut-based granola, and/or 2 teaspoons nut butter of choice

¼ cup fresh blueberries and/or chopped apple

1. Place the oats in a fine-mesh strainer and rinse under cool running water until clear to remove impurities.

2. Coat a 3-quart or larger slow cooker with avocado oil spray or a thin layer of healthy oil to prevent sticking.

3. Combine all the ingredients except the toppings in a medium bowl and transfer to the prepared slow cooker. For daytime cooking, set the slow cooker for 2 hours on high. To cook the oatmeal overnight, set the slow cooker for 4 hours on low and go to sleep; most slow cookers will automatically turn off after the cook time or switch to "keep warm" until morning.

4. If the oatmeal is thicker than you like, stir in extra warm water or milk until it reaches your desired consistency.

5. To serve, scoop ½ to ¾ cup of the oatmeal into a bowl and top with the walnuts, flax seeds, granola, and/or nut butter along with the blueberries.

LIFE KITCHEN TIPS:

Slow cooker oatmeal makes an easy breakfast when hosting overnight guests. You can prepare it the night before, and everyone awakens to the smell of apple pie! I also find it helpful to prepare this recipe on Sunday night to make breakfast on Monday morning easy for the whole family, with leftovers that will keep for 2 to 3 days in the refrigerator. Reheat leftovers with extra plant-based milk of your choice on the stovetop over medium heat for 5 minutes or in the microwave for 90 to 120 seconds on high.

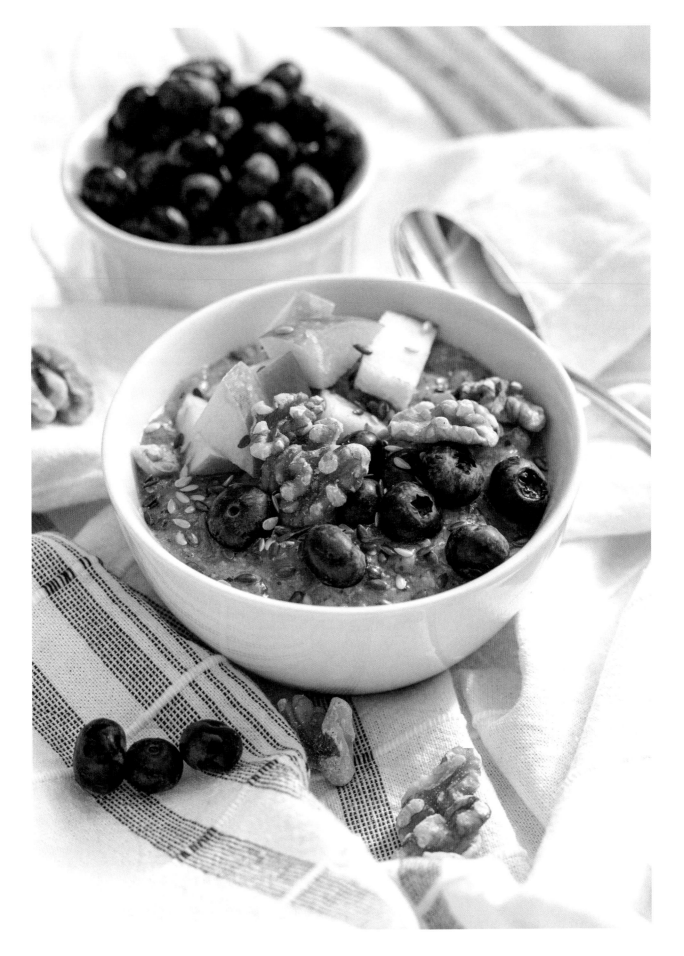

CELEBRATION GRANOLA

MAKES 5 cups
(20 servings)

PREP TIME: 15 minutes

COOK TIME: 50 minutes

This granola is a winner at my house. It quickly got the name Celebration Granola because my kids were uncharacteristically excited to eat granola and its flavors are reminiscent of the fall and winter holidays. And why not start your day with a breakfast that feels special? The combination of spices with blackstrap molasses creates a deeply sweet, satisfying flavor, and the molasses along with nuts and seeds provides an excellent source of plant-based iron, which is essential for all of us, but particularly for growing children and menstruating women. In the *Dr. Katie Detox,* one of our favored pairings is this granola with full-fat coconut yogurt and fresh berries, figs, or persimmons; it creates a small yet satiating breakfast that goes the distance.

---

1 cup raw walnuts

1 cup raw pecans

½ cup raw shelled pumpkin seeds

½ cup raw shelled sunflower seeds

1 cup rolled oats

1 cup unsweetened shredded coconut

1 tablespoon ground cinnamon

2 teaspoons ginger powder

¼ teaspoon ground cardamom

½ teaspoon fine sea salt

½ cup melted virgin coconut oil

¼ cup blackstrap molasses

1 tablespoon honey

1 teaspoon pure vanilla extract

SERVE EACH ¼-CUP PORTION WITH:

⅓ cup full-fat coconut yogurt

¼ cup berries or diced fresh fruit of choice

1. Preheat the oven to 275°F, using the convection setting if your oven has one. Line two rimmed baking sheets with parchment paper.

2. Put the nuts and seeds in a food processor and pulse until roughly chopped. Transfer to a large bowl and stir in the oats, coconut, spices, and salt.

3. Combine the melted coconut oil, molasses, honey, and vanilla extract in a separate cup or bowl. If the mixture is not pourable, warm it over medium-low heat on the stovetop or in the microwave for 10 seconds. Pour over the dry ingredients and mix thoroughly.

4. Spread the granola on the prepared baking sheets. Bake for 45 to 50 minutes, until lightly browned, stirring every 15 minutes to ensure even baking. Remove from the oven and allow to cool completely over several hours. The granola will be soft when warm but will get crunchy as it cools. Store in a large glass jar in the pantry. The granola will stay fresh for up to 2 weeks.

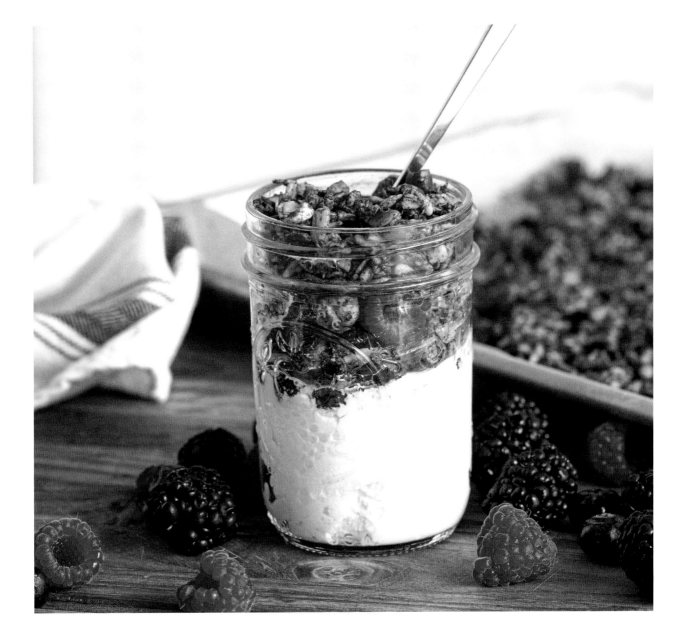

LIFE KITCHEN TIPS:

Using the oven's convection setting gives you granola that is perfectly crispy; in my oven, 45 minutes is just right. Regular baking takes a few minutes longer and results in a somewhat softer texture, but the granola is still delicious. Letting granola cool completely before storing helps keep it crunchy, allowing excess moisture from baking to evaporate as it cools. If your granola is not crunchy when completely cool, it needs to bake for 10 to 15 minutes longer. I use unbleached parchment paper as a makeshift funnel to easily move the granola into a canning jar for storage.

VARIATION:

Celebration Granola Bars. *The secrets to getting granola to stick together in larger chunks for homemade granola bars are adding one egg white while mixing and not stirring during baking. To make granola bars, evenly spread the granola mixture (with one egg white added) over one rimmed baking sheet so that it's about ½ inch thick and bake as directed opposite, without stirring. Once the granola is completely cool, cut into bars.*

SWEET & SAVORY BUTTERNUT SQUASH & SPINACH PORRIDGE

SERVES 4

PREP TIME: 5 minutes

COOK TIME: 30 minutes

It's hard to find ways to build vegetables into traditionally sweet breakfasts, but the combination of naturally sweet squash with a mild, soft green like spinach makes this porridge an easy sell for the whole family. The fiber-rich combination of chewy red quinoa, hearty steel-cut oats, and vegetables along with the satiating fat and protein of almond butter and pumpkin seeds is a well-rounded start to the day. I like to use red quinoa in this recipe for its chewiness and color, but any color of quinoa will work just fine.

½ cup steel-cut oats

½ cup quinoa

3 cups unsweetened plant milk, plus more if needed

½ cup unsweetened canned butternut squash puree

Pinch of kosher salt

2 cups shredded spinach

1 tablespoon ground or whole flax seeds

1 teaspoon ground cinnamon

½ teaspoon pure vanilla extract

TOP EACH SERVING WITH:

1 tablespoon natural almond butter

1 tablespoon raw shelled pumpkin seeds

1 teaspoon unsweetened dried cranberries, or ½ teaspoon honey

1. Place the oats and quinoa in a fine-mesh strainer and rinse under cool running water until clear to remove impurities.

2. Bring the milk to a boil in a medium saucepan over high heat. When boiling, add the oats, quinoa, puree, and salt. Continue to boil for 2 minutes, then reduce the heat to low. Simmer for 15 to 20 minutes, until the porridge is thickened and the milk is absorbed.

3. Remove the porridge from the heat and stir in the spinach, flax, cinnamon, and vanilla. Add more milk as needed to reach the desired consistency.

4. Divide the porridge into bowls. Top with the almond butter, pumpkin seeds, and dried cranberries or honey.

LIFE KITCHEN TIPS:

If you don't have canned butternut squash puree, canned pumpkin works great. We make this recipe fun for the whole family by "decorating" the porridge with a variety of toppings; if you don't have the ones I listed, consider hemp seeds, Celebration Granola (page 238), roasted cashews, and dried tart cherries as some yummy alternatives.

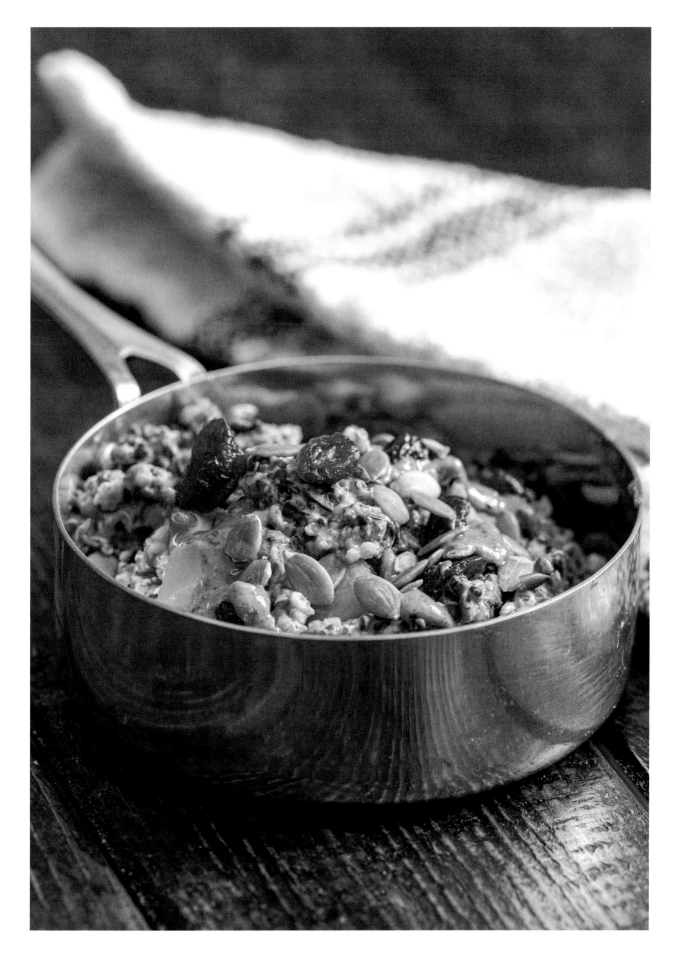

SWEET POTATO PANCAKES

MAKES 10 pancakes

PREP TIME: 10 minutes, plus 20 minutes for batter to rest

COOK TIME: 32 minutes

Using the natural fiber-rich sweetness of sweet potatoes and berries is the best way to enjoy a sweet breakfast that sustains your blood sugar balance. Sweet potatoes are an excellent source of beta-carotene, the plant pigment that gives them their undeniably beautiful orange glow. Beta-carotene is a powerful provitamin antioxidant that in the body is converted to vitamin A, known to support eye health and prevent cellular damage by combating unstable free radicals. Oat bran is especially rich in beta-glucans, a type of soluble fiber that binds cholesterol-rich bile and improves bowel movements. In fact, the 1¾ cups of oat bran in this recipe has an impressive 25 grams of fiber! Cloves are an antimicrobial, detoxifying, antioxidant-rich aromatic spice that gives these pancakes their deep flavor.

1¾ cups gluten-free oat bran

2 teaspoons baking powder

½ teaspoon fine sea salt

1 teaspoon ground cinnamon

⅛ teaspoon ground cloves

1 cup mashed cooked sweet potatoes (about one 8-ounce sweet potato)

¼ cup melted virgin coconut oil, plus more for the pan

2 cups unsweetened plant milk of choice

1 teaspoon pure vanilla extract

TOP EACH SERVING WITH:

2 tablespoons Coconut Whipped Cream (page 334), or 1 tablespoon nut butter of choice

⅓ cup Warm Berry Compote (page 296), freshly made or rewarmed

1. In a large bowl, whisk together the dry ingredients. In a separate bowl, stir together the mashed sweet potatoes, melted coconut oil, milk, and vanilla extract. Pour over the dry ingredients and stir until well combined. Allow the batter to rest in the refrigerator for 20 minutes. It will thicken.

2. Heat a large skillet or griddle over medium-low heat; lightly coat the surface with about ½ tablespoon of coconut oil. Scoop about ¼ cup of the batter onto the pan to make 6-inch pancakes, leaving a bit of space between them. Cook for about 5 minutes, until the edges are golden and the pancakes can be easily lifted with a spatula. Flip and cook for a few minutes more, until cooked through and golden brown. Repeat with the remaining batter, using more coconut oil as needed. You can keep the cooked pancakes warm in a 200°F oven.

3. Serve 2 or 3 pancakes with the coconut whipped cream or nut butter and the compote.

LIFE KITCHEN TIPS:

> *Oat bran is coarser than oat flour and requires more liquid in this recipe. If you don't have oat bran, you can substitute 2 cups of gluten-free oat flour for the oat bran and use a little less plant milk. These pancakes reheat well in the toaster, so making a larger batch on the weekends could make your weekday breakfasts quick and easy.*

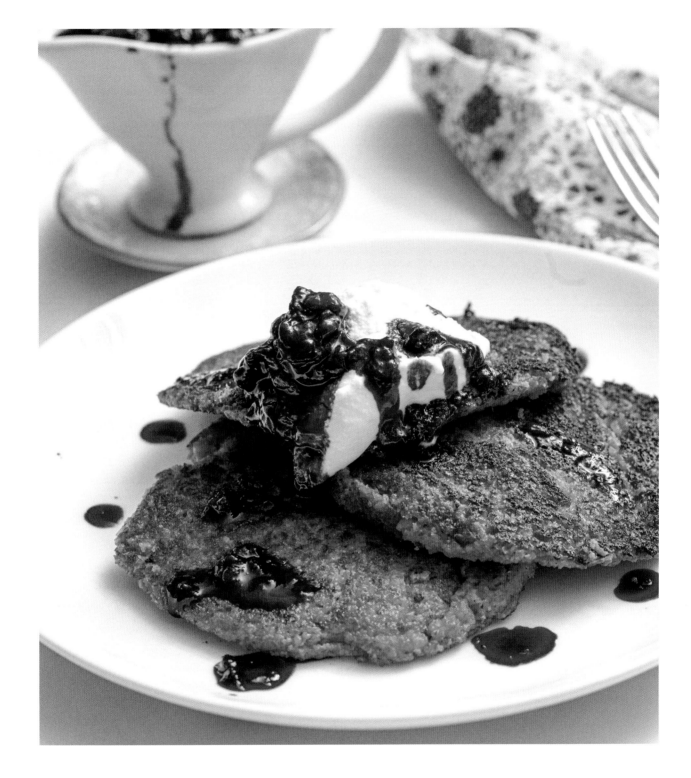

VARIATION:

_____

Breakfast for Dinner. *To make a savory pancake for any time of day, omit the cinnamon and vanilla and sprinkle sliced scallions on the pancake batter after pouring it onto the pan. Serve 2 to 3 pancakes with 1 tablespoon of cashew butter drizzle and garnish with 1 tablespoon of shelled hemp seeds and additional sliced scallions.*

MORNING GLORY MUFFINS

MAKES 10 muffins

PREP TIME: 15 minutes

COOK TIME: 25 minutes

My family loves baked goods, but most muffins are too sweet and leave you hungry and wanting more soon after due to a sharp rise in blood sugar and insulin. These delightful, satiating muffins are the result of literally a dozen batches that my amazing nanny, Angie, and I trialed over the course of a month, and we're confident that this is one of the best muffins out there. The hearty fiber of an apple and carrots combined with the satiating fat of omega-3–rich walnuts, coconut, and ground flax seeds will carry you long into the day. I prefer using a raisin medley to get different varieties and colors of raisins, creating a beautiful muffin that just begs to be enjoyed. These muffins freeze well, so you can make a batch on the weekend and have options for weekdays when you may be more pressed for time.

½ cup raisins

1½ cups hot water

3 tablespoons ground flax seeds

1½ cups oat flour

2 teaspoons baking powder

¼ teaspoon baking soda

½ teaspoon fine sea salt

1½ teaspoons ground cinnamon

1 teaspoon ground cardamom

½ cup unsweetened shredded coconut

½ cup melted virgin coconut oil

2 tablespoons honey

1 teaspoon pure vanilla extract

½ cup chopped toasted walnuts

1¼ cups grated carrots (about 3 carrots)

1 medium apple, peeled and grated

TOP EACH MUFFIN WITH:

1 tablespoon nut butter of choice

¼ cup seasonal berries, crushed, or Warm Berry Compote (page 296)

1. Soak the raisins in the hot water for 10 minutes. (This plumps the raisins and makes the "raisin water" for the flax eggs.) Once done, reserve ¾ cup of the soaking water and drain the raisins.

2. Preheat the oven to 350°F. Line a 12-cup muffin tin with 10 liners.

3. Make the flax eggs: In a small bowl, whisk together the ground flax seeds with the reserved raisin water and let it sit in the refrigerator for 10 minutes to thicken.

4. Meanwhile, put the oat flour, baking powder, baking soda, salt, cinnamon, cardamom, and shredded coconut in a large bowl and whisk to combine.

5. When the flax eggs are ready, add the melted coconut oil, honey, and vanilla extract to the bowl with the flax eggs and stir well. Add the wet ingredients to the flour mixture and stir just until combined. Fold in the plumped raisins, walnuts, carrots, and apple.

6. Scoop the batter evenly into the lined muffin cups, filling each nearly to the top. Bake for 20 to 25 minutes, until the tops of the muffins are firm and golden. Transfer the pan to a wire rack to cool for about 15 minutes, then remove the muffins and let them cool to room temperature. Serve with the nut butter and crushed berries or compote.

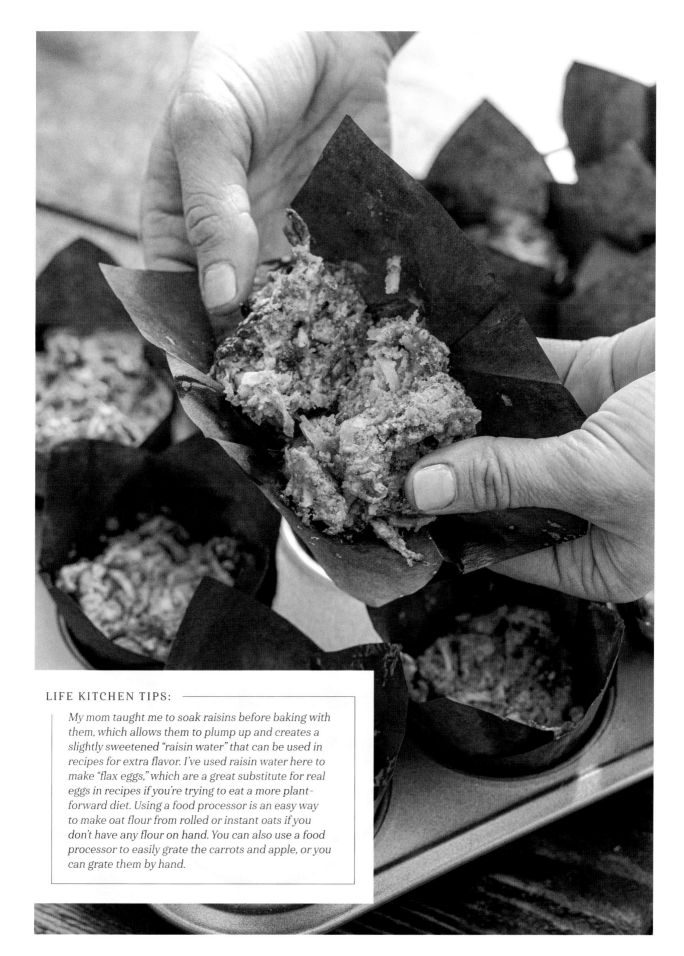

LIFE KITCHEN TIPS:

My mom taught me to soak raisins before baking with them, which allows them to plump up and creates a slightly sweetened "raisin water" that can be used in recipes for extra flavor. I've used raisin water here to make "flax eggs," which are a great substitute for real eggs in recipes if you're trying to eat a more plant-forward diet. Using a food processor is an easy way to make oat flour from rolled or instant oats if you don't have any flour on hand. You can also use a food processor to easily grate the carrots and apple, or you can grate them by hand.

OMEGA AVOCADO TOAST

SERVES 2

PREP TIME: 5 minutes (not including time to make bread)

COOK TIME: 5 minutes

Almost everyone loves avocado toast, so why not use it as a vehicle to deliver hearty vegetables and anti-inflammatory omega-3 fats? Shelled hemp seeds, also called hemp hearts, are a powerhouse of nutrition, packing all nine essential amino acids along with minerals (iron, magnesium, and zinc), omega-3–rich fats, and fiber into a lovely, nutty little package. While related to the cannabis plant, hemp seeds have nothing to do with the psychoactive compound THC found in marijuana and in normal quantities are not potent enough to cause the effects of CBD, making them safe and nutritious for the whole family.

---

4 slices Whole-Grain Nut & Seed Bread (page 294)

1 Hass avocado, halved, pitted, and peeled

Coarse or flaky sea salt and freshly ground black pepper

1 cup roasted vegetables of choice (page 286)

2 teaspoons tahini

2 tablespoons raw shelled hemp seeds or dukkah from Spiced Nut Mix (page 326)

1 radish, thinly sliced, for garnish

Crushed red pepper, for garnish (optional)

Toast the bread slices. Mash the avocado flesh with a fork, then spread it on the toast. Sprinkle the avocado spread with salt and pepper to taste. Top with a single layer of roasted vegetables. Drizzle with the tahini and sprinkle with the hemp seeds or dukkah. Garnish with the radish slices and crushed red pepper, if desired. Serve right away.

LIFE KITCHEN TIP:

Toasting the bread before topping it with avocado and vegetables not only creates a more rigid delivery vehicle for all of your plant goodness, but it tastes better, too. Toasting bread is similar to the caramelization of roasting vegetables or the browning of meat and happens due to the Maillard reaction, a chemical change that creates new flavors and aromas from the combination of amino acids and sugars in food when heated.

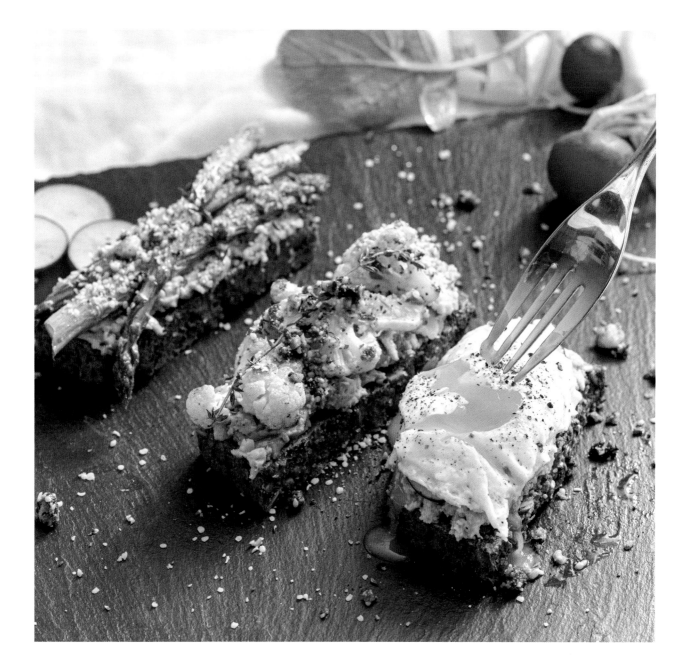

VARIATIONS:

- Top the seasoned avocado spread with thinly sliced radishes, an over-easy or poached egg, and shelled hemp seeds.

- Top the seasoned avocado spread and roasted vegetables with thinly sliced browned tofu and dukkah from the Spiced Nut Mix (page 326).

- Top the seasoned avocado spread with high-quality smoked wild salmon, thinly sliced cucumbers, shelled hemp seeds, juice of a lemon wedge, capers, and chopped fresh dill.

- Don't have avocado? Spread the toast with unsalted natural cashew butter instead and top with roasted vegetables, shelled hemp seeds, and crushed red pepper.

*To make this recipe *Dr. Katie Detox* friendly, omit the crushed red pepper.

RECOVERY SMOOTHIE

SERVES 1

PREP TIME: 10 minutes

This recipe is written by a woman who changed my life: my sleep therapist. Dr. Shelby Harris teaches Cognitive Behavioral Therapy for Insomnia (CBT-I), which revolutionized my relationship with sleep. I wrote a guest chapter in her book *The Women's Guide to Overcoming Insomnia.*[1] She created this smoothie to enhance muscle recovery after exercise, combined with the magic of a good night's sleep.

"As a sleep psychologist, I'm passionate about getting the most out of my sleep at night. I also love to exercise for stress relief and have completed fifteen marathons. Three years ago, I started weight training twice weekly to help with injury prevention and bone density. I used to think that a simple exercise session did not require any fuel afterward, but when I thoughtfully added this post-workout smoothie rich with protein, healthy fats, and replenishing carbohydrates, I found that I felt even better overall and recovered faster from a challenging long run, speedwork, or weightlifting session. Sleep is also important for muscle building, performance improvement, and restoration. During the deepest stages of sleep, most of which happens during the first third of the night, our bodies generate new cells and restore themselves from the day's work. Enjoying this smoothie in the morning after a good night's sleep is the best recipe for me to get the most out of my workouts."

Since cacao nibs have a little caffeine in them, omit the nibs if you are enjoying this smoothie later in the day to preserve your sleep architecture at night.

---

1 cup unsweetened plant milk

½ cup organic silken tofu

1½ heaping cups baby spinach

½ heaping cup frozen banana slices (about ½ medium banana)

1 tablespoon unsalted natural cashew butter

Juice of 1 lemon wedge (optional) (see Tips)

1 teaspoon unsweetened cacao nibs, or 1 heaping tablespoon Celebration Granola (page 238), for garnish (optional)

Put all of the ingredients in a blender and pulse until smooth. Garnish with the cacao nibs or granola, if desired.

LIFE KITCHEN TIPS:

> *Eat your bananas while they are still a little green on the stem to optimize their taste and balance their effect on your blood sugar. This is the ideal time to freeze them as well. Adding a squeeze of lemon juice preserves this smoothie's green color if you're making it ahead of time.*

---

[1] S. Harris, *The Women's Guide to Overcoming Insomnia: Get a Good Night's Sleep Without Relying on Medication* (New York: W. W. Norton Books, 2019): 175–97.

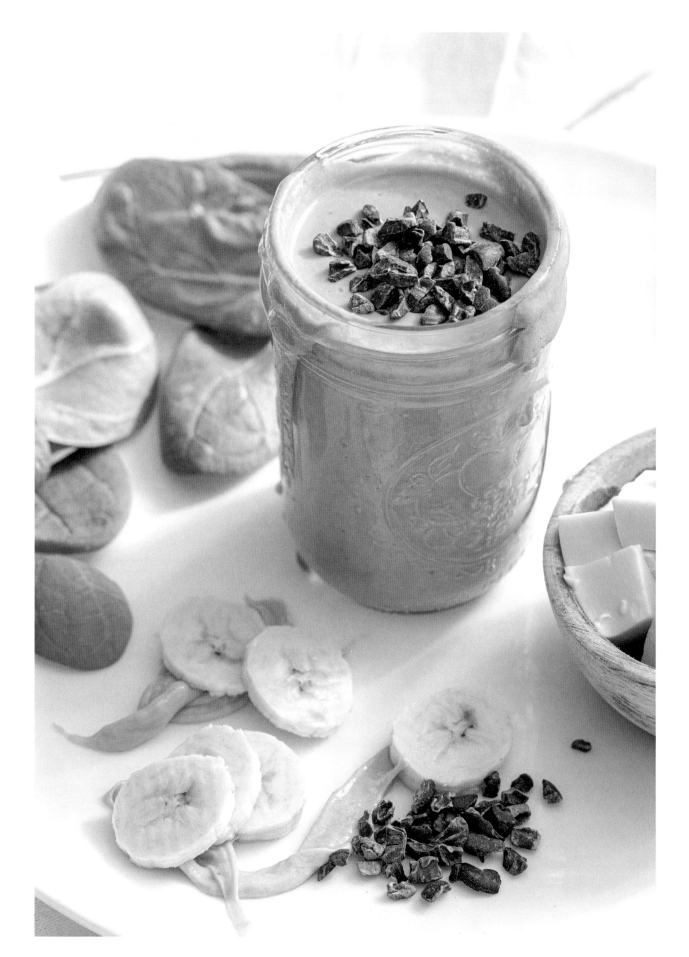

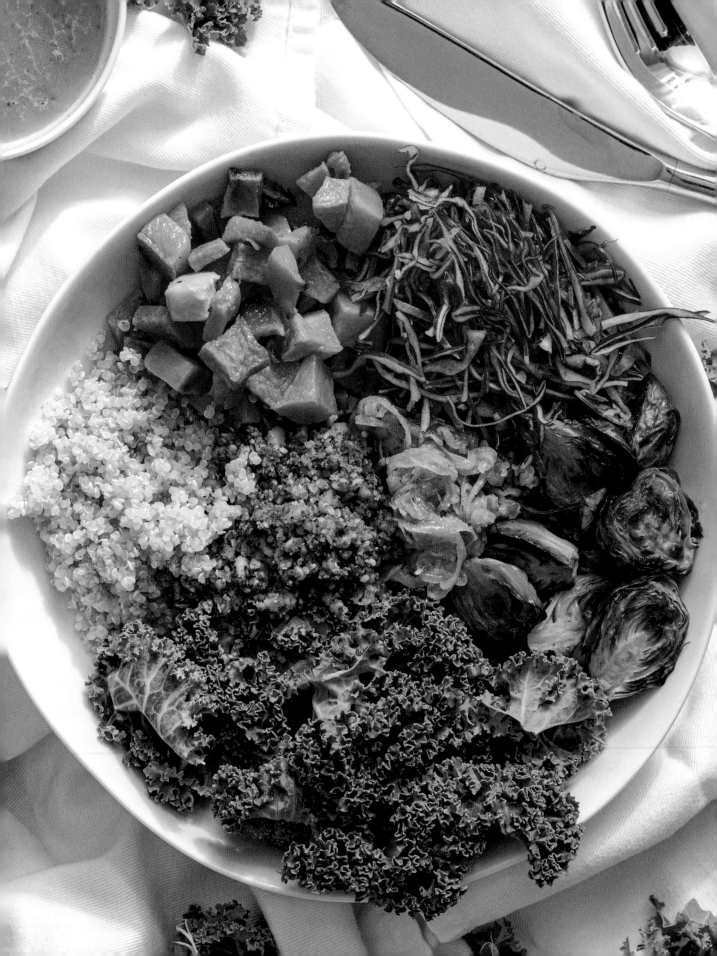

MIDDAY RECIPES

BREAK FOR NOURISHMENT
THAT WILL CARRY YOU
THROUGH YOUR DAY

KALE & QUINOA GREEK SALAD

SERVES 6
PREP TIME: 30 minutes
COOK TIME: 20 minutes

Almost nothing brings me more joy than a lunchtime break with a satisfying mouthful of hearty kale salad. Kale salads are a busy person's best friend because they hold up well in the refrigerator for several days, so you can prepare a large batch and have leftovers. While all parsley offers an anti-inflammatory benefit, I like curly parsley in this salad because it also holds up well. Featuring quinoa cooked with bone broth, this salad is a powerhouse of nutrition. Quinoa is a complete plant-based protein, meaning it has all of the essential amino acids your body needs to maintain its muscle mass, but when prepared with protein-rich broth, it's extra supportive. The olives and feta add a salty depth of flavor that keeps you from reaching for the salt shaker, which is good for blood pressure management along with magnesium-rich kale.

SALAD:

¼ cup minced red onions

⅔ cup quinoa

1 cup organic chicken bone broth

6 cups destemmed and chopped kale

2 cups chopped fresh curly parsley

2 cups cubed roasted beets or halved grape tomatoes

2 cups chopped celery

1 (15-ounce) can chickpeas, drained and rinsed

½ cup pitted halved Kalamata olives

½ cup toasted pine nuts

¼ cup crumbled organic feta cheese (optional)

GREEK DRESSING:

⅓ cup extra-virgin olive oil

2 tablespoons red wine vinegar

4 cloves garlic, minced

1 tablespoon minced fresh oregano, or 1 teaspoon dried oregano leaves

1½ tablespoons Dijon mustard

¼ teaspoon freshly ground black pepper

¼ teaspoon fine sea salt

1. Place the onions in a bowl of cool water to soak. Set aside.

2. Rinse and cook the quinoa according to the Hearty Whole Grains recipe (page 290) using the bone broth. Allow to cool before adding the quinoa to the salad.

3. Meanwhile, prepare the dressing: Put the ingredients in a lidded jar and shake to combine. Place the kale and parsley in a large bowl, pour the dressing over them, and massage for 30 seconds, or until the kale is softened.

4. Drain the onions and add them to the kale and parsley along with the quinoa, beets, celery, chickpeas, olives, pine nuts, and feta, if using. Toss to combine.

* To make this salad *Dr. Katie Detox* friendly, use beets instead of tomatoes and omit the feta.

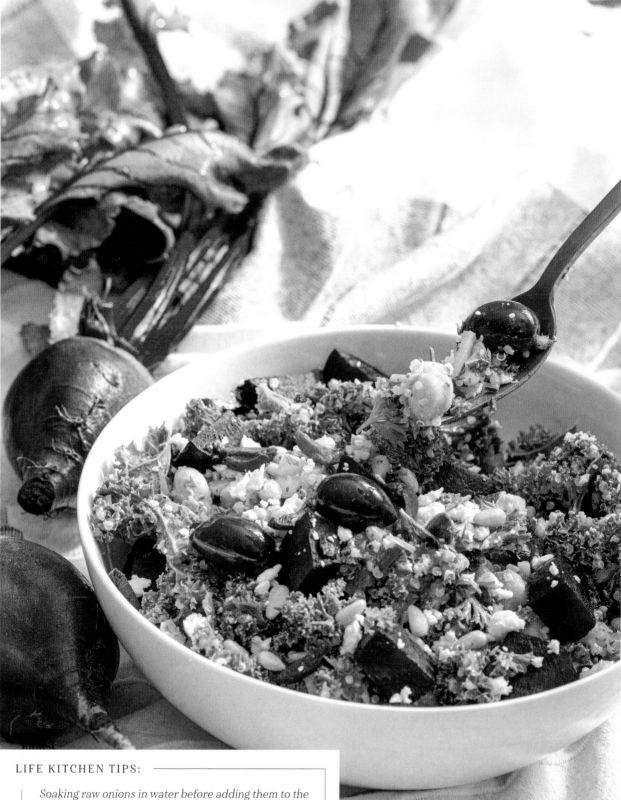

ARUGULA & LENTIL SALAD

SERVES 4

PREP TIME: 25 minutes

COOK TIME: 20 minutes

I really wanted to call this a "Menstrual Health Salad" because it's perfect during the first few days of the menstrual period when female hormones need support. Celery works as a diuretic, which helps with uncomfortable bloating, and provides a salty, satisfying crunch. Pumpkin seeds and walnuts (along with the flax seeds on the Coriander & Flax Roasted Eggplant) are plant-based sources of omega-3 fatty acids, which support estrogen from the start of the period to ovulation. Bitter greens, like arugula, watercress, radicchio, endive, and dandelion, are great for enhancing the body's natural detoxification. And kombu is a sea vegetable that eases digestion and bloating from plant proteins. In short, you'll feel better after you eat this salad! If you're curious about seed cycling and its effects on menstrual health, check out the Spiced Nut Mix recipe on page 326.

---

1 cup green or brown lentils

1 (2-inch) piece kombu

2 cloves garlic, minced

1 bay leaf

2 cups water

Grated zest and juice of ½ lemon

½ teaspoon fine sea salt

¼ teaspoon freshly ground black pepper

8 cups arugula (about 5 ounces)

½ cup chopped celery

¼ cup toasted shelled pumpkin seeds

¼ cup chopped toasted walnuts

1 crisp apple, cored and chopped

½ batch Coriander & Flax Roasted Eggplant (page 280)

WHITE BALSAMIC LEMON DRESSING *(makes ¹/₂ cup)*:

¼ cup extra-virgin olive oil

Juice of ½ lemon

2 tablespoons white balsamic vinegar

1 teaspoon whole-grain or Dijon mustard

½ to 1 teaspoon honey, to taste

¼ teaspoon fine sea salt

1. Rinse the lentils in a strainer under running water. Combine the rinsed lentils, kombu, garlic, bay leaf, and water in a medium saucepan. Bring to a rapid simmer over medium-high heat, then reduce the heat to low and simmer, uncovered, for about 20 minutes, until the liquid is absorbed and the lentils are tender. Stir in the lemon zest and juice, salt, and pepper while the lentils are still warm. Allow the seasoned lentils to cool, then discard the kombu and bay leaf.

2. Whisk the dressing ingredients together in a small bowl.

3. Combine the lentils, arugula, celery, pumpkin seeds, walnuts, apple, and eggplant in a large bowl and toss with enough dressing to coat. Leftover dressing will keep in the refrigerator for up to a week.

* To make this salad Dr. Katie Detox friendly, substitute mushrooms for the eggplant as explained on page 280.

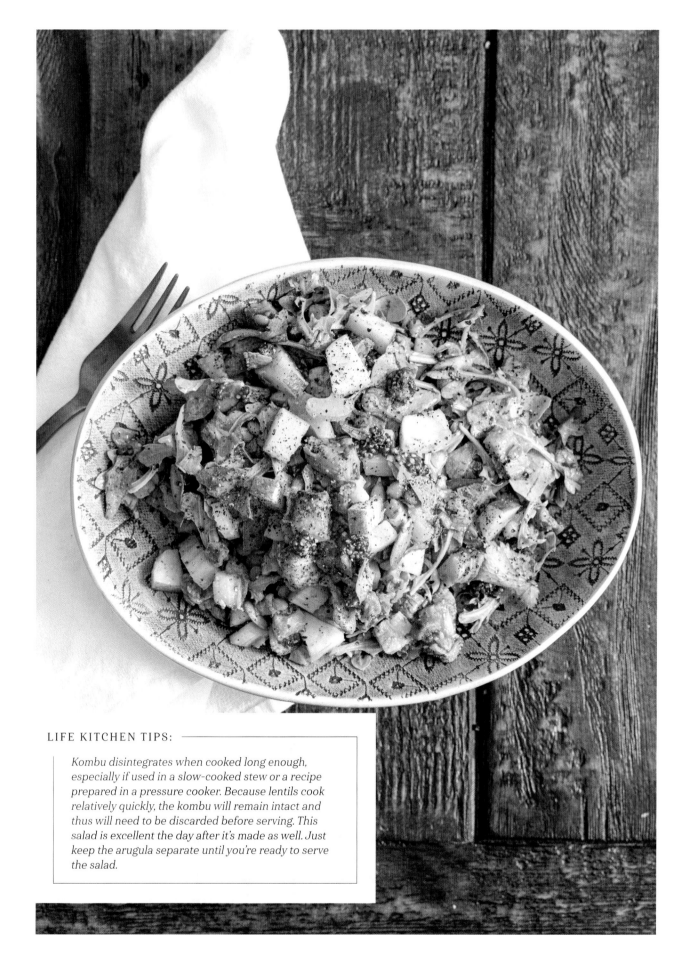

LIFE KITCHEN TIPS:

Kombu disintegrates when cooked long enough, especially if used in a slow-cooked stew or a recipe prepared in a pressure cooker. Because lentils cook relatively quickly, the kombu will remain intact and thus will need to be discarded before serving. This salad is excellent the day after it's made as well. Just keep the arugula separate until you're ready to serve the salad.

CREAMY ROASTED BROCCOLI SOUP

SERVES 8
PREP TIME: 15 minutes
COOK TIME: 25 minutes

This soup is a pleaser for the whole family and reheats well, making it ideal for a leftover lunch on a busy day. Kids love the mild flavor, and adults love the nod to a traditionally decadent cream-based soup that comes from the pureed cannellini beans. Beans also pack a punch of plant-based protein and filling fiber to keep you satiated. Getting adequate dietary iodine has become harder since so many of us have switched from traditional iodized salt to less-refined kosher and natural sea salts, so adding iodine-rich sea vegetable flakes to this soup is an easy way to incorporate an essential mineral for thyroid health. Kombu is also helpful for reducing intestinal discomfort from legumes.

---

2 heads broccoli (about 1¼ pounds)

¼ cup plus 2 tablespoons extra-virgin olive oil, divided

1¼ teaspoons fine sea salt, divided

½ teaspoon freshly ground black pepper

5 cloves garlic, minced, divided

2 medium yellow or white onions, chopped

3 cups organic chicken bone broth

1 to 3 cups water (see Tips)

1 red-skinned potato, peeled and cut into 1-inch pieces

1 (29-ounce) can cannellini beans, drained and rinsed

1 (3-inch) piece kombu

Juice of 1 lemon

1 teaspoon dulse or kelp granules

3 to 4 tablespoons nutritional yeast (see Tips)

TOP EACH SERVING WITH:

A few roasted broccoli florets (from above)

¼ cup Whole Grain Nut & Seed Croutons or Crackers (page 295)

¼ cup microgreens

1 tablespoon shelled hemp seeds or toasted sunflower seeds

Crushed red pepper (optional)

1. Preheat the oven to 400°F and line a rimmed baking sheet with parchment paper.

2. Remove and discard the tough lower stalk of each head of broccoli and peel the remaining stalk. Chop the peeled stalks into ½-inch pieces and the florets into 1-inch pieces to yield about 8 cups. Toss the broccoli with ¼ cup of the olive oil, ½ teaspoon of the salt, the pepper, and four-fifths of the minced garlic, then spread out on the prepared baking sheet. Roast for 20 minutes, until golden brown and tender. Set aside.

3. Meanwhile, heat the remaining 2 tablespoons of oil in a stockpot over medium heat. Add the onions and sauté until translucent, about 10 minutes. Add the remaining minced garlic and sauté for a minute more, until fragrant.

4. Add the bone broth and water and bring to a boil. Add the potato pieces, beans, remaining ¾ teaspoon of salt, and the kombu and reduce the heat to medium-low. Simmer for about 10 minutes, until the potatoes are tender.

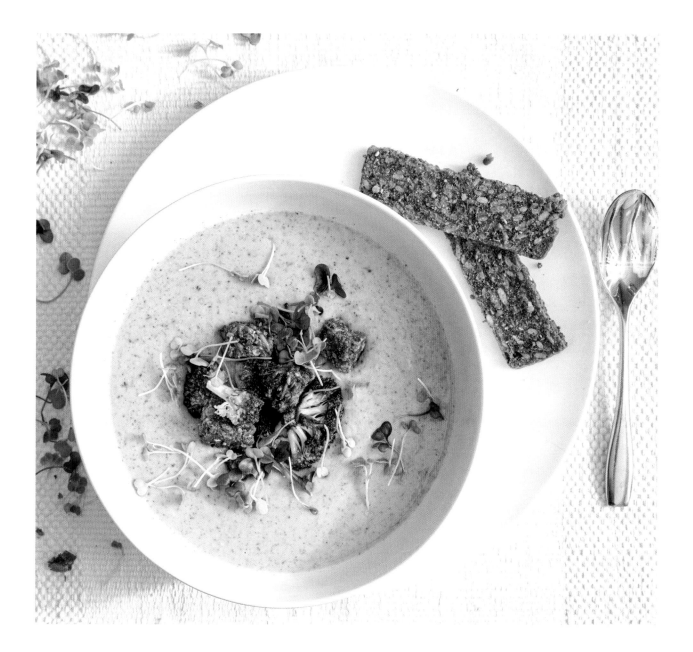

5. Remove the soup from the heat and stir in the lemon juice, dulse, nutritional yeast, and half of the roasted broccoli.

6. Puree the soup with an immersion blender until smooth. If you don't have an immersion blender, carefully transfer the soup in batches to a countertop blender. Once smooth, add all of the remaining roasted broccoli stems and about half of the remaining roasted florets and pulse lightly to leave a few chunkier pieces, if desired.

7. Ladle the soup into bowls and garnish with the remaining roasted broccoli florets, the croutons or crackers, microgreens, and seeds. Sprinkle with crushed red pepper, if desired.

*To make this soup *Dr. Katie Detox* friendly, omit the crushed red pepper.

ROOTS & GREENS SALAD

SERVES 4

PREP TIME: 25 minutes (not including time to cook quinoa)

COOK TIME: 25 minutes

Roots & Greens came to life as a collaboration with my dear friend Lisa Clarke, the chef of Soirée Catering and the *Dr. Katie Detox.* We chose the title based on the gorgeous plant ingredients, but now I think Roots & Greens perfectly describes my grounded Irish friend who always greets the day with optimism. I met Lisa at a playdate with our toddlers in 2013, she's since become my go-to gal for all food needs from catering my annual Hygge party to being the muscle behind the meal delivery for our Dr. Katie Detoxers. This light, bright salad uses a sweet lemon dressing to enhance the natural sweetness of the caramelized onions and vegetables. It is midday nourishment that will put a spring in your step and keep you humming all afternoon.

---

2 tablespoons extra-virgin olive oil, divided

2 cups shaved Brussels sprouts

¼ teaspoon fine sea salt, divided

¼ teaspoon freshly ground black pepper, divided

2 cups peeled and ½-inch-diced butternut squash

1 red onion, thinly sliced

6 cups destemmed and roughly chopped kale

1 cup chopped purple cabbage

1 cup cooked and cooled quinoa from Hearty Whole Grains (page 290)

½ cup toasted sliced almonds or dukkah from Spiced Nut Mix (page 326)

SWEET LEMON DRESSING:

¼ cup extra-virgin olive oil

Juice of 1 lemon

2 tablespoons white balsamic vinegar

1 tablespoon plus 1 teaspoon honey

Fine sea salt and freshly ground black pepper, to taste

1. Preheat the oven to 425°F. Line two rimmed baking sheets with parchment paper.

2. In a medium bowl, toss ½ tablespoon of the olive oil with the shaved Brussels sprouts, ⅛ teaspoon of the salt, and ⅛ teaspoon of the pepper and spread in an even layer on one baking sheet. Using the same bowl, toss ½ tablespoon of the olive oil with the butternut squash, the remaining ⅛ teaspoon of the salt, and the remaining ⅛ teaspoon of the pepper and spread in an even layer on the second baking sheet. Place both baking sheets in the oven and roast for 10 to 25 minutes, until golden brown. Check the Brussels sprouts after 10 minutes since they will roast quickly, and continue to roast the squash until soft in the center. (Alternatively, roast the Brussels sprouts and squash using the method for Easy Roasted Vegetables on page 286.)

3. In a large skillet, heat the remaining tablespoon of olive oil over medium-low heat and add the sliced onion. Allow to cook slowly, stirring every so often to prevent burning, until the onion slices turn a rich brown color.

4. While the onion is caramelizing, place the kale and cabbage in separate bowls. Whisk the dressing ingredients together in a small bowl and pour over the kale and cabbage. Massage the kale and cabbage with the dressing for 30 seconds.

5. Divide the salad components among four bowls and top with the caramelized onions and nuts.

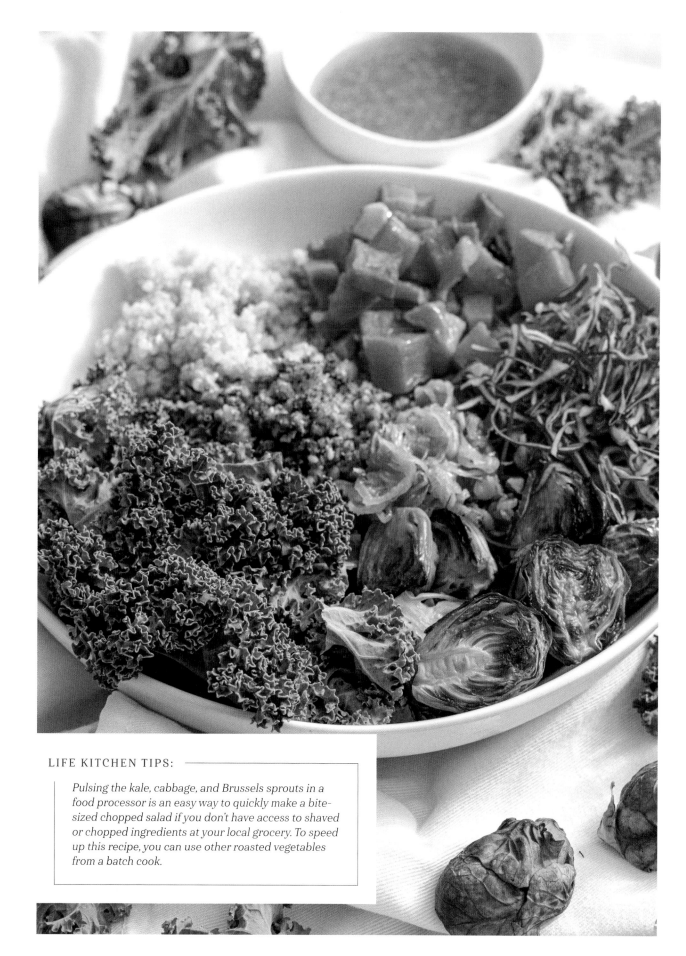

LIFE KITCHEN TIPS:

Pulsing the kale, cabbage, and Brussels sprouts in a food processor is an easy way to quickly make a bite-sized chopped salad if you don't have access to shaved or chopped ingredients at your local grocery. To speed up this recipe, you can use other roasted vegetables from a batch cook.

INTENSIVE SALAD SHAKER

SERVES 2

PREP TIME: 25 minutes (not including time to cook millet)

Salad shakers are one of the many beloved and bespoke recipes in the five-day get-down-to-business *Dr. Katie Detox Intensive.* Integrative Health Coach Courtney Evans concocted the very first salad shaker, and when I saw it brought to life by Chef Lisa Clarke, I was starstruck by the pure beauty of how fresh ingredients could come together to create a truly artistic presentation in an ordinary mason jar. Our Detoxers love salad shakers so much that they've texted us, "Nothing can go wrong on Salad Shaker Day!" And it's true—even if I get buried at work in a mountain of patient care, I know my thirty-minute midday break will be celebrated with the pure delight of a salad shaker.

⅓ cup cooked and cooled millet from Hearty Whole Grains (page 290)

⅔ cup shelled edamame

⅓ cup pitted Kalamata olives

⅓ cup shredded cooked beets

⅓ cup chopped artichoke hearts

⅓ cup shredded purple cabbage

⅓ cup diced cucumbers

4 watermelon radishes, cut into julienne or thinly sliced

⅔ cup shredded or chopped romaine lettuce

⅓ cup shredded carrots

⅓ cup toasted shelled pistachios

¼ cup dried unsweetened cranberries

2 tablespoons shelled hemp seeds

¼ cup Carrot Ginger Dressing (page 298), for serving

1. Divide the ingredients evenly between two 28-ounce mason jars, layering them in the order listed, starting with the millet and finishing with the hemp seeds. Leave some room at the tops of the containers for shaking.

2. When ready to serve, add 2 tablespoons of the dressing to each salad shaker and shake until thoroughly combined.

LIFE KITCHEN TIPS:

Buying frozen shelled edamame and a package of precooked beets makes kitchen prep a lot easier. Batch-cooking the millet according to the Hearty Whole Grains recipe is also helpful and provides easy leftovers for another meal. You can make enough salad shakers and dressing for several days and store them in the refrigerator until ready to serve.

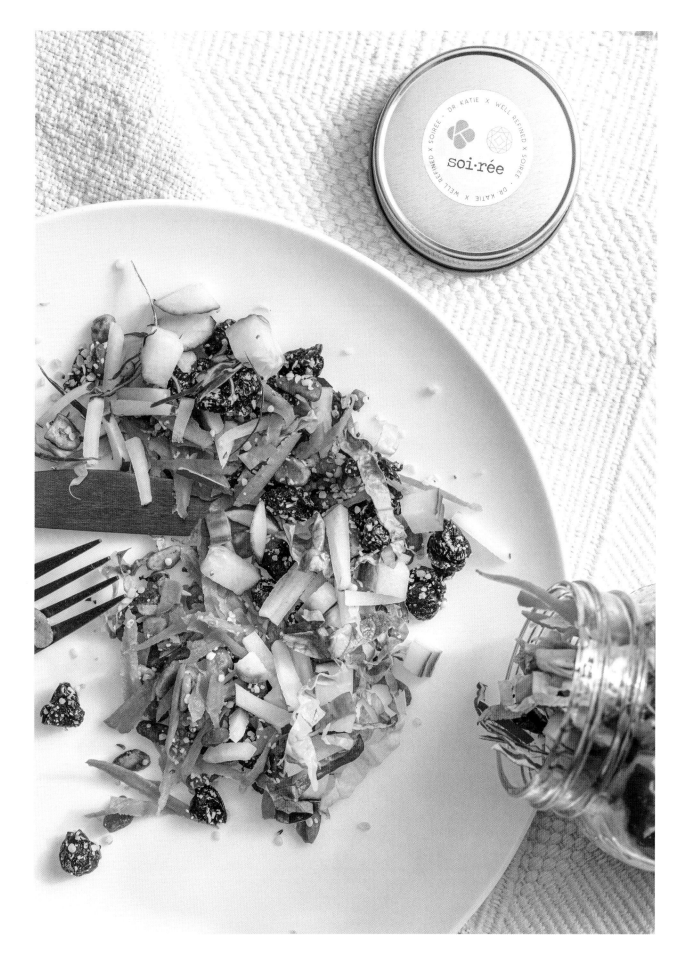

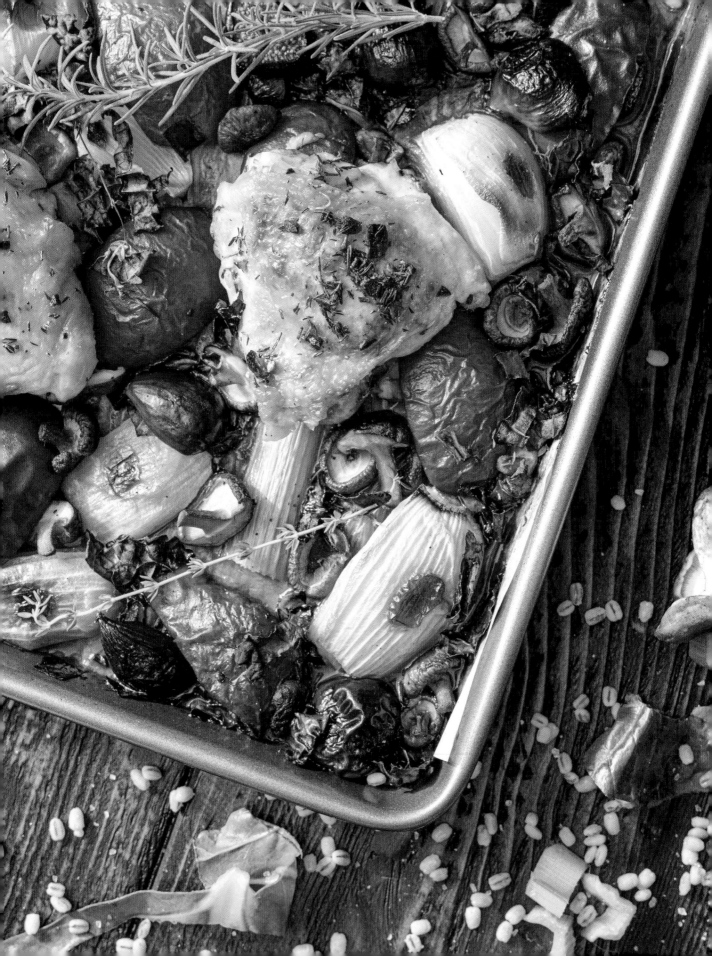

SUPPER RECIPES

 END YOUR DAY FEELING
SATIATED BEFORE REST

SHEET PAN ROASTED CHICKEN WITH PEARS, FIGS & SWISS CHARD

SERVES 4

PREP TIME: 20 minutes

COOK TIME: 30 minutes

I love a sheet pan dinner, especially on a Sunday evening when hosting friends, because it allows me to be present with my guests while our food is in the oven. I recommend leaving the skin on the chicken to retain moisture while roasting but then removing it prior to eating to avoid the inflammatory animal fat. Fresh figs are a gorgeous seasonal fruit rich in vitamin B_6 and copper, both essential for brain health and mood maintenance. I like Mission figs because they are sweeter and juicier than other varieties.

---

3 tablespoons extra-virgin olive oil

2 cloves garlic, minced

4 tablespoons fresh rosemary leaves, or 4 teaspoons dried, divided

4 tablespoons fresh thyme leaves, or 4 teaspoons dried, divided

½ teaspoon kosher salt

½ teaspoon freshly ground black pepper

2 medium yellow onions, quartered

4 stalks celery, cut into 4-inch lengths

2 cups shiitake mushrooms, sliced

1 large bunch Swiss chard, stems roughly chopped into ½-inch pieces and leaves sliced into ribbons

2 cups fresh Mission figs, halved

4 small pears, cored and halved or quartered

4 bone-in, skin-on organic chicken thighs (about 1½ pounds)

⅔ cup barley or farro

1. Preheat the oven to 350°F. Line a rimmed baking sheet with parchment paper.

2. Whisk together the olive oil, garlic, half of the rosemary and thyme, the salt, and pepper.

3. Toss the vegetables and fruit in a large bowl with the olive oil mixture. Arrange the celery stalks evenly on the prepared baking sheet, then spread the remaining produce around the pan, placing the onions, figs, and pears cut side down.

4. Lift the skin gently from the chicken and rub both the skin and the underlying meat with the remaining half of the herbs. Replace the skin and nestle the chicken into the vegetables on the baking sheet.

5. Roast for 30 minutes, or until the vegetables are tender and the chicken skin is golden brown and the meat is cooked through. When done, the juices of the chicken should run clear, and the internal temperature should be close to 165°F. You may need to remove the Swiss chard leaves or other produce and cook the chicken longer depending on the size of the chicken thighs.

6. Meanwhile, cook the barley or farro according to the Hearty Whole Grains recipe (page 290).

7. To serve, remove and discard the chicken skin. Divide the vegetables and barley or farro among four plates and top with the chicken.

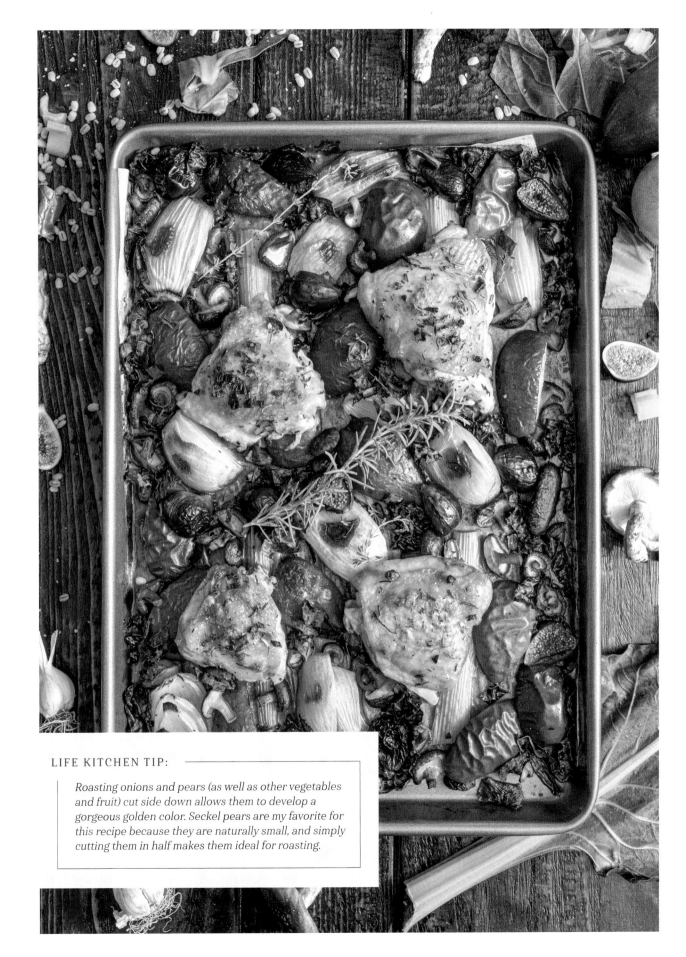

THAI COCONUT CURRY NOODLE SOUP

SERVES 6

PREP TIME: 30 minutes, plus time to press tofu

COOK TIME: 30 minutes

Here's some cultural fusion for you! We love Thai curry at my house, and it's a favorite treat to order as takeout. My kids will eat anything with noodles in it. We often use soba as our noodle of choice because it's wheat free, is a nice source of the B vitamin thiamine, and has a hearty texture. *Soba* is Japanese for buckwheat, and it's hot on the Japanese food scene, making appearances everywhere from street food walk-ups to fine dining restaurants. It is traditionally served on New Year's Eve in Japan because its long noodles signify a long life. *Soba* is usually served cold or in a warm soy-based broth that isn't very hearty, but this recipe combines the richness of coconut milk and fiber-rich vegetables, filling your tummy and sending satiety signals to your brain before retiring for the evening.

---

1 (14-ounce) package organic extra-firm tofu

2 tablespoons virgin coconut oil, divided

1 bunch scallions, sliced, white bottoms and green tops separated

4 cloves garlic, minced

1 tablespoon grated fresh ginger

2 cups finely diced carrots

2 cups chopped shiitake mushrooms

4 cups chopped bok choy (about 1 pound), white stems and green tops separated

1½ teaspoons fine sea salt

1 tablespoon plus 1 teaspoon Intensive Thai Spice Mix (page 302), divided

4 cups chicken bone broth

1 cup water

1 tablespoon coconut aminos

1 tablespoon fish sauce

½ (8-ounce) package 100% buckwheat soba noodles

1 (13.5-ounce) can full-fat, unsweetened coconut milk

¼ cup chopped fresh basil leaves

¼ cup chopped fresh cilantro leaves, plus more for garnish

1 lime, cut into 6 wedges

1. Press the tofu for a minimum of 10 minutes and up to 24 hours (see page 221 for tips).

2. Heat a soup pot over medium heat. Melt 1 tablespoon of the coconut oil in the pot, then add the white parts of the scallions and sauté until translucent. Add some water if the bottom of the pot seems dry.

3. Add the garlic, ginger, and carrots and sauté for a few minutes more. Add the mushrooms, bok choy stems, salt, and 1 tablespoon of the Thai spice mix and stir to combine.

4. Pour in the broth and water and bring the soup to a boil over high heat. Lower the heat to medium, add the coconut aminos and fish sauce, and continue to cook until the vegetables begin to soften but are not fully cooked, about 10 minutes.

5. Meanwhile, cut the pressed tofu into ½-inch cubes and toss with the remaining teaspoon of Intensive Thai spice mix. Heat the remaining tablespoon of coconut oil in a large skillet over medium heat. Sear the tofu for about 5 minutes per side, until golden brown. Remove the pan from the heat.

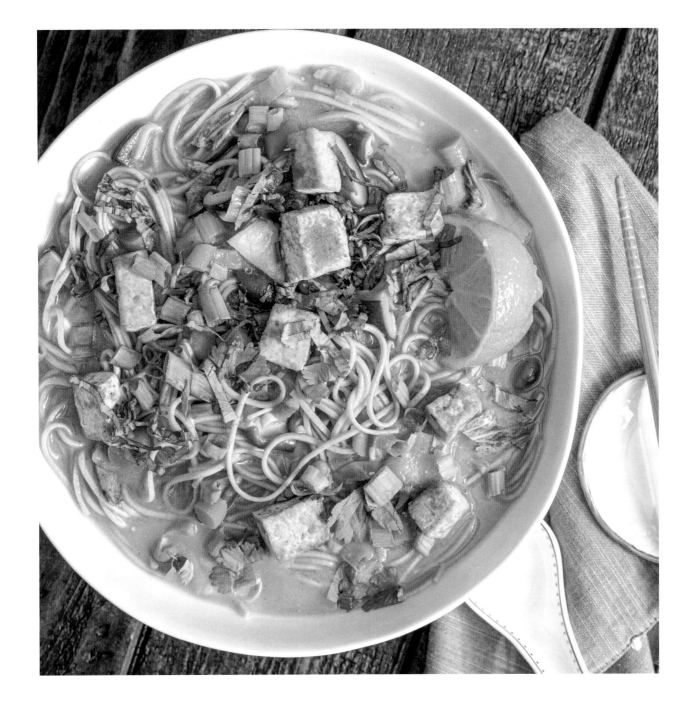

Consider eating this soup with chopsticks. I find that chopsticks slow me down when eating, helping my brain to recognize satiety signals more easily. Enjoy this soup as a leftover by adding fresh soba noodles when reheating.

6. When the vegetables are beginning to soften but not fully cooked, add the soba noodles to the soup and cook for the length of time suggested in the package instructions, usually about 8 minutes.

7. When the soba and vegetables are tender, remove the pot from the heat. Add the bok choy leaves, seared tofu, coconut milk, basil, and cilantro and stir to combine. Garnish each serving with the green scallion tops and additional cilantro and serve with a wedge of lime.

ALMOND FURIKAKE CRUSTED HALIBUT WITH ROASTED VEGETABLES, BLACK RICE & COCONUT LIME CREAM

SERVES 4

PREP TIME: 15 minutes

COOK TIME: 45 minutes

I was introduced to furikake when I had dinner at Jun's house for the first time in 2001. My future mother-in-law, Keiko, served me a little bowl of warm white rice with tiny black specks in it that were salty, spicy, and a bit reminiscent of the umami flavor of fish. Because a lot of commercially available furikake contains sugar and monosodium glutamate (MSG), I was inspired to reimagine a furikake using almonds, sesame seeds, and roasted nori. Roasted nori is an amazing source of iodine and comes in snack packs, making it easy to keep fresh for small-batch furikake or a midday nibble. This recipe, with its crisp furikake coating, is my healthier take on fried fish, combining the omega-3s in skin-on halibut with a bright, satiating coconut cream sauce served on a bed of antioxidant-rich black rice and roasted vegetables. Black rice is often packaged as "forbidden rice" because in ancient China it was reserved for the aristocracy, but I love its chewy texture so much that it's made its way into my family's everyday meals.

---

1 (1-pound) skin-on wild halibut fillet, cut into 4 portions

4 cups Brussels sprouts, halved if small or quartered if large

4 tablespoons melted virgin coconut oil, divided

1 (2½-pound) kabocha squash, cut into ½-inch cubes (about 4 cups)

¼ teaspoon garlic powder

1 teaspoon fine sea salt, divided, plus more for the fish

½ teaspoon freshly ground black pepper, divided

1 cup black rice

1½ cups water

1 cup full-fat, unsweetened canned coconut milk, divided

1 tablespoon plus 1 teaspoon coconut aminos

Grated zest and juice of ½ lime, plus lime wedges for serving if desired

½ teaspoon arrowroot flour

½ small bunch scallions, green tops sliced, for garnish

ALMOND FURIKAKE:

2 tablespoons finely ground almonds or almond meal

2 tablespoons black sesame seeds

4 (2 by 3-inch) sheets roasted nori, crumbled

¼ teaspoon fine sea salt

½ teaspoon crushed red pepper

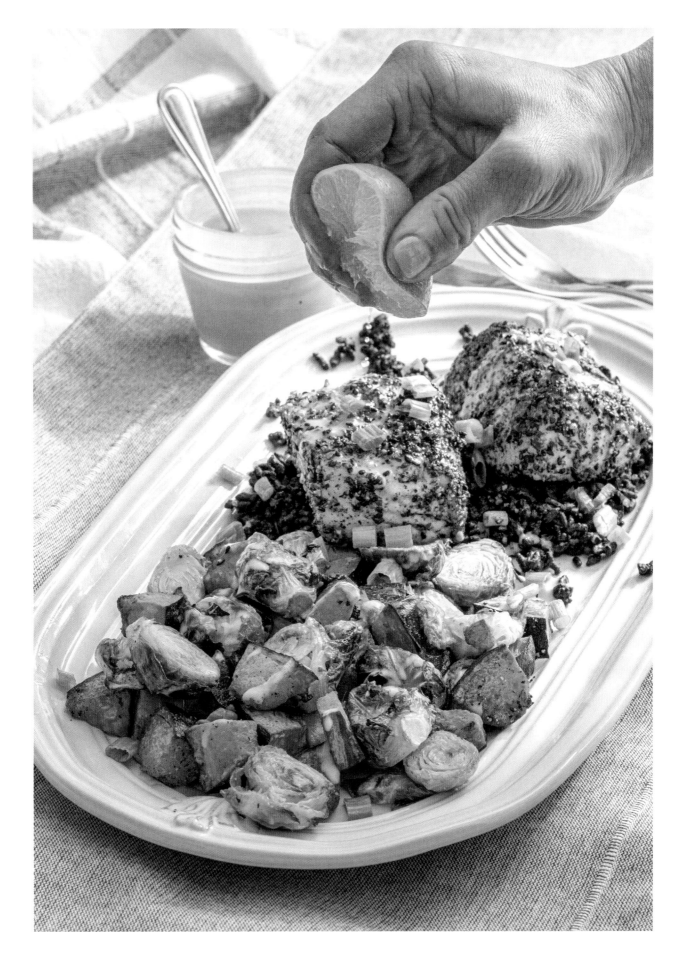

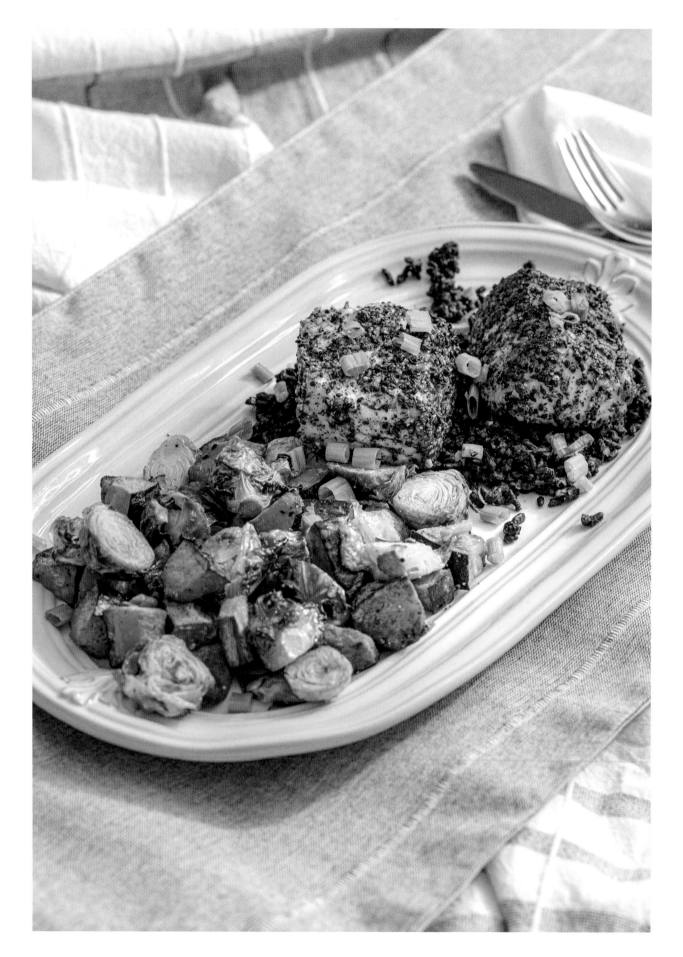

Buying pre-peeled and chopped squash makes life easier, but you can make a whole squash easier to cut by microwaving it on high in 30-second intervals, rotating the squash between intervals, until the squash is slightly warm and a serrated knife more easily cuts the flesh. I leave the skin on most squashes, including kabocha, delicata, and acorn, for ease and added nutrition. (The only squash skins I don't recommend consuming are spaghetti squash and any skin that's extra shiny, which might have been treated with wax.) Pulsing whole almonds and roasted nori in a food processor is an efficient way to make the furikake ingredients.

1. Preheat the oven to 425°F. Line two rimmed baking sheets with parchment paper.

2. Sprinkle the halibut with a little salt to season it. Set aside while you prepare the vegetables.

3. Place the Brussels sprouts in a large bowl. Toss with 2 tablespoons of the melted coconut oil, the garlic powder, ¼ teaspoon of the salt, and ¼ teaspoon of the pepper. Spread out on one of the baking sheets, cut side down.

4. Place the kabocha squash in the same bowl. Toss with 1 tablespoon of the coconut oil, ¼ teaspoon of the salt, and the remaining ¼ teaspoon of pepper. Spread out on the second baking sheet.

5. Place both baking sheets in the oven, stirring the Brussels sprouts and squash after 20 minutes to ensure even roasting and to remove any smaller pieces that are completely roasted. Continue roasting for 5 to 10 minutes more, until tender.

6. Combine the rice, water, ½ cup of the coconut milk, and the remaining ½ teaspoon of salt in a medium saucepan. Cover, bring to a boil, and then lower the heat and simmer for 30 to 35 minutes, until the liquid is absorbed. Allow it to continue steaming with the lid on for another 10 minutes, then fluff the rice with a fork and add 1 teaspoon of the coconut aminos, half of the lime zest, and half of the lime juice. Keep warm until ready to serve.

7. Meanwhile, combine the ingredients for the furikake in a shallow dish. Dredge the halibut on all sides in the furikake until thoroughly coated.

8. Heat the remaining tablespoon of coconut oil in a large skillet over medium-high heat. Using tongs, place the halibut skin side up in the hot pan. Allow it to sear for about 2 minutes, until browned, then flip. Continue browning on all sides, finishing with the skin side down. Continue cooking the fish until it's firm to the touch and just barely opaque on the inside, 3 to 5 more minutes, depending on the thickness of your fillet. Remove the fish from the pan.

9. In a separate small saucepan, combine the remaining ½ cup of coconut milk with the remaining tablespoon of coconut aminos, the remainder of the lime zest and juice, and the arrowroot flour. Warm over medium-low heat until the sauce is just about to bubble, whisking as needed to combine. Remove from the heat.

10. Divide the vegetables evenly among four plates alongside ½ cup of rice and a piece of halibut. Drizzle the coconut lime sauce over everything and top with the scallions. For an extra kick of lime, squeeze a lime wedge over the top before serving, if desired.

*To make this dish *Dr. Katie Detox* friendly, omit the crushed red pepper in the furikake.

TEMPEH "BLT" COLLARD WRAPS

MAKES 6 wraps

PREP TIME: 15 minutes, plus time to marinate tempeh

COOK TIME: 30 minutes

I didn't like tempeh the first time I had it, which just goes to show that even adults need to trial a new food a few times before deciding whether it's a keeper. Tempeh is made from fermented soybeans and sometimes grains and is found in the refrigerated section of the grocery store. I prefer pure soy tempeh because it's rich in both protein and fiber, with a 4-ounce portion boasting 22 grams of protein and 12 grams of fiber. Because it's a whole soy, it has the right ratio of daidzein and genistein isoflavones, making it an anti-inflammatory powerhouse. Tempeh's ultimate glory comes from being fermented, which means that it's naturally rich in healthy probiotic bacteria and is full of calcium, magnesium, and phosphorus, making it great for bone health.

---

2 (8-ounce) packages organic soy tempeh

⅓ cup tamari

⅓ cup dark maple syrup

¼ cup avocado oil

2 teaspoons smoked paprika

¼ teaspoon freshly ground black pepper

For serving:

6 large collard leaves, large stems removed

3 cups shredded lettuce

3 cups cooked whole grain of choice (see Hearty Whole Grains, page 290)

2 ripe tomatoes, sliced

2 medium Hass avocados, sliced

Lemony Basil Cashew Cream (page 300) (optional)

Thinly sliced fresh basil (optional)

1. Cut the tempeh into ½-inch slices and, if you desire a more mild-tasting tempeh, boil or steam it for 10 to 15 minutes.

2. In a medium bowl, whisk together the tamari, maple syrup, avocado oil, paprika, and pepper. Place the tempeh in a shallow glass dish and pour the marinade over the tempeh. Refrigerate for at least 1 hour or up to 2 days.

3. When ready to bake, preheat the oven to 375°F and line a rimmed baking sheet with parchment paper. Place the tempeh on the prepared baking sheet, leaving some space between the pieces. Bake for 30 minutes, until browned, using a spatula to flip the tempeh after 20 minutes.

4. Leave the serving components deconstructed until ready to eat. To construct the wraps, arrange one-sixth of the tempeh, ½ cup of lettuce, ½ cup of whole grain, a few tomato slices, one-third of an avocado, and a drizzle of cashew cream, if desired, down the center of each collard leaf. Roll the leaf around the fillings to form a wrap.

*To make this wrap *Dr. Katie Detox* friendly, omit the tomatoes or replace them with roasted beet slices or thinly sliced apple or cucumber.

ALTERNATIVE:

Instead of a collard wrap, omit the whole grain and serve the tempeh on a piece of toasted Whole-Grain Nut & Seed Bread (page 294) or crusty sourdough bread to create a satiating sandwich.

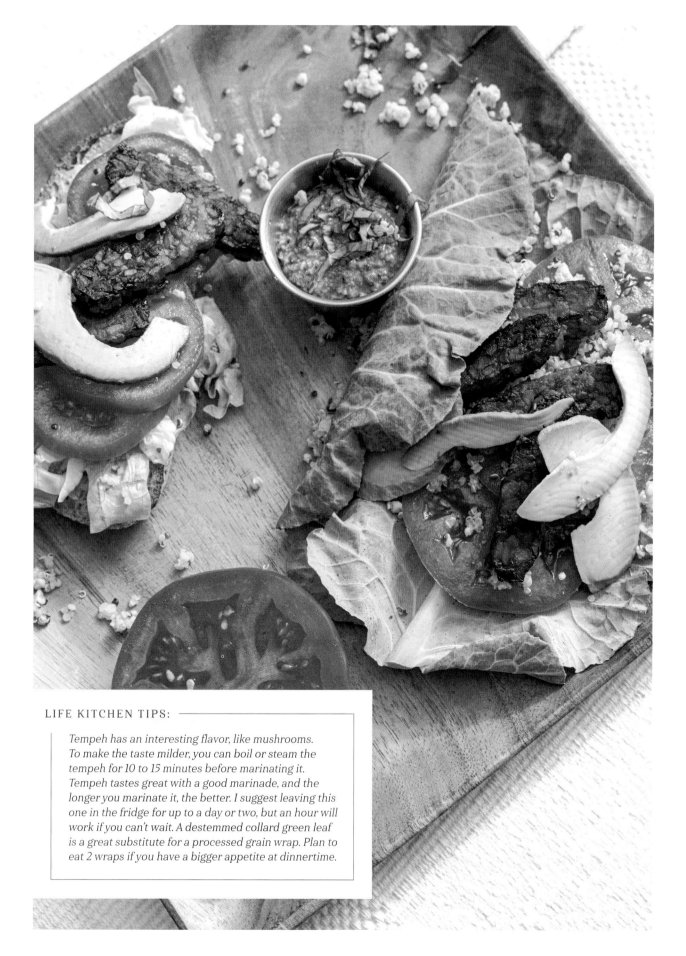

ROASTED SALMON WITH MISO SHALLOT JAM

SERVES 4

PREP TIME: 25 minutes

COOK TIME: 20 minutes

Wild-caught salmon is one of the most potent sources of anti-inflammatory omega-3 fatty acids, with one 3.5-ounce serving having up to 2,000 milligrams.[2] At my house, we try to have wild omega-3–rich fish twice weekly. This recipe is a great alternative to traditional barbecue or teriyaki sauce because it uses miso, a fermented soybean paste. The salty, earthy, umami flavor of miso works well in combination with the sweetness from coconut aminos on any plant or animal protein. I encourage you to try this Miso Shallot Jam on beef, chicken, pork, tempeh, and tofu. This recipe is relatively quick, so you could make an otherwise boring weeknight dinner feel a little fancier without much effort if you paired it with a simple salad or sautéed greens. On those days when you have a little more time to spend in the kitchen, I highly suggest pairing this dish with Crispy Parsley (page 282) and Harvest Wild Rice with Apples, Sage & Goji Berries (page 284).

---

1 tablespoon avocado oil

4 (5-ounce) skin-on wild salmon fillets

Fine sea salt and freshly ground black pepper

Miso Shallot Jam:

1 tablespoon avocado oil

¼ cup minced shallots

2 cloves garlic, minced

⅓ cup orange juice (from ½ to 1 medium orange)

1 teaspoon white miso

1 teaspoon tamari or soy sauce

1 teaspoon rice wine vinegar

1 tablespoon coconut aminos

1. Preheat the oven to 425°F. Grease a rimmed baking sheet with the avocado oil.

2. Season the salmon on both sides with salt and pepper, being mindful to salt the skin side more. Place the fillets skin side up on the prepared baking sheet.

3. Make the jam: In a small saucepan, heat the avocado oil over low heat. Add the shallots and cook until softened, 2 to 3 minutes. Add the garlic and cook for 30 seconds more, just until fragrant. Add the orange juice, miso, tamari, vinegar, and coconut aminos and whisk until combined. Bring to a simmer and cook, stirring every minute or so, until the sauce has thickened, 5 to 6 minutes. Season with pepper and remove the pan from the heat.

4. Turn the oven to broil and broil the fish skin for 2 to 5 minutes, until golden and crispy. Then flip the fillets over and spoon about half of the jam on top. Return the oven to 425°F and roast the salmon until it begins to look opaque in the center when gently flaked, 6 to 10 minutes, depending on thickness. When done, immediately remove the fillets from the pan and drizzle them with the remaining jam. Serve with the side(s) of your choice.

---

[2] "Omega-3 fatty acids: fact sheet for health professionals," National Institutes of Health, last updated March 26, 2021, https://ods.od.nih.gov/factsheets/Omega3FattyAcids-HealthProfessional/

*To make this dish Dr. Katie Detox friendly, use pomegranate juice instead of orange juice.

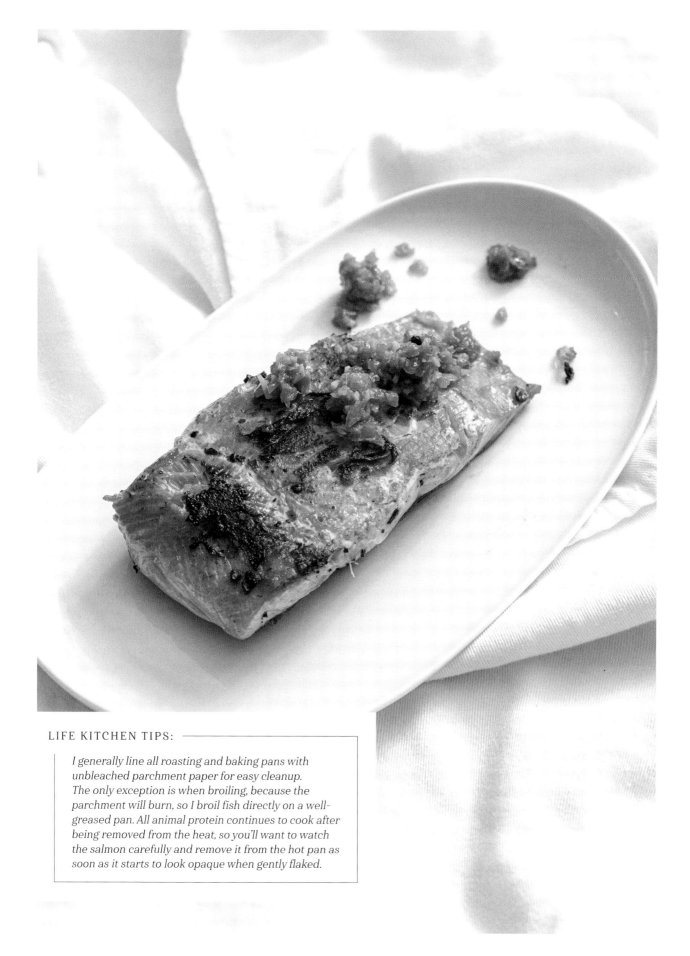

MUSHROOM BURGERS WITH PARSNIP FRIES

MAKES 6 burgers

PREP TIME: 15 minutes

COOK TIME: 40 minutes

This recipe is a favorite among our Dr. Katie Detoxers, and for good reason: the texture and deep, slightly sweet flavor of the mushroom burger paired with the complex taste of slightly spicy, nutty roasted parsnip fries will have you in literal heaven. The mastermind behind this unique recipe is Integrative Health Coach Courtney Evans of *Well Refined*, my partner in the *Dr. Katie Detox.* Not only is she a flavor genius in the kitchen, but she takes an insightful, soulful approach to finding the deeper meaning of health with her clients, which extends to our relationship as well. We like the phytonutrient profile of mushrooms because they contain a lot of fiber, especially in the form of beta-glucans, which have been linked to improved cholesterol levels and regulation of blood sugar along with the mineral chromium, not to mention they are immune-boosting and have anti-cancer properties. This recipe takes a little time, but I guarantee you will be a happy camper at the dinner table.

---

2 cups brown rice

6 medium parsnips (about 1½ pounds), unpeeled

¼ cup plus 2 teaspoons avocado oil, divided

1 teaspoon garlic powder

1½ teaspoons fine sea salt

1 teaspoon turmeric powder

½ teaspoon freshly ground black pepper

3 tablespoons nutritional yeast

2 tablespoons extra-virgin olive oil

2 shallots, chopped

3 cups chopped mushrooms (any type)

2 tablespoons coconut aminos

¼ cup balsamic vinegar

½ teaspoon dark maple syrup

2 cloves garlic, minced

½ cup crushed raw walnuts

¼ cup ground flax seeds

1 cup gluten-free chickpea crumbs, divided (see Tips)

For serving:

6 large radicchio leaves

2 medium Hass avocados, halved, pitted, peeled, and mashed, or ⅓ cup Lemony Basil Cashew Cream (page 300)

Crushed red pepper (optional)

1. Preheat the oven to 425°F. Line a rimmed baking sheet with parchment paper.

2. Cook the rice according to the Hearty Whole Grains recipe (page 290). Keep warm.

3. Cut the parsnips in half crosswise, then slice lengthwise into thin strips like shoestring fries. Toss the parsnips with ¼ cup of the avocado oil, garlic powder, salt, turmeric, pepper, and nutritional yeast. Transfer the seasoned parsnips to the prepared baking sheet and roast for 25 to 40 minutes, until golden brown, flipping halfway through.

4. Meanwhile, heat a sauté pan over medium heat. Add the olive oil and shallots and sauté for 1 to 2 minutes, then add the mushrooms and cook until softened. Stir in the coconut aminos, vinegar, maple syrup, and minced garlic, then transfer the mixture to a food processor.

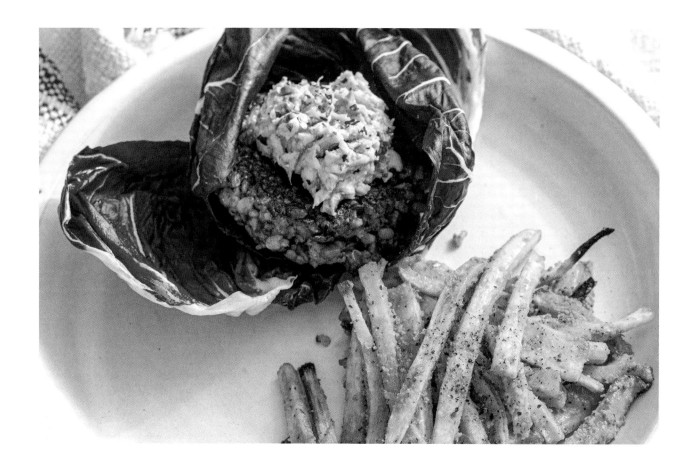

LIFE KITCHEN TIPS:

To shorten your prep time, rewarm rice from a prior batch-cook when making the burger patties. I often make the patties ahead and store them uncooked in the fridge for 2 or 3 days, browning only those that I need for a meal. If you can't find packaged chickpea crumbs, you can make your own using a food processor. Preheat the oven to 350°F. Drain and rinse two 15-ounce cans of chickpeas and pulse in the food processor until chunky. Spread the pulsed chickpeas into a single layer on a rimmed baking sheet and roast until they're completely dry, about 20 minutes. Then return them to the food processor and pulse until they have a breadcrumb-like texture. You should have about 1½ cups of crumbs. Store extras in an airtight container in the freezer for up to 3 months.

5. To the food processor, add the walnuts, ground flax seeds, ½ cup of the chickpea crumbs, and the warm brown rice and pulse until combined. Transfer to a medium bowl and add the remaining chickpea crumbs. Form the mixture into six burger patties, about ½ inch thick.

6. Heat the remaining 2 teaspoons of avocado oil in the same sauté pan or a grill pan over medium heat. Cook the burgers for 4 to 5 minutes on each side, until golden brown. Serve the burgers on radicchio leaves topped with smashed avocado or a dollop of cashew cream and a sprinkle of crushed red pepper, if desired. Serve the hot parsnip fries alongside the burgers.

*To make this recipe *Dr. Katie Detox* friendly, omit the crushed red pepper.

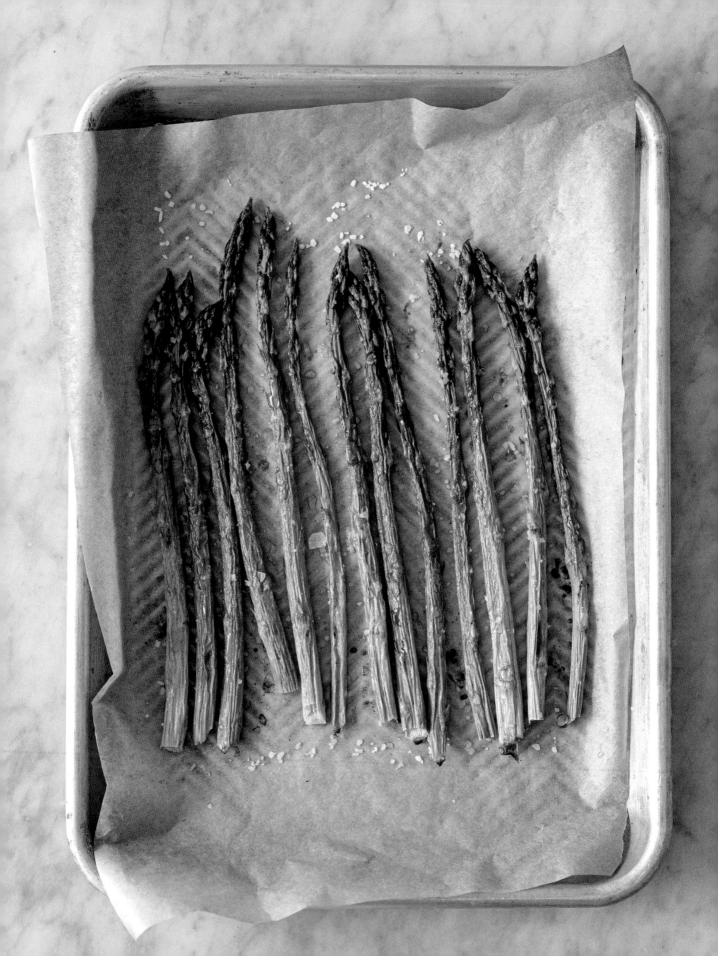

BATCH COOKING & SIDES

TO MAKE KITCHEN PREPARATIONS EASIER

CORIANDER & FLAX ROASTED EGGPLANT

SERVES 4

PREP TIME: 10 minutes

COOK TIME: 30 minutes

This recipe was inspired by a beloved patient who came to her acupuncture appointment bearing warm roasted eggplant dusted in crushed coriander seeds. I gobbled it right up! Coriander is the dried seed from the same plant that yields cilantro, but surprisingly, they have different flavors. Coriander seeds have a sweet aromatic flavor with citrus undertones and offer an anti-inflammatory boost to any vegetable medley. Coriander historically has been used as a medicinal treatment for gastrointestinal maladies, but newer evidence suggests that it reduces oxidative stress and free radicals and may be useful for preventing cancer, controlling blood sugar, and lowering LDL cholesterol. The ground flax seeds not only add anti-inflammatory omega-3 fat but also create a great texture akin to breadcrumbs that I find so pleasing.

---

2 medium eggplants (about 1½ pounds)

¼ cup extra-virgin olive oil

1 heaping tablespoon coriander seeds, toasted and crushed

1 tablespoon ground flax seeds

½ teaspoon garlic powder

Grated zest of ½ lemon, plus more for garnish if desired

½ teaspoon fine sea salt

¼ teaspoon freshly ground black pepper

Handful of fresh parsley leaves, for garnish (optional)

1. Preheat the oven to 425°F. Line a rimmed baking sheet with parchment paper.

2. Cut the eggplants into ½-inch cubes and place in a large bowl. Combine the olive oil, coriander, ground flax seeds, garlic powder, lemon zest, salt, and pepper in a small bowl, then pour over the eggplant. Toss the eggplant to evenly coat.

3. Move the spiced eggplant to the prepared baking sheet and roast for 30 minutes, until golden brown, stirring halfway through to encourage even roasting. Garnish with extra lemon zest and fresh parsley before serving, if desired.

*To make this recipe *Dr. Katie Detox* friendly, substitute 1 pound of chopped shiitake mushrooms for the eggplant. Adjust the oven temperature to 350°F and roast for 15 to 25 minutes, until golden brown and a little crispy.

LIFE KITCHEN TIPS:

As with all seeds, toasting coriander seeds brings out their aromatic flavor and doesn't need to be any more complicated than using a small skillet and shaking the pan a bit to prevent burning. Toast whole seeds on the stovetop over medium-low heat for 3 to 5 minutes, until lightly colored and fragrant, and then crush them with a wine bottle or small ceramic dish. It's worth the extra effort, but ground coriander works, too. If your eggplant is too spongy, you didn't roast it long enough or didn't use enough olive oil.

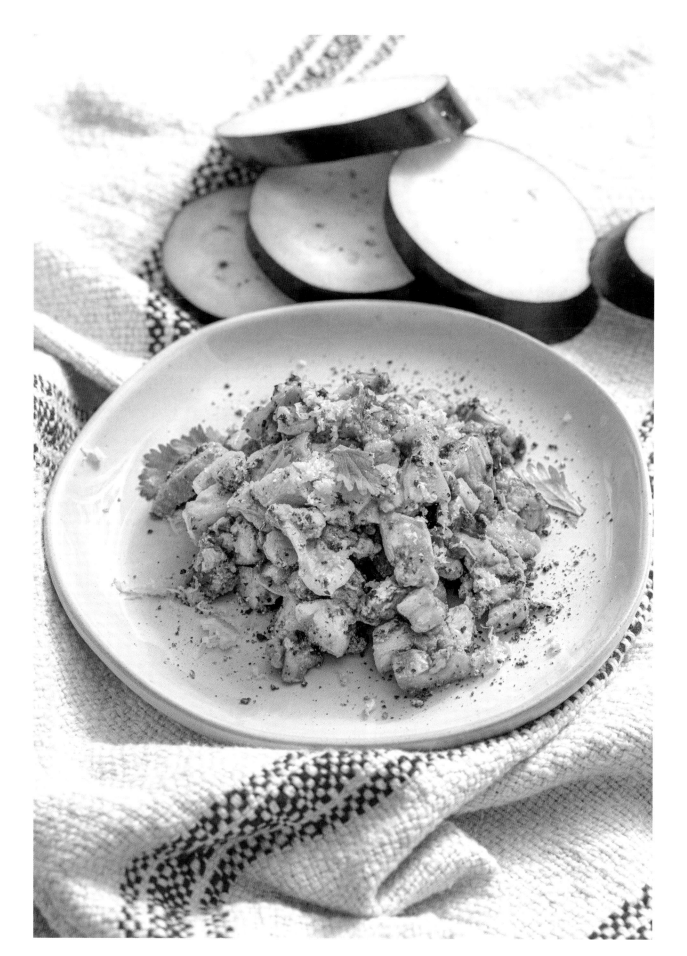

CRISPY PARSLEY

SERVES 3 to 4
PREP TIME: 5 minutes
COOK TIME: 12 minutes

Parsley is my favorite anti-bloat herb because it works as a natural diuretic, allowing the kidneys to rid the body of unnecessary water. And guess what? You can sauté or roast curly parsley just like any other green. You'll never go wrong having parsley in your refrigerator since it's useful in so many recipes. In fact, I think parsley is sorely underrated in the kitchen and certainly when it comes to medicinal plants. Parsley is rich in vitamins A, C, and especially K. Combined with garlic, it makes this dish a tonic that's great in your quest to prevent cardiovascular disease, regulate blood sugar, and fight infection due to the antibacterial properties in its essential oils. Those on vitamin K–blocking blood thinners like warfarin want to include a consistent amount of vitamin K–rich greens like parsley in their daily diet to prevent issues with medication management.

6 bunches curly parsley (about 1 pound)

2 cloves garlic, minced

1 tablespoon extra-virgin olive oil

Kosher salt and freshly ground pepper

1. Preheat the oven to 425°F. Line a rimmed baking sheet with parchment paper.

2. Soak the parsley in water to remove the grit, then dry with paper towels or a salad spinner. Roughly chop the leaves into bite-sized pieces and discard the stems. You should have about 8 cups.

3. Place the parsley and garlic on the prepared baking sheet and toss with the olive oil and a sprinkle of salt and pepper. Roast for 5 to 12 minutes to the desired level of crispiness, being careful not to let the parsley burn.

LIFE KITCHEN TIP:

> *A salad spinner is one of my favorite kitchen tools because it allows you to wash and dry produce thoroughly, removing the sand and grit that often finds its way into curly greens like parsley and kale.*

ALTERNATIVE STOVETOP PREPARATION:

In a sauté pan over medium heat, warm the olive oil. Add the parsley, garlic, and a sprinkle of salt and pepper and cook until the parsley is cooked and fragrant and the garlic is lightly browned, about 5 minutes. Serve immediately. Note that the parsley will still be delicious but will not be quite as crispy as when cooked in the oven.

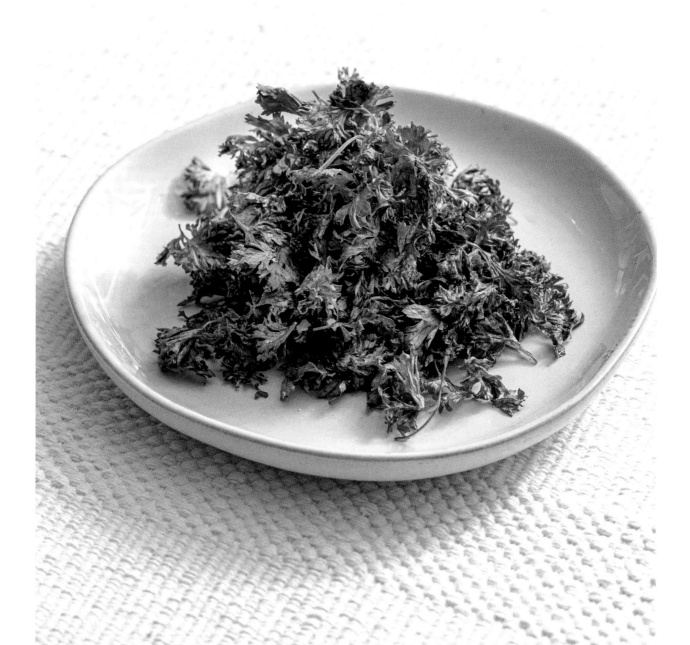

HARVEST WILD RICE WITH APPLES, SAGE & GOJI BERRIES

DR. KATIE DETOX FRIENDLY

SERVES 4

PREP TIME: 15 minutes

COOK TIME: 45 minutes

This recipe made its first appearance alongside our roasted turkey at Christmas dinner after my husband and I both decided we didn't like the traditional bread stuffing we had made at Thanksgiving. Any whole grain will work, but I like the flavor and nuttiness of long-grain wild rice. Interestingly, wild rice is not actually rice at all, but a species of grass grown near fresh water that produces a seed that is cooked like rice. Wild rice has about thirty times more antioxidant activity than white rice, and a lot more fiber, too.[3] It's also a complete protein, meaning it has all the essential amino acids that our bodies cannot make, but similar to other whole grains, it has only about 4 grams of protein per half-cup serving. If you want to add protein and more immune-boosting nourishment, cook your whole grains in bone broth.

1 cup wild rice

Fine sea salt

1 tablespoon ghee or unsalted butter

1 medium yellow onion, chopped

4 cloves garlic, minced

1 medium crunchy green apple, finely chopped (do not peel)

1 teaspoon toasted sesame oil

1 teaspoon white miso

½ cup chopped fresh parsley

1 tablespoon chopped fresh sage

1 tablespoon chopped fresh thyme

¼ cup dried goji berries

Freshly ground black pepper

1 scallion, chopped, for garnish

Recommended pairings:

Crispy Parsley (page 282)

Roasted Salmon with Miso Shallot Jam (page 274)

1. Cook the rice with a tiny pinch of salt according to the Hearty Whole Grains recipe (page 290) until it cracks open and begins to curl, about 45 minutes. Drain the excess water and fluff the rice with a fork. (You can prepare the wild rice in advance and rewarm it before adding it in Step 2.)

2. When the rice is nearly done, heat the ghee in a large skillet over medium heat. Sauté the onion and garlic until tender, about 1 minute. Add the apple, sesame oil, miso, herbs, and goji berries and sauté for another minute or so. Add the cooked rice and season with salt and pepper to taste. Garnish with the chopped scallion.

*To make this dish *Dr. Katie Detox* friendly, use unsweetened dried cranberries or chopped unsweetened dried apricots instead of goji berries.

---

[3] Y. Qiu, Q. Liu, and T. Beta, "Antioxidant activity of commercial wild rice and identification of flavonoid compounds in active fractions," *Journal of Agricultural and Food Chemistry* 57, no. 16 (2009): 7543–51.

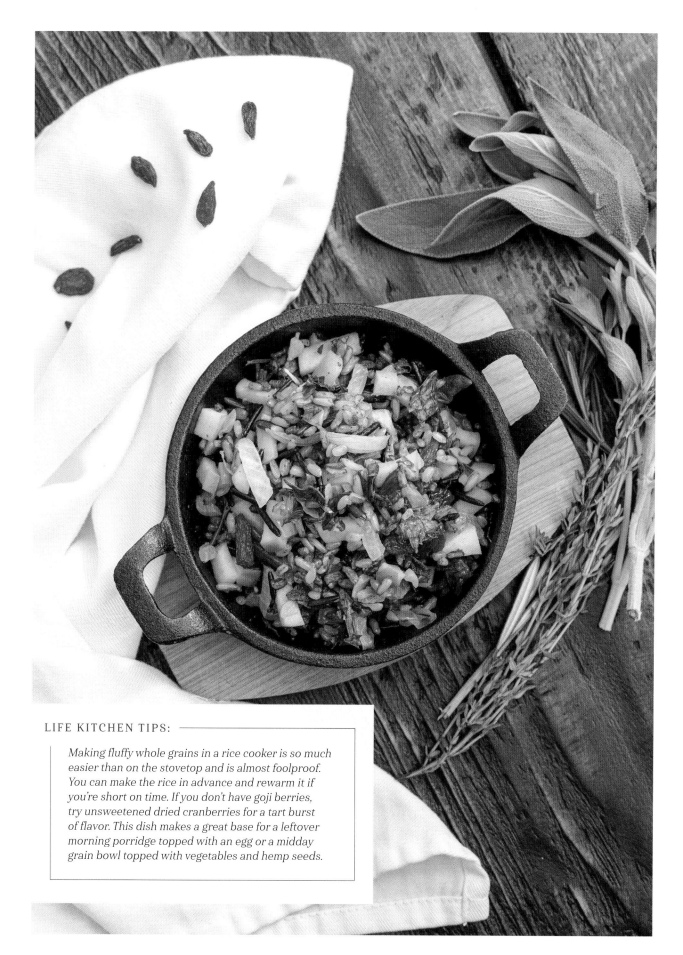

LIFE KITCHEN TIPS: ───

Making fluffy whole grains in a rice cooker is so much easier than on the stovetop and is almost foolproof. You can make the rice in advance and rewarm it if you're short on time. If you don't have goji berries, try unsweetened dried cranberries for a tart burst of flavor. This dish makes a great base for a leftover morning porridge topped with an egg or a midday grain bowl topped with vegetables and hemp seeds.

EASY ROASTED VEGETABLES

SERVES 2 or more

PREP TIME: 10 to 20 minutes

COOK TIME: 5 to 40 minutes (depending on type of vegetable)

Roasted vegetables are the cat's meow, the cream of the crop, the best thing since sliced bread. Gone are the days of boiling, where you lose many of the phytonutrients. It's okay to steam your vegetables or eat them raw, but the tastiest way to enjoy any vegetable is roasted because the heat of the oven caramelizes the natural sugar in the plant, creating that perfect crispy golden color. You don't need a recipe to roast vegetables, just a general technique of cutting uniform pieces to allow them to cook evenly and a guideline on timing. For more tips on preparing vegetables, see pages 215 and 216.

The yield of this recipe will vary depending on the type of vegetable you roast and the amount of that vegetable that fits on the baking sheet. One serving of roasted vegetables is ½ cup, and I recommend at least eight servings of vegetables per day for the average person. I like to roast a few pans at a time so that I have a variety of roasted veggies to enjoy throughout the week.

Vegetable(s) of choice

Extra-virgin olive oil, avocado oil, or melted virgin coconut oil, ghee, or butter

Fine sea salt and freshly ground black pepper

Dried or fresh herbs and/or spices of choice (optional)

Fresh herbs, for garnish (optional)

1. Preheat the oven to 425°F (or 400°F if using the convection setting; see Tips for notes on roasting temperature). Line a rimmed baking sheet with parchment paper.

2. Prepare the vegetables according to the chart below. Many slender vegetables, such as asparagus and green beans, can be left whole. Bulkier vegetables should be cut into 1-inch pieces. Make sure to dry all vegetables thoroughly.

3. Place the vegetables in a mound on the prepared baking sheet. Drizzle with enough oil or fat to lightly coat, usually 1 to 4 tablespoons per baking sheet, and season with salt and pepper along with herbs or spices, if desired. Using your hands or a pair of tongs, mix to evenly coat the vegetables in the fat and seasonings, then spread the vegetables out, leaving some space between pieces to encourage browning.

4. Roast until the vegetables are crispy and a little brown on the outside and tender on the inside, using the cooking time guidelines listed in the chart below. Turn the vegetables once or twice during cooking. Garnish with fresh herbs before serving, if desired.

*To make vegetables that are *Dr. Katie Detox* friendly, avoid nightshades like bell peppers, eggplant, potatoes, and tomatoes.

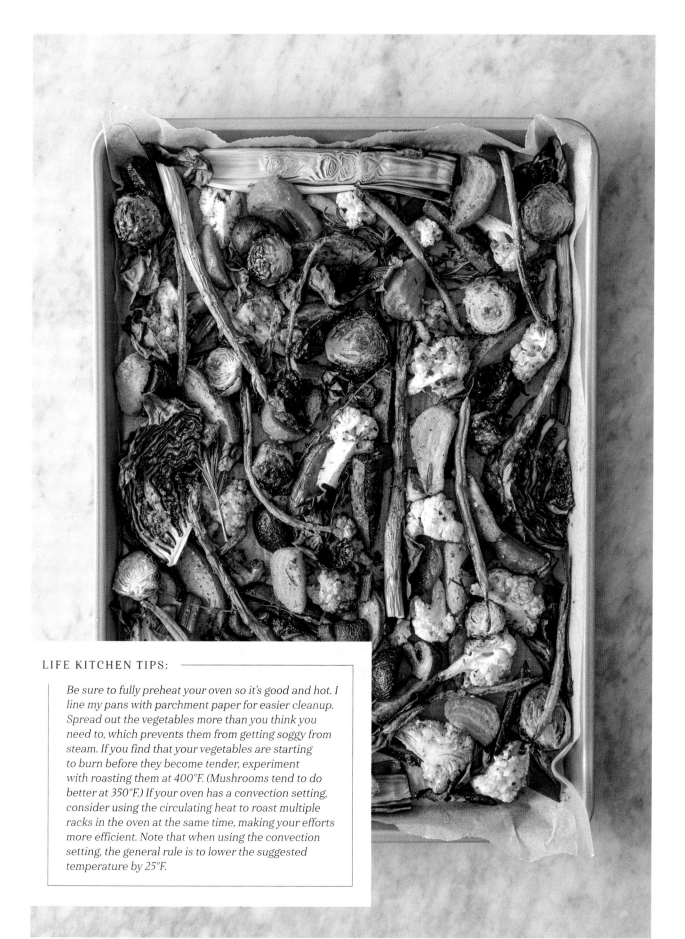

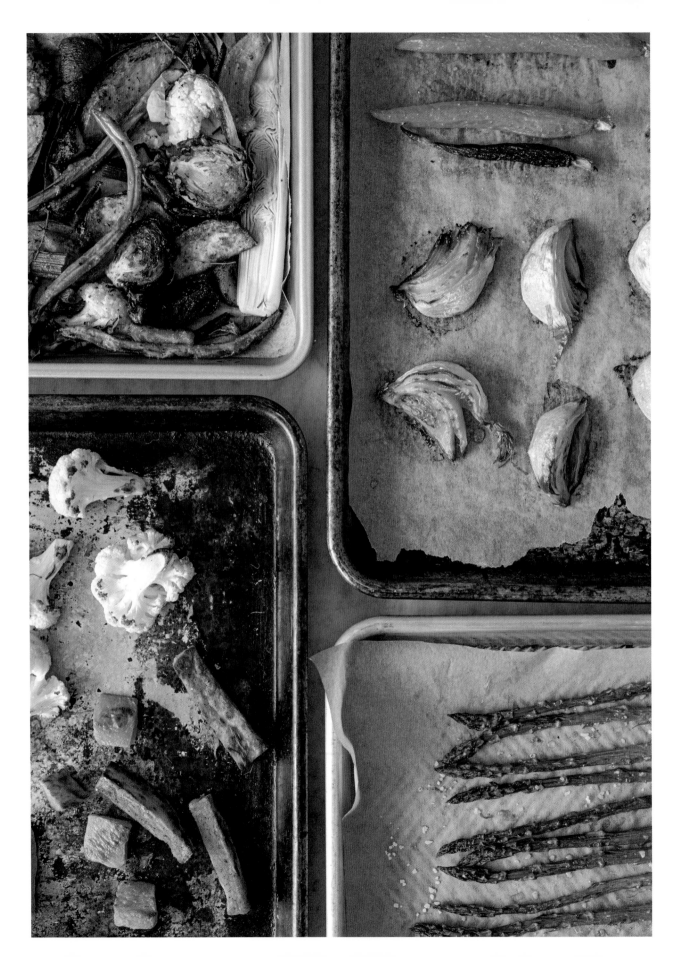

Vegetable (cut into 1-inch pieces unless otherwise noted)	Roasting Time at 425°F (conventional setting) / 400°F (convection setting)
Asparagus, whole	8 to 12 minutes
Beets	25 to 40 minutes
Bell peppers	20 to 30 minutes
Broccoli florets and peeled stems	8 to 20 minutes
Brussels sprouts, halved	15 to 25 minutes
Cabbage, cut into wedges	40 to 55 minutes
Carrots and parsnips, whole if slender	25 to 40 minutes
Cauliflower florets and peeled stems	20 to 40 minutes
Eggplant	20 to 40 minutes
Fennel	25 to 35 minutes
Green beans, whole	12 to 15 minutes
Leafy greens (kale, Swiss chard, collard greens, curly parsley), chopped or cut into ribbons	5 to 15 minutes
Leeks, sliced in half lengthwise	15 to 20 minutes
Mushrooms	15 to 25 minutes at 350°F
Onions, quartered	20 to 30 minutes
Potatoes	25 to 35 minutes
Radishes, whole or halved	20 to 30 minutes
Sweet potatoes	25 to 35 minutes
Summer squash (like zucchini)	20 to 35 minutes
Tomatoes (or whole cherry or grape tomatoes)	15 to 25 minutes
Winter squash (like butternut, delicata, or kabocha)	25 to 40 minutes

HEARTY WHOLE GRAINS

MAKES 2 to 4 cups, depending on type of whole grain

PREP TIME: 5 minutes

COOK TIME: 20 to 45 minutes

Batch-cooking grains on the weekends is a great way to have ready-to-go helpers later in the week when you're busy or tired. You can easily scale up this recipe using the ratios shown in the chart on page 293. A rice cooker is an almost foolproof way to make whole grains, so I suggest investing in one for your kitchen. I've included instructions for using both a rice cooker and a pan on the stovetop. Cooking grains in nourishing bone broth is my favorite way to add flavor and get powerful immune-boosting nutrients and protein from natural collagen, an important structural component in the body. If you prefer to use water to cook your grains, adding a teaspoon of extra-virgin olive oil, virgin coconut oil, or toasted sesame oil at the end of cooking provides blood sugar anchoring to this fiber-rich carbohydrate. You can also find satiating nutritional balance by cooking grains in a mixture of canned unsweetened coconut milk and water, since coconut milk is rich in fat and delivers a yummy sweet flavor. For more on whole grains, see pages 110 to 114.

---

1 cup whole grain of choice

1½ to 4 cups bone broth, vegetable stock, canned full-fat, unsweetened coconut milk, or water, depending on type of whole grain (see chart, page 293)

Small pinch of fine sea salt (optional)

1 teaspoon healthy oil of choice (optional)

1. In a large strainer or colander, rinse the whole grain well under cool water until the water runs mostly clear.

2. If using a rice cooker, combine the rinsed whole grain, liquid, and a small pinch of salt, if desired, in the rice cooker. Turn on the rice cooker and choose the correct cooking setting. The rice cooker will automatically turn off when done. Keep the lid on to allow the grain to continue steaming for 10 to 15 minutes to prevent stickiness and encourage fluffiness.

   If using the stovetop method, combine the rinsed whole grain, liquid, and a small pinch of salt, if desired, in a medium saucepan and bring the liquid to a boil. Reduce the heat to medium-low, cover, and simmer until the grain is tender and the water is absorbed, 20 to 45 minutes, depending on the grain used. Remove the pan from the heat, keeping the lid on to allow the grain to continue steaming for 10 to 15 minutes to prevent stickiness and encourage fluffiness.

3. Add a teaspoon of healthy oil to the cooked grain, if desired. Using a rice cooker spoon or wooden spatula, fluff the rice before serving.

*To make this recipe *Dr. Katie Detox* friendly, avoid grains with gluten.

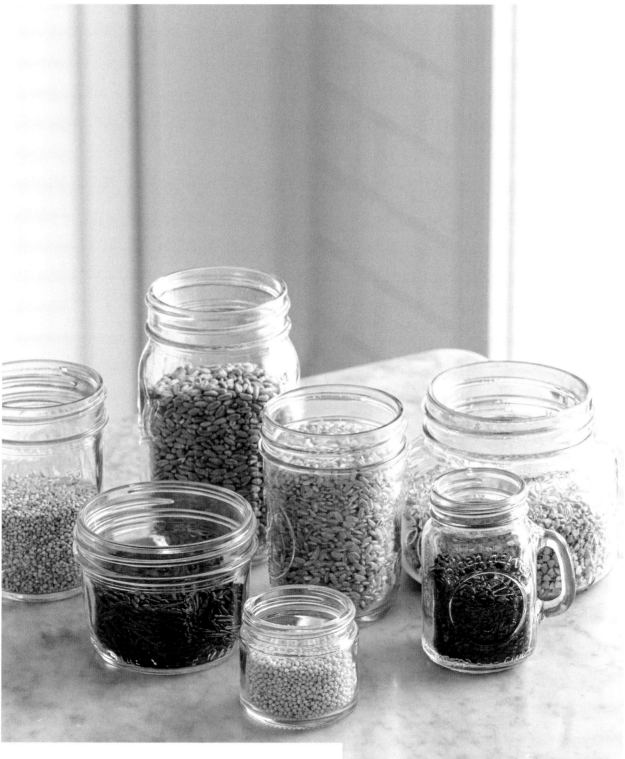

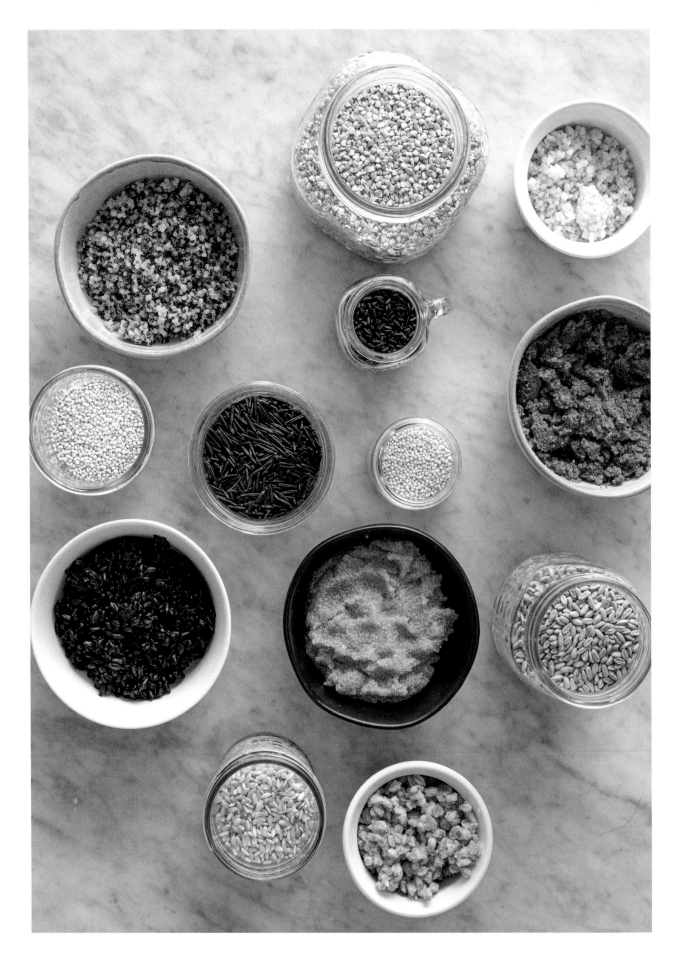

Whole Grain	Gluten-Free?	Protein Per Serving (½ Cup Cooked)	Whole Grain: Liquid Ratio	Yield from 1 Cup Whole Grain
Amaranth	✓	5g	1:3	2 cups
Barley, pearled		2g	1:2.5	3½ cups
Brown rice	✓	2g	1:2	3 cups
Buckwheat groats	✓	3g	1:2	4 cups
Bulgur		3g	1:2	3 cups
Farro		4g	1:3	3 cups
Kamut		6g	1:3	3½ cups
Millet	✓	3g	1:2	4 cups
Quinoa	✓	4g	1:1.5	3 cups
Steel-cut oats		5g	1:3	3½ cups
Teff	✓	5g	1:4	2½ cups
Wheat berries		6.5 g	1:3	2 cups
Wild and black rice	✓	3g	1:3	3 cups

WHOLE-GRAIN NUT & SEED BREAD

MAKES 1 loaf (16 slices)

PREP TIME: 15 minutes, plus 2 hours to rest

COOK TIME: 70 minutes

This bread's taste and versatility will have you at hello. And of course, who doesn't love bread? I had a variation of this bread for the first time more than a decade ago at my friend Cathrin's house in Brooklyn. She paired her mom Ulli's seed bread with a bit of salted butter alongside a warm bowl of homemade soup on a cold winter's day, and it totally hit the spot. Nuts, seeds, and whole grains combine to create a fiber-rich, slow-burning carbohydrate with grounding healthy fats that will satiate your belly instead of spiking your blood sugar. This bread is the ultimate treat in the "slow carb, not low carb" game and lends itself to many variations depending on your mood.

1½ cups oat flour

1 cup raw shelled sunflower seeds

½ cup unblanched almond flour, almond meal, or hazelnut flour

½ cup whole flax seeds

4 tablespoons raw shelled pumpkin seeds, divided

3 tablespoons ground flax seeds

2 tablespoons chia seeds

1 teaspoon fine sea salt

1½ cups warm water

3 tablespoons melted virgin coconut oil or extra-virgin olive oil

1 tablespoon honey or dark maple syrup (optional)

1. Line an 8½ by 4½-inch loaf pan with parchment paper, leaving some paper overhanging the sides.

2. Place all the dry ingredients except for 1 tablespoon of the pumpkin seeds in a large bowl and stir well to combine. Whisk together the water, oil, and honey, if using, and add to the dry ingredients. Using a large spoon, mix well until everything is completely soaked and the dough becomes thick. (If the dough is too thick to stir, add 1 to 2 teaspoons of water until the dough is manageable. It should be stiff but still possible to stir or spread without too much resistance.)

3. Scoop the dough into the prepared loaf pan and smooth the top with the back of a spoon, then press the remaining tablespoon of pumpkin seeds firmly on top. Let the dough sit at room temperature for at least 2 hours, all day, or even overnight to firm up. When the dough is ready, it will retain its shape even when you use the parchment paper to pull it away from the sides of the pan.

4. When ready to bake, preheat the oven to 350°F. Place the pan in the oven and bake for 50 minutes. Grabbing hold of the overhanging parchment paper, remove the bread from the pan. Then place it upside down directly on the oven rack and bake for another 10 to 20 minutes, until the bread sounds hollow when tapped. Let cool completely before slicing. Store in an airtight container for up to 3 days or in the freezer for up to a month.

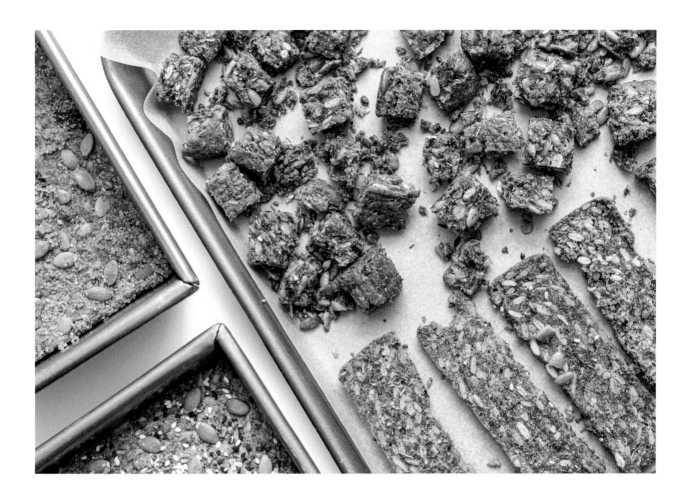

LIFE KITCHEN TIPS:

If you don't have oat flour or nut flour, pulsing rolled oats or whole nuts in a food processor works well to make homemade flour. The longer the dough sits, the better the bread because the resting time allows the flax and chia seeds to bind it together, making a less crumbly bread. I recommend the all-day or overnight method if you have time. This bread won't rise because there's no leavening agent. Store the bread you'll eat within 3 days in a tightly sealed container and freeze the rest in slices for quick and easy toast, like the Omega Avocado Toast (page 246) or in crouton form on top of any salad or the Creamy Roasted Broccoli Soup (page 256).

VARIATIONS:

Spiced Raisin Bread. *Soak ½ cup of chopped raisins in the 1½ cups of warm water called for in the recipe. Add 2 teaspoons of ground cinnamon, ¼ teaspoon of ground nutmeg, and ¼ teaspoon of ground cardamom to the dry mixture, and add the soaked raisins and raisin soaking water to the wet ingredients when mixing in Step 2. Consider using leftovers for a whole-grain French toast.*

Everything Bagel Bread. *Add 1 tablespoon of everything bagel seasoning while mixing and a few extra shakes on top before baking.*

Crackers. *Slice the bread into thin strips and let them dry out overnight, or toast thin slices in a toaster. Drizzle with a few tablespoons of extra-virgin olive oil and sprinkle with garlic powder, dried thyme leaves, salt, and pepper, tossing to evenly coat. Bake on a parchment paper–lined rimmed baking sheet at 375°F for 15 minutes, or until golden brown.*

Croutons. *Cut the bread into cubes and let them dry out overnight, or toast slices in a toaster and then cut into cubes. Drizzle with a few tablespoons of extra-virgin olive oil and sprinkle with garlic powder, dried thyme leaves, salt, and pepper, tossing to evenly coat. Bake on a rimmed baking sheet at 375°F for 15 minutes, tossing once about halfway through, until golden brown.*

WARM BERRY COMPOTE

MAKES 1½ cups (4 to 5 servings)

PREP TIME: 15 minutes

COOK TIME: 10 minutes

A warm berry compote is so easy to make and elevates any breakfast or dessert to the next level of delight. The combination of phytonutrient-rich berries and warming spices supports your constitution and makes your house smell great. I pair this compote with Sweet Potato Pancakes (page 242), but also consider adding a bit on top of a Morning Glory Muffin (page 244), Slow Cooker Apple Pie Oatmeal (page 236), Sweet & Savory Butternut Squash & Spinach Porridge (page 240), or Extra-Dark Chocolate Avocado Mousse (page 320). It also pairs well with a dollop of Coconut Whipped Cream (page 334) for a sweet fix or a smear of nut butter on a slice of Whole-Grain Nut & Seed Bread (page 294).

2½ cups frozen berries of choice

2 tablespoons water

1 teaspoon ground cinnamon

⅛ teaspoon ground cloves

⅛ teaspoon ground nutmeg

½ teaspoon pure vanilla extract

½ teaspoon dark maple syrup

⅛ teaspoon fine sea salt

½ teaspoon arrowroot flour (optional)

Put the frozen berries, water, spices, vanilla extract, maple syrup, and salt in a small saucepan. Bring the mixture just to a simmer over medium heat, then turn the heat down to low and continue to cook until the berries are soft and the juice is thickened, about 10 minutes. If you would like a thicker compote, mix in the arrowroot in the last minute of cooking. Store leftovers in a lidded glass container in the refrigerator for up to 3 days.

LIFE KITCHEN TIP:

Arrowroot flour is a great alternative to traditional flour and cornstarch for thickening.

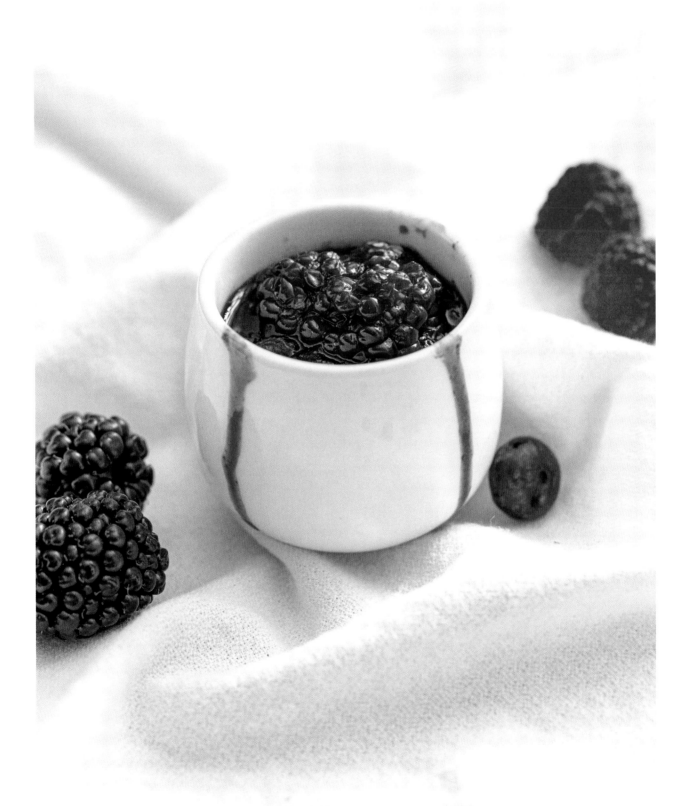

CARROT GINGER DRESSING

MAKES about 2½ cups (20 servings)

PREP TIME: 10 minutes

My delightful sister-in-law, Aya, helped me perfect this delightful salad dressing. One benefit is that it incorporates the power of miso, a probiotic-rich fermented paste with a salty flavor, and the prebiotic goodness of onions. The good little bacteria in your gut (probiotics) love the fiber-rich carbohydrates of prebiotic-rich foods and break them down to create short-chain fatty acids (SCFAs). SCFAs are anti-inflammatory messengers that preserve the integrity of the intestinal lining, help us recognize fullness by releasing gut-specific satiety hormones, and support immunity in part by keeping the gut pH normal. Alliums (the family that includes onions, garlic, leeks, shallots, and chives) are particularly amazing because they have been associated with decreasing cancer risk, in addition to antimicrobial effects.[4]

1½ cups roughly chopped carrots

⅓ cup roughly chopped yellow onions

1½ tablespoons grated fresh ginger

⅓ cup avocado oil

5 tablespoons unfiltered apple cider vinegar

1 tablespoon dark maple syrup

1 tablespoon white miso (see Tips)

1 teaspoon toasted sesame oil

¼ teaspoon fine sea salt

Freshly ground black pepper to taste

Recommended pairing:

Intensive Salad Shaker (page 260)

Pulse all the ingredients in a blender, adding a little water as needed to achieve a relatively smooth consistency. Serve in 2-tablespoon portions over any salad. Leftover dressing will keep in the refrigerator for up to 5 days.

LIFE KITCHEN TIPS:

Storing grated or peeled ginger in a plastic bag in the freezer is an easy way to have fresh ginger on hand. Grated ginger defrosts on the countertop in minutes. Miso comes in several varieties. White miso has the mildest flavor and is the type I prefer for this dressing. Consider using the leftover dressing as a marinade or topping to brighten up grilled chicken or roasted fish, or as a dressing on shredded cabbage to make a delicious slaw.

---

[4] H. L. Nicastro, S. A. Ross, and J. A. Milner, "Garlic and onions: their cancer prevention properties," *Cancer Prevention Research* (Philadelphia, Pa.) 8, no. 3 (2015): 181–9.

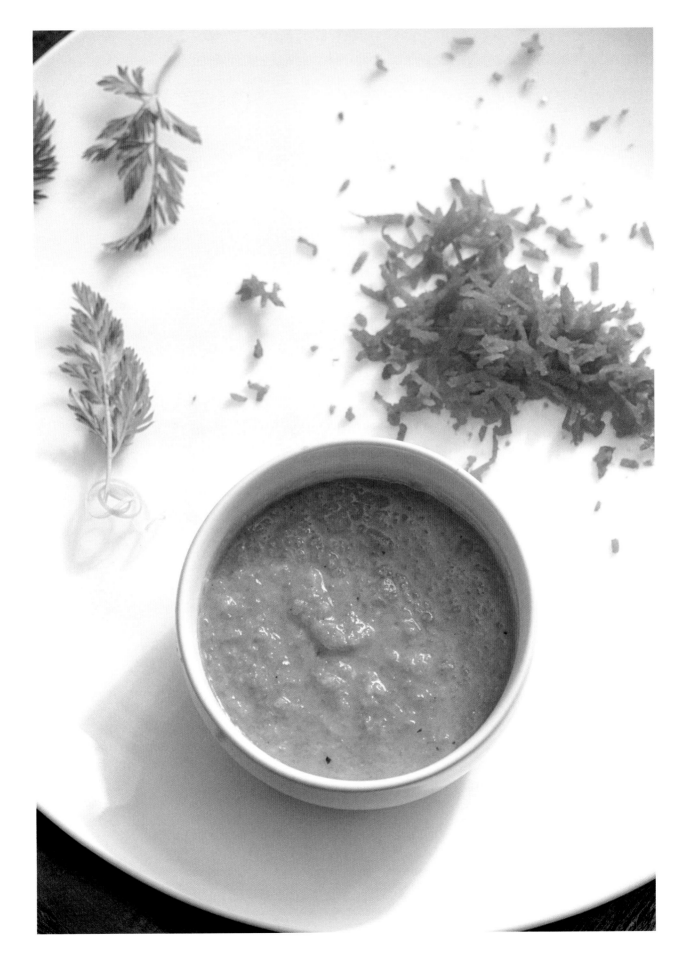

LEMONY BASIL CASHEW CREAM

MAKES about 1 cup (8 servings)

PREP TIME: 15 minutes, plus 30 minutes to soak cashews

Cashews are fantastic for replicating the creaminess of dairy and eggs in recipes. This gorgeous green cream is delightful on everything from a piece of toasted Whole-Grain Nut & Seed Bread (page 294) as a snack to a dip with crackers or vegetables to a pesto alternative served with homemade pasta, or—best of all—as a mayonnaise alternative in the Tempeh "BLT" Collard Wraps (page 272) and Mushroom Burgers (page 276). This sauce combines creamy cashews with basil, a fragrant anti-inflammatory herb. Basil's health benefits come from its inherent essential oils along with vitamin K, which is important for blood clotting, as well as vitamin A and lutein, both essential for eye health.

½ cup raw cashews

Grated zest and juice of 1 lemon

1 cup fresh basil leaves, loosely packed

½ cup extra-virgin olive oil

1 teaspoon nutritional yeast

⅛ teaspoon fine sea salt

¼ teaspoon freshly ground black pepper

For garnish (optional):

Grated lemon zest

Thinly sliced fresh basil

1. Soak the cashews in boiling water for 30 minutes or in room-temperature water for 2 hours until soft, then drain.

2. Put the soaked cashews and the remaining ingredients in a high-powered blender and blend until smooth. Serve in 1-tablespoon dollops topped with extra lemon zest and basil, if desired. Store leftovers in a lidded glass container in the refrigerator for up to 5 days.

LIFE KITCHEN TIPS:

The longer you soak the cashews, the creamier your blended cashews will be. I often allow my cashews to soak in the refrigerator for most of a day or overnight. If you prefer a thinner sauce for drizzling, add 1 tablespoon of water when blending.

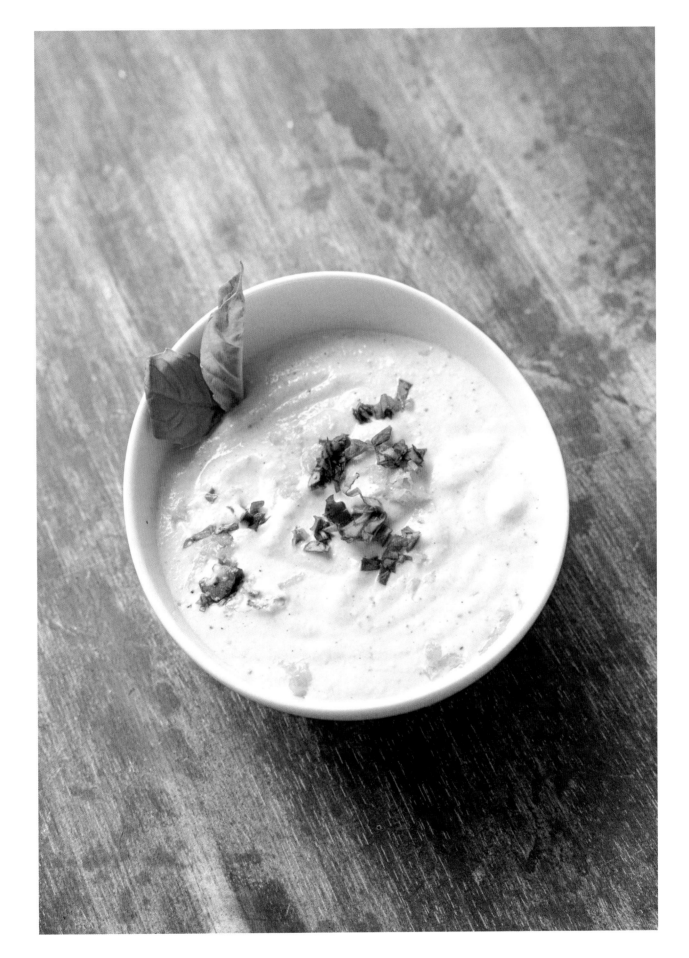

INTENSIVE THAI SPICE MIX

MAKES about
8 teaspoons

PREP TIME: 10 minutes

It's tough to find an all-around Thai spice mix that doesn't have nightshade spices in it. Nightshades are the class of plants that includes bell peppers, hot peppers, cayenne pepper, paprika, eggplant, potatoes (but not sweet potatoes), tomatoes, tomatillos, and goji berries. They contain the alkaloid solanine, which can be irritating to some people with osteoarthritis or inflammatory arthritis or who have a general sensitivity. How do you know if you're sensitive to nightshades? Go nightshade-free for three weeks and see if your achy joints, digestive woes, or sense of inflammation improves. I recommend making a batch of this spice mix and enjoying it in multiple recipes, including the Thai Coconut Curry Noodle Soup (page 266) and Golden Daydream Latte (page 308). You can also use it as an alternative to the spices used to make the snack mix in the Spiced Nut Mix recipe (page 326), and then combine the prepared snack mix with dried fruit, dark chocolate pieces, and cacao nibs to make our *Dr. Katie Detox Intensive* Trail Mix. It's also great just as a little pick-me-up on an otherwise bland piece of chicken, fish, tofu, or tempeh.

2 teaspoons ginger powder

2 teaspoons turmeric powder

1 teaspoon ground coriander

1 teaspoon ground cumin

½ teaspoon ground cardamom

½ teaspoon mustard powder

½ teaspoon kosher salt

¼ teaspoon freshly ground black pepper

¼ teaspoon ground cinnamon

¼ teaspoon ground cloves

Combine all the ingredients in a bowl. Store the mixture in a lidded glass container in a cool, dry place; it will keep for 3 to 6 months if you used newly opened ingredients.

LIFE KITCHEN TIP:

We love to repurpose in the kitchen. Instead of throwing away an empty spice container, refill it easily by making a homemade funnel with a piece of parchment paper and pouring each spice down the hatch. It works great!

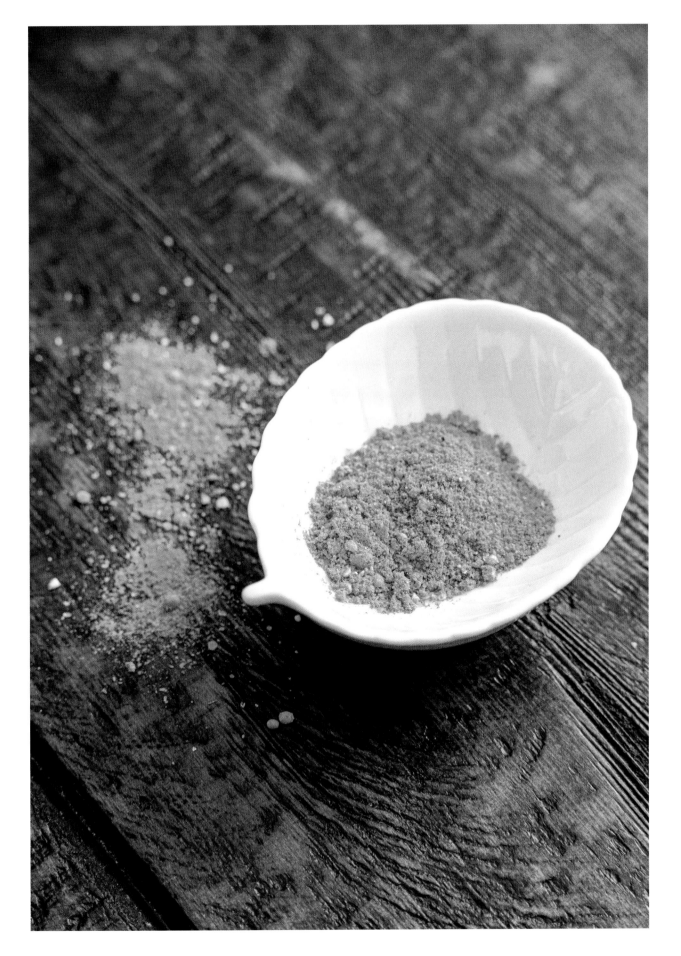

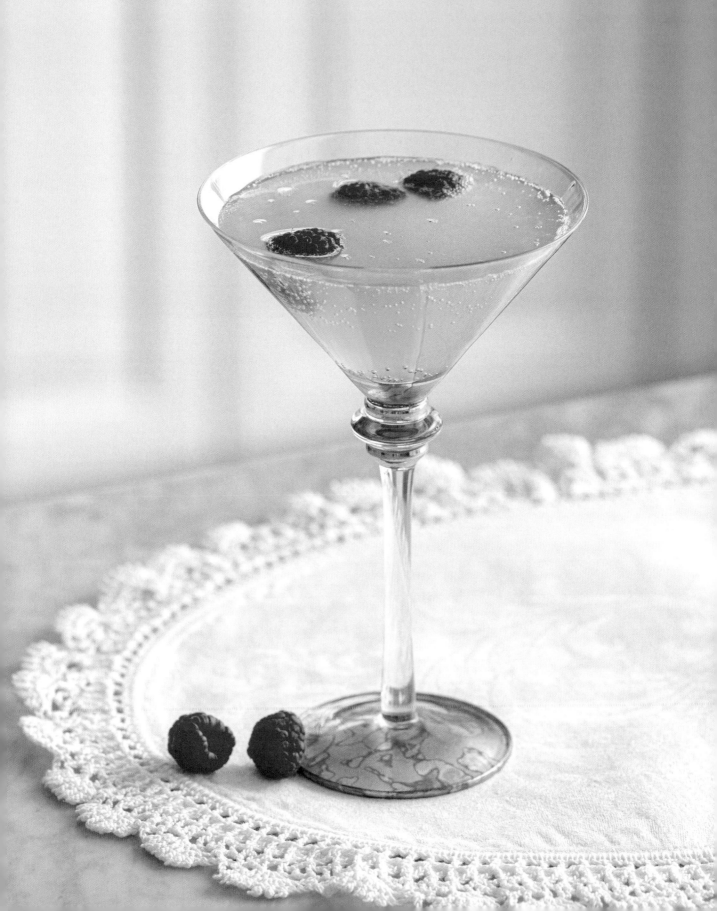

SIPS

TAKE A LOAD OFF AND NOURISH YOUR SOUL

DR. KATIE LIFE WATER

SERVES 6

PREP TIME: 2 minutes

Dr. Katie Life Water got its notoriety during one of my ten-day Dr. Katie Detoxes where my health coach and I spend ten days helping others to gently improve their daily rhythms surrounded by a community of support. Many of the Detoxers complained about their boredom with plain water, so I suggested my favorite way to enjoy water with lemon and a smidgen of flaky salt. Although acidic to taste, once metabolized, lemons produce alkaline by-products in the body, which are thought to lessen the work of the kidneys and bones to balance our pH. Salt, while problematic in large amounts and in processed foods, is essential for electrolyte balance in the body and helps to replace the salt naturally lost when sweating. My favorite salt to use here is Maldon sea salt flakes, but you could also use kosher salt or Himalayan pink salt.

1 liter water

1 lemon, cut into 6 wedges

Flaky sea salt

Fill a liter-sized glass or metal drinking container with the water. Squeeze the juice of 1 lemon wedge into the water. Add the juiced wedge and a smidgen of salt and shake to combine.

LIFE KITCHEN TIPS:

When cutting a lemon for serving purposes, I find it helpful to cut off the ends first. Then I cut the lemon into wedges, avoiding or chopping off the white inner membrane, which makes your wedges look pretty and easy to squeeze.

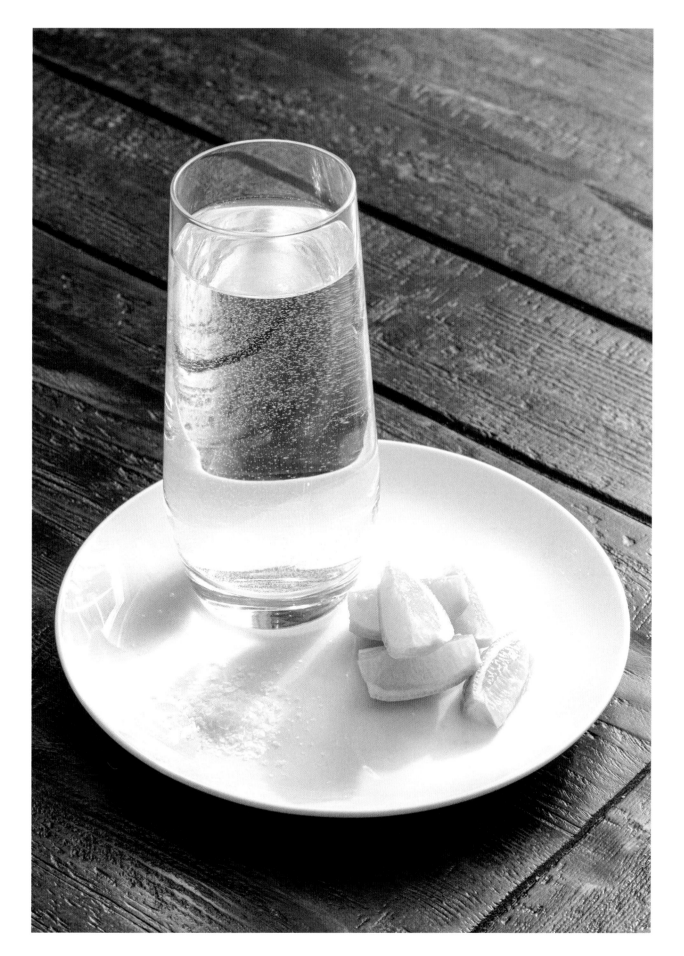

GOLDEN DAYDREAM LATTE

SERVES 1

PREP TIME: 10 minutes

COOK TIME: 1 minute

This is the beverage I turn to on a weekend afternoon when I want something satiating that soothes my body and soul without revving me up or calming me down. Turmeric lattes are all the rage these days; this version ups the ante with my Intensive Thai Spice Mix, which combines many more anti-inflammatory spices and has almost infinite uses. Cinnamon balances the blood sugar in combination with the anchoring fat from coconut milk, so this drink will keep you full until dinnertime. I love using Medjool dates because they combine satiating fiber with incredible sweetness, so a little goes a long way.

½ cup full-fat, unsweetened canned coconut milk

8 ounces hot water

½ teaspoon Intensive Thai Spice Mix (page 302)

1 small Medjool date, pitted

½ teaspoon pure vanilla extract

3 shakes of ground cinnamon (optional)

1. Warm the coconut milk in the microwave for 30 to 60 seconds on high or in a small saucepan on the stovetop over medium heat.

2. Put the warmed milk, hot water, spice mix, date, vanilla, and cinnamon in a blender and blend until smooth and frothy, about 20 seconds. Pour into a 12-ounce cup to serve.

LIFE KITCHEN TIPS:

Look for canned coconut milk that doesn't contain guar gum, a stabilizing agent added to many foods that can cause digestive woes. I keep coconut milk at room temperature so that a good shake before opening allows it to be mixed thoroughly. I store extra milk in the refrigerator in a lidded glass container for use in coffee or for making whole grains.

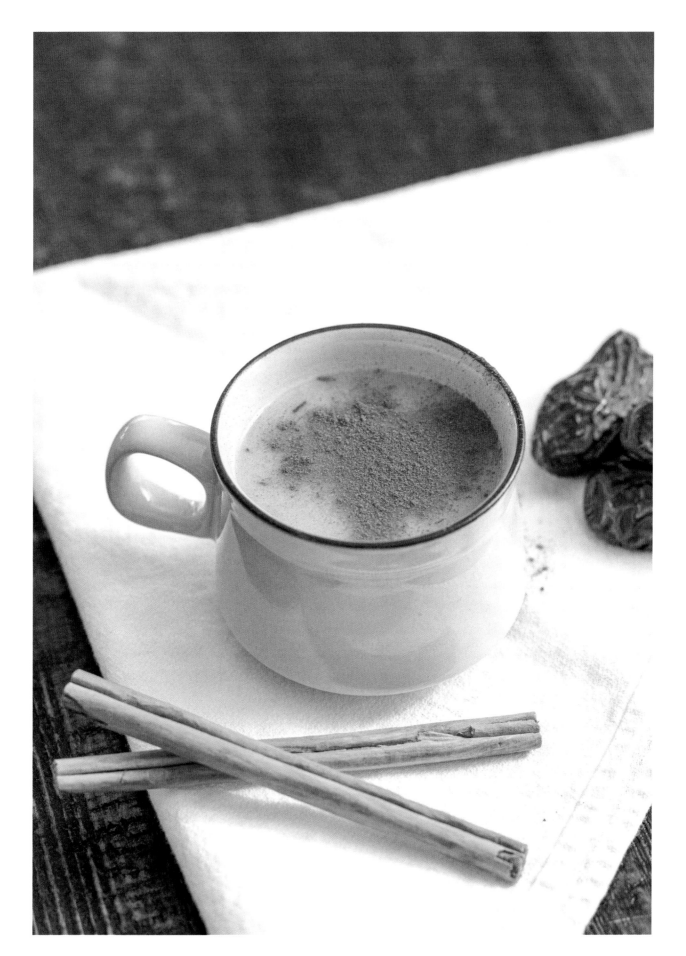

MACA CACAO HOT CHOCOLATE

SERVES 1

PREP TIME: 10 minutes

COOK TIME: 2 minutes

Maca and cacao are antioxidant-rich superfoods that make the perfect early-afternoon pick-me-up. This uplifting drink combines unrefined raw cacao nibs with the beautiful Peruvian cruciferous root vegetable maca. Maca is known in herbal medicine for being a vitality-enhancing adaptogen, a designation given to plants and herbs that help us adapt to stress. I like maca for those days when my body is feeling like it needs a little boost but I don't want the jolt of caffeine. The malty flavor of maca combined with the fiber of cacao nibs and Medjool date along with the anchoring of tahini and spice of black pepper gives this hot chocolate depth and texture that will satiate and energize you. As with all adaptogens, I recommend you consult your Integrative Medicine doctor about maca before adding it to your diet.

1 cup creamy unsweetened plant milk of choice, such as macadamia milk

2 teaspoons maca powder

2 teaspoons cacao nibs

2 teaspoons cacao or cocoa powder

1 teaspoon tahini

¼ teaspoon ground cinnamon (optional)

1 small Medjool date, pitted

½ teaspoon pure vanilla extract

Sprinkle of fine sea salt

2 turns of freshly ground black pepper

TOPPINGS (*optional*):

Coconut Whipped Cream (page 334)

Grated dark chocolate

1. Warm the plant milk in the microwave for 60 to 120 seconds on high or in a small saucepan on the stovetop over medium heat.

2. Pour the warmed milk into a high-powered blender, then add the maca powder, cacao nibs, cacao powder, tahini, cinnamon (if using), date, vanilla, salt, and pepper. Blend for about 20 seconds, until smooth and frothy. Pour into an 8-ounce cup and serve with a dollop of coconut whipped cream and grated dark chocolate, if desired.

LIFE KITCHEN TIPS:

If you don't have Medjool dates, substitute ½ to 1 teaspoon of grade A dark maple syrup. If you don't have a high-powered blender, you can warm all of the ingredients in a pan, allowing the cacao nibs to soften, and use either a regular countertop blender or an immersion blender to blend.

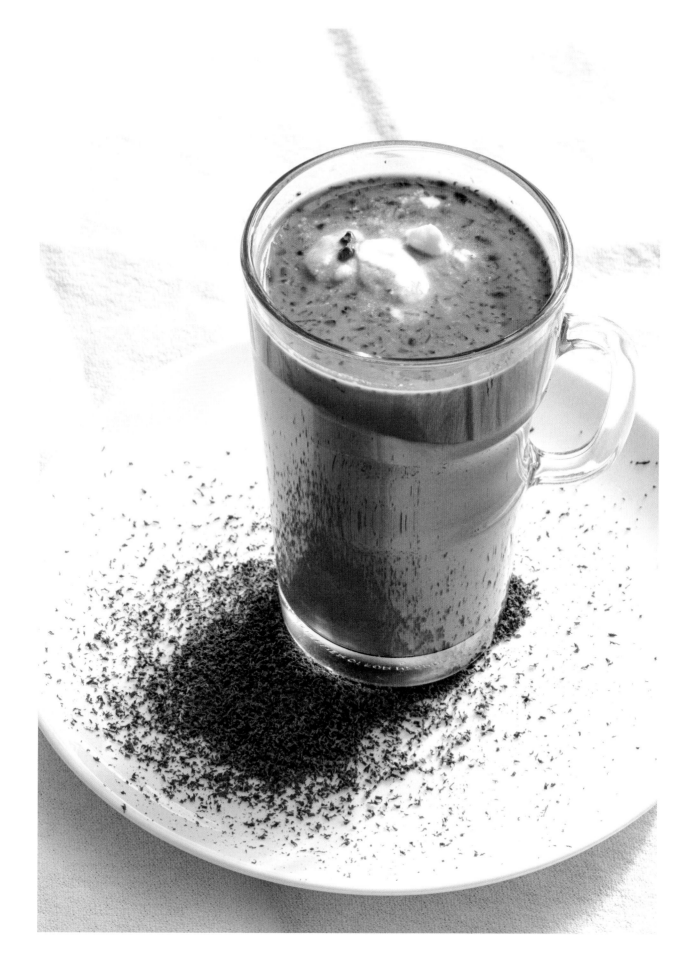

CHAMOMILE LAVENDER ANTIOXIDANT DREAM MILK

SERVES 1

PREP TIME: 10 minutes

COOK TIME: 1 minute

Lull yourself to sleep with this dreamy combination of relaxing chamomile and lavender and antioxidant-rich black sesame seeds in soothing warm coconut milk. I like black sesame butter (tahini) as an alternative to the usual tahini because black sesame seeds have extra antioxidants and a more potent sesame flavor compared to white sesame seeds. Cinnamon not only adds a sweet flavor but also regulates blood sugar, making this drink the perfect nightcap after a busy day. Though any type of cinnamon can be used, I prefer Ceylon; this "true" cinnamon has a sweeter, milder flavor and is lower in coumarin than traditional cassia cinnamon, which may be harmful in larger, more regular doses.

---

2 bags chamomile lavender tea (see Tips)

1 cup hot water

½ cup full-fat, unsweetened canned coconut milk

1 tablespoon black sesame seeds or black sesame butter

¼ teaspoon honey

Pinch of fine sea salt

3 shakes of ground cinnamon

1. Steep the tea bags in the hot water for 10 minutes, covering the tea to keep it warm.

2. Meanwhile, warm the coconut milk in the microwave for 30 to 60 seconds on high or in a small saucepan on the stovetop over medium heat.

3. Put the steeped tea, warmed coconut milk, sesame seeds, honey, salt, and cinnamon in a blender and blend for about 20 seconds, until smooth and frothy. Pour into a 16-ounce cup to serve.

LIFE KITCHEN TIPS:

Steeping 2 bags of chamomile lavender tea in a cup of hot water for 10 minutes brings out its stomach-calming, stress-relieving, and sleep-promoting properties. I like Traditional Medicinals teas because they're high-quality, affordable, and available at many stores. If you'd like to make your own tea, steep 1 teaspoon of dried chamomile and ½ teaspoon of dried lavender in 1 cup of hot water for 10 to 15 minutes. A high-powered blender makes the creamiest drink, but a regular blender or immersion blender will work, too.

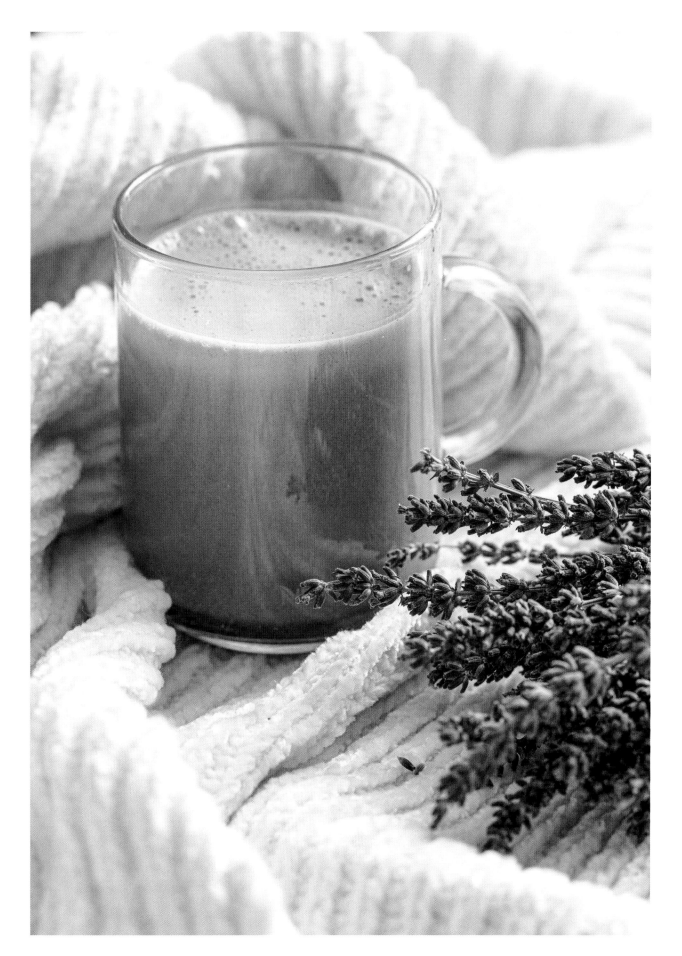

SPICED APPLE TODDY

SERVES 1

PREP TIME: 5 minutes, plus 5 minutes to steep

Apple cider vinegar, or ACV, is not for the faint of heart. Its characteristic sour and biting flavor is off-putting to many, but it is so good for your whole body. ACV is made by fermenting the sugar of apples with yeast to make alcohol and then further fermented with bacteria into potent acetic acid, which is where most of its health benefits come from. You may notice that raw, unfiltered organic ACV looks a bit murky from sediment in the bottle. This substance is called the mother and consists of proteins, enzymes, and friendly bacteria, so just shake the bottle before using. ACV is known to be antimicrobial, meaning it fights viruses and bacteria and kills germs, making this beverage a go-to during cold and flu season. ACV may help with indigestion due to low stomach acid and may help stabilize blood sugar by improving insulin sensitivity. It may also lower cholesterol levels and increase satiety, helping some people to lose weight, but definitive studies are still in the works.

---

1 bag honeybush, hibiscus, or turmeric tea

1 cup hot water

1 to 2 tablespoons unfiltered apple cider vinegar

Juice of ½ lemon

4 shakes ground cinnamon

2 shakes ground nutmeg

2 shakes ginger powder

Drizzle of honey

FOR GARNISH:

1 apple slice or lemon wedge

1 cinnamon stick

Using a 12-ounce cup, steep the tea in the hot water according to the package directions, keeping the cup covered to retain heat if you're serving a hot toddy. Add the remaining ingredients to the cup and stir. Garnish with an apple slice or lemon wedge and a cinnamon stick.

LIFE KITCHEN TIPS:

Use your external environment to guide your decision about whether to have a piping hot toddy or cold toddy served over ice. If you're new to ACV, start with 1 or 2 teaspoons and work your way up to 1 to 2 tablespoons in this beverage.

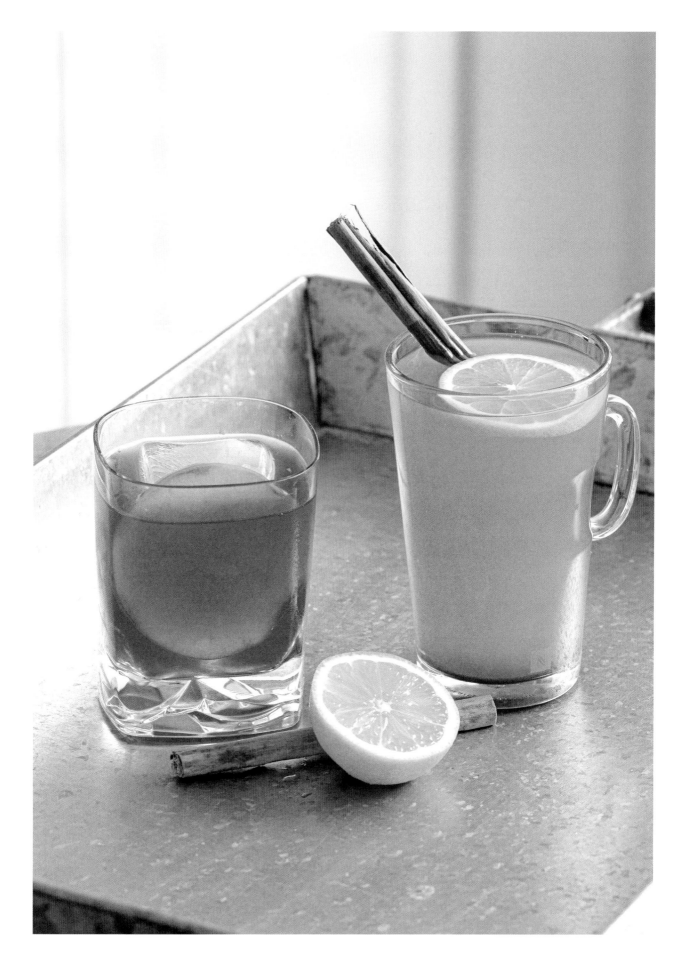

DK-TINI

SERVES 6

PREP TIME: 2 minutes

This idea came my way on just the right day at just the right time from my friend Alison, who's always looking at recipes and figuring out how to make them a little more "DK-friendly." She dropped off this combo on my doorstep as a celebratory treat to my team after we completed the marathon of Community Photography Day, which is how I managed the pressure of making more than forty recipes camera-ready over the course of two days. What better way to enjoy a cocktail than with the supportive powers of kombucha, an effervescent tangy drink made of fermented black tea and fruit juice that reinforces our gut's natural microbiome? A few raspberries not only look gorgeous and festive, but you'll appreciate their inherent sweetness in contrast to the dryness of the sparkling wine.

1 (16-ounce) bottle kombucha, chilled

1 (750-ml) bottle *brut* sparkling wine, chilled

18 raspberries

Divide the kombucha and sparkling wine among 6 festive 8-ounce glasses and drop in 3 raspberries per glass. Toast to your wellness!

*To make this drink *Dr. Katie Detox* friendly, eliminate the sparkling wine . . . so really you're just drinking kombucha topped with raspberries.

LIFE KITCHEN TIPS:

When drinking kombucha and alcohol, the less sugar the better. Buy a kombucha with 8 grams or less of sugar per 8-ounce portion and brut sparkling wine, which is the driest type of bubbly, to avoid unnecessary added sweetness. Leftover kombucha will keep in a sealed glass container in the refrigerator for a few days; leftover sparkling wine should be sealed with a specially designed champagne stopper and stored in the refrigerator for a few days.

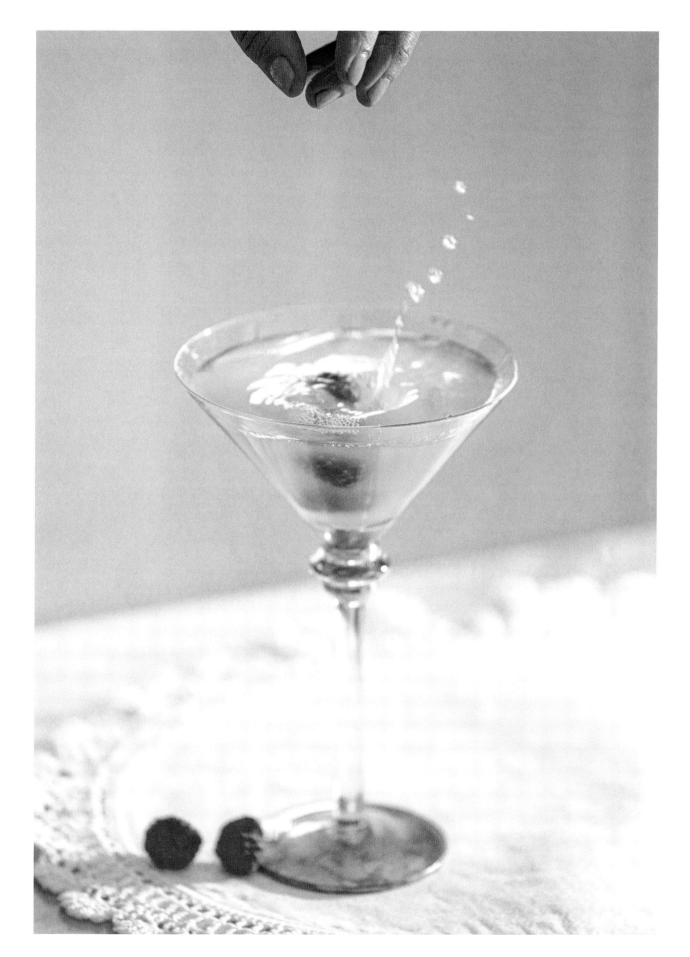

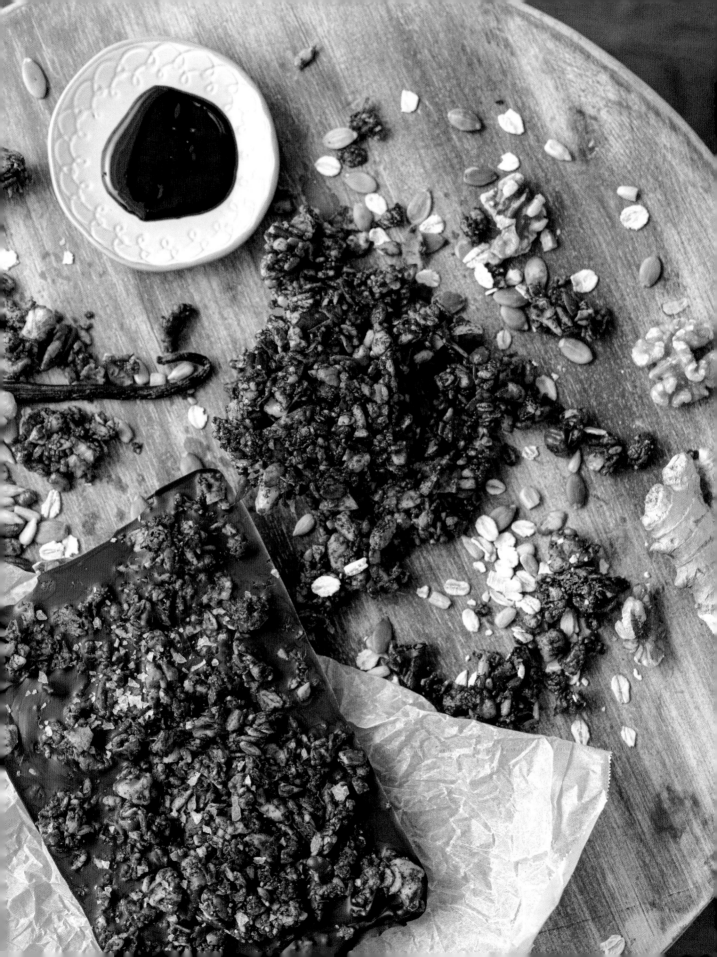

SNACKS & DELIGHTS

FOR WHEN YOU JUST NEED A LITTLE SOMETHING

EXTRA-DARK CHOCOLATE AVOCADO MOUSSE

SERVES 4

PREP TIME: 10 minutes

COOK TIME: 1 minute

It's no secret how much I love extra-dark chocolate. I have a little almost every day…usually around 3 p.m. when the day starts to feel long and a little cocoa and caffeine pick-me-up beckons. When I say dark, I mean in the 85% to 95% cacao range, which ensures that I get more of the antioxidants and flavanols without so much sugar. My favorite bar of chocolate is Theo because it's widely available and super smooth, but any brand you like will work just fine. This recipe uses the humble avocado to create a creamy dairy-free mousse that will satisfy your chocolate craving and fill your belly, since avocados are a delicious source of healthy monounsaturated fats and fiber.

---

1 (3-ounce) bar dark chocolate (85% to 95% cacao)

2 very ripe Hass avocados, peeled and pitted

1 to 2 tablespoons dark maple syrup, to taste

Seeds scraped from ½ to 1 vanilla bean, or 2 teaspoons pure vanilla extract

Pinch of kosher salt

½ cup Coconut Whipped Cream (page 334), for garnish

¾ cup fresh berries of choice, for garnish

1. Break the chocolate bar into small pieces and place in a microwave-safe bowl. Microwave on high in 20- to 30-second intervals, stirring after each interval, until the chocolate is melted. Alternatively, melt the chocolate pieces in a heatproof bowl set over a pan of simmering water, stirring occasionally, until smooth.

2. Put the melted chocolate, avocados, maple syrup, vanilla seeds or extract, and salt in a food processor and pulse until smooth.

3. Divide the mousse among bowls and top with the coconut whipped cream and berries.

LIFE KITCHEN TIPS:

When buying avocados, purchase them at a variety of ripenesses and then keep them on the counter. Once they get to the point where they give just a smidge under pressure from your thumb, you can transfer them to the refrigerator, where they will remain at the perfect ripeness for many days. Store leftover cut avocado covered in the refrigerator with the pit intact to prevent browning. Squeezing a little lemon juice on the flesh also helps to prevent browning.

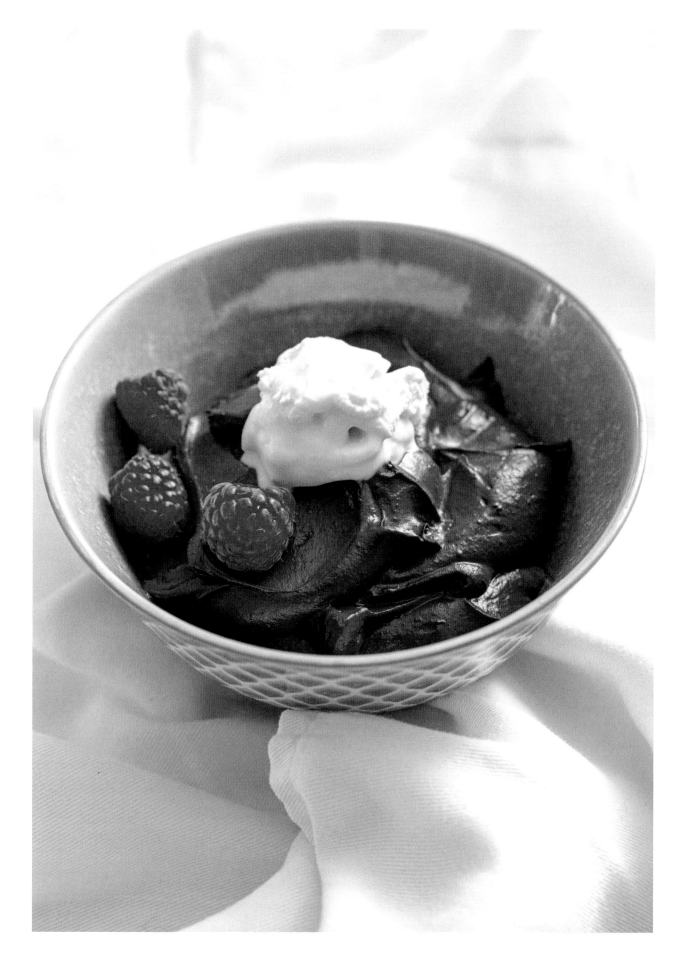

SWEET BEET HUMMUS WITH CRUNCHY VEGETABLES

SERVES 4

PREP TIME: 10 minutes

COOK TIME: 40 minutes

It's hard to argue with something that Nature makes bright red. Beets are full of nutritious, colorful antioxidants combined with a nice helping of vitamin C, iron, magnesium, folic acid, and fiber. And you know how much I like fiber! If you notice that your urine or stool changes color after you eat beets, you're not alone. Some people cannot break down the color compound betanin, also present in rhubarb and Swiss chard. Beets are rich in natural nitrates, which the body converts to nitric oxide, allowing for natural relaxation of blood vessels and better blood flow and blood pressure control. Thank you, Hippocrates, who said, "Let food be thy medicine, and medicine be thy food." Beets are sweet, so this hummus is well balanced with the addition of savory tahini and spices alongside crunchy vegetables.

---

1 medium beet

1 (15-ounce) can chickpeas, drained and rinsed

2 cloves garlic, peeled

2 tablespoons tahini

2 tablespoons extra-virgin olive oil

Juice of 1 lemon

3 tablespoons warm water

½ teaspoon ground coriander

½ teaspoon ground cumin

¼ teaspoon fine sea salt

⅛ teaspoon freshly ground black pepper

Dukkah from Spiced Nut Mix (page 326) or toasted pine nuts, for garnish

Finely chopped fresh parsley, for garnish

8 cups assorted sliced or trimmed raw vegetables, like carrots, celery, cauliflower, snap peas, green beans, and radishes, for serving

1. Preheat the oven to 425°F.

2. Wrap the beet in parchment paper followed by aluminum foil, then roast it on a rimmed baking sheet for 30 to 40 minutes, until tender. Allow to cool and remove and discard the skin. (The skin should easily rub off under cool water.)

3. Put the beet with the remaining ingredients in a food processor and pulse until smooth. Add warm water as needed to get to the desired consistency. Garnish with a sprinkle of dukkah or pine nuts and parsley and serve with an array of vegetables. The hummus will keep for up to 3 days in the refrigerator.

LIFE KITCHEN TIPS:

I like the brand Eden Organic for canned beans because they are pressure cooked with the sea vegetable kombu, which eases digestion for many people. I find this especially important when making hummus. If your digestive system doesn't do well with raw vegetables, consider blanching your vegetables for a minute in boiling water or steaming them for a few minutes until slightly softened. If you prefer a super smooth hummus, try boiling the drained and rinsed chickpeas in water with 1 teaspoon of baking soda for 15 minutes. You'll have to drain the chickpeas again, but the baking soda further softens the chickpeas, giving you expertly prepared hummus that will impress any palate.

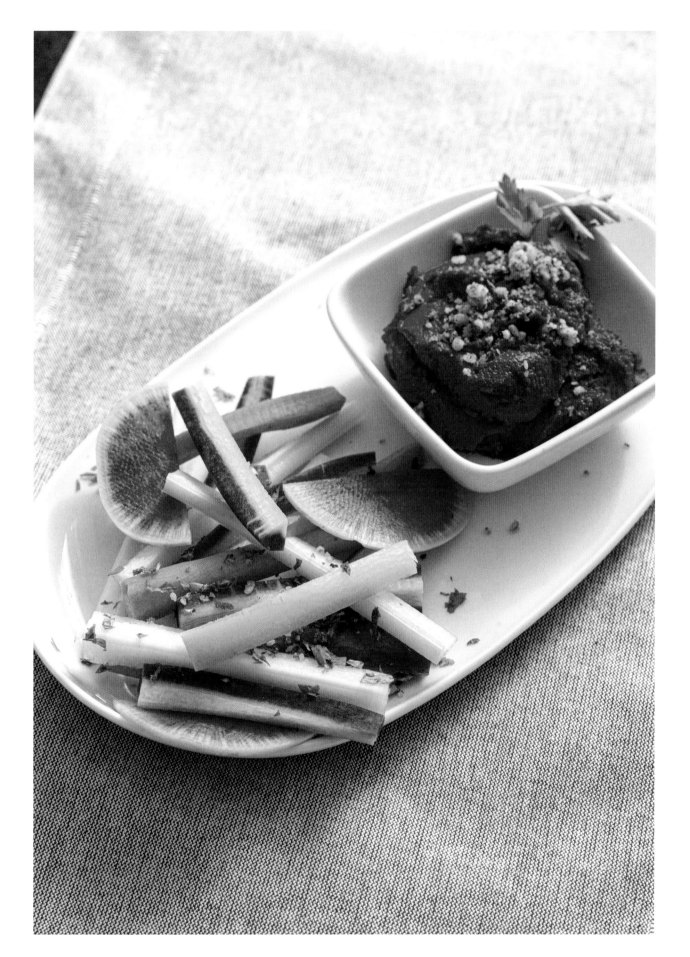

CELEBRATION GRANOLA BARK

SERVES 20

PREP TIME: 2 minutes, plus 1 hour to harden (not including time to make granola)

COOK TIME: 10 minutes

Chocolate bark is a mainstay in the *Dr. Katie Detox* because it takes an already delicious bar of extra-dark chocolate to the next level. Maybe you'll be so inspired by the idea of dark chocolate bark that you'll create your own yummy version with toasted nuts and seeds, a bit of unsweetened dried fruit, and an extract like almond or peppermint.

1 pound dark chocolate, preferably 85% cacao or higher

½ cup Celebration Granola (page 238)

Flaky sea salt (optional)

1. Line a 9 by 13-inch rimmed baking sheet or baking pan with parchment paper, allowing it to overhang the sides.

2. Break the chocolate into small pieces and place in a heatproof bowl. Set the bowl over a pan of simmering water and stir occasionally until the chocolate is melted and smooth, about 10 minutes. Once the chocolate has melted, pour it onto the prepared pan and spread out to the edges using a rubber spatula. Sprinkle with the granola and flaky sea salt, if desired.

3. Let sit at room temperature for at least 2 hours or in the fridge for 1 hour to harden. Then chop into the desired shapes of approximately ¼-cup servings.

4. Serve chilled or at room temperature. Store in the refrigerator in a tightly sealed container for up to a week. Alternatively, you can wrap individual pieces in parchment paper and store in a larger lidded container in the freezer for up to a month.

LIFE KITCHEN TIPS:

Adding a smidgen of salt enhances the flavor because it helps your body recognize the sweetness that's present in the food. This is especially useful when working with bitter dark chocolate.

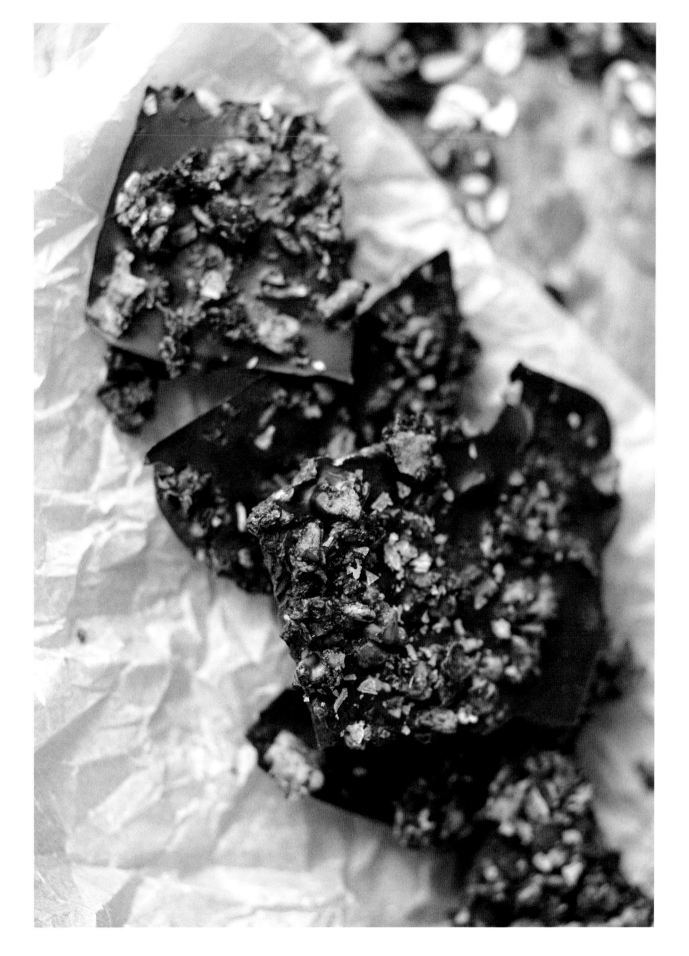

SPICED NUT MIX— TWO WAYS

MAKES 1¼ cups (5 servings)

PREP TIME: 15 minutes

COOK TIME: 9 or 12 minutes (depending on version)

This recipe can be either a traditional dukkah or a spiced nut mix for elevated snacking. Dukkah is an Egyptian condiment that combines nuts, spices, and herbs, usually a flavorful base of finely chopped hazelnuts with coriander and cumin, and enhances almost any dish. I use it to garnish several recipes in this book, like the Omega Avocado Toast (page 246), Roots & Greens Salad (page 258), and Sweet Beet Hummus (page 322). I use Brazil nuts in my dukkah because they are rich in selenium, an essential mineral that supports thyroid hormone health. I encourage you to be creative and make your own version of this recipe depending on your *Wellness Intuition*.

FOR THE DUKKAH:

½ cup raw Brazil nuts

½ cup raw hazelnuts

2 tablespoons extra-virgin olive oil, divided

2 tablespoons finely chopped fresh mint leaves

FOR THE SNACK MIX:

1 cup raw walnuts, pecans, and/or cashews

1 tablespoon extra-virgin olive oil

1 tablespoon honey

FOR BOTH THE DUKKAH AND THE SNACK MIX:

2 tablespoons white sesame seeds

2 teaspoons ground coriander

1 teaspoon ground cumin

1 teaspoon ground fennel

⅛ teaspoon ground allspice

⅛ teaspoon freshly ground black pepper

⅛ teaspoon kosher salt

Directions for Dukkah:

1. Heat a large skillet over medium-low heat, then pour in the Brazil nuts, hazelnuts, and 1 tablespoon of the olive oil. Cook, stirring often with a wooden spoon, until the nuts begin to toast and smell fragrant, 3 to 5 minutes. Add the sesame seeds and continue stirring until the seeds are lightly browned and toasted, about 3 minutes. Add the spices and salt and continue to stir over the heat for 1 to 2 minutes more, until fragrant and well mixed.

2. Remove the nut mixture from the pan and allow it to cool completely. Transfer to a food processor and pulse with the remaining tablespoon of olive oil and mint leaves until it resembles a coarse meal, with the nuts about the size of peas. Store in a lidded container in the refrigerator for up to 3 days, adding a few tablespoons to recipes as desired.

Directions for Snack Mix:

1. Preheat the oven to 350°F and line a rimmed baking sheet with parchment paper.

2. Put the nuts, olive oil, honey, sesame seeds, spices, and salt in a large bowl and stir until well coated. Transfer to the prepared baking sheet and roast in the oven for 10 to 12 minutes, stirring after 5 minutes, until golden brown.

3. Remove from the oven and allow to cool completely on the baking sheet, then transfer to a lidded container. Store in the refrigerator for up to 3 days. Serve in ¼-cup portions.

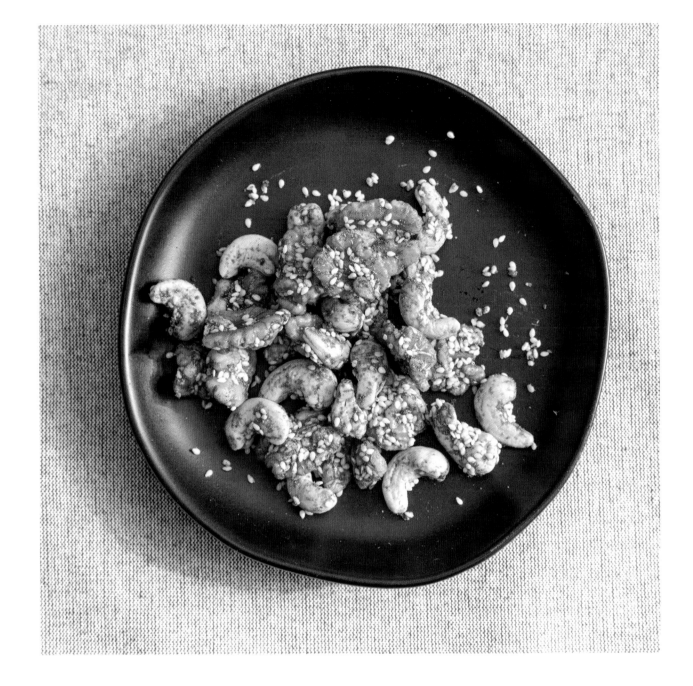

LIFE KITCHEN TIPS:

When making this recipe as a snack mix, I like to use walnuts, pecans, and/or cashews as an alternative to hazelnuts and Brazil nuts because their natural grooves pick up the spice mixture well. Dry roasting works nicely if using whole aromatics (spices). If using ground spices like in this recipe, adding oil prevents them from burning and awakens their flavor. If you won't be using all of your dukkah or snack mix within 3 days, consider freezing it.

MENSTRUAL HEALTH TIP:

If you menstruate, you could tie this recipe to your cycle by using seeds instead of nuts, called seed cycling. Seed cycling is a tasty way to support estrogen and progesterone. To seed cycle, you prioritize 1 tablespoon each of pumpkin and flax seeds during the follicular phase of your cycle from menstrual period until ovulation. During the luteal phase that follows ovulation, you prioritize 1 tablespoon each of sesame and sunflower seeds. (And if you're postmenopausal, you can use the moon cycle to guide your seed cycling, prioritizing pumpkin and flax seeds from new moon to full moon and sesame and sunflower seeds from full moon to the next new moon.)

THE CHOCOLATIEST OF COOKIES

MAKES 24 to 30 cookies

PREP TIME: 20 minutes, plus up to 2 hours to cool

COOK TIME: 10 minutes

Dark chocolate is like an authentic lifelong friendship: it's delicately sweet, incredibly deep and grounding, and satiating for the soul. This recipe came by way of my best friend, Stephanie. We met over twenty years ago in our all-girls residence hall at the University of Michigan, and I remember the exact day she said to me, "I just *really* don't understand why you love chocolate so much." And I, of course, replied, "I just *really* don't understand why you *don't* love chocolate. It's the best food on the planet!" Fast-forward a few years, through several cross-country moves, a few kids, different jobs, and significant health challenges, and we're both in committed relationships with our college boyfriends whom we inundate with plant-rich cooking…and she's come around to adoring dark chocolate, too. We joke about what time of day it's socially acceptable to start eating dark chocolate (we've settled on 10 a.m.) and frequently send little packages of new brands to try back and forth between Chicago and Connecticut. Dark chocolate is the rich vehicle for me to express my gratitude for my friendship with this amazing woman.

1½ cups rolled oats

1 cup oat flour

1 (3-ounce) bar dark chocolate (85% cacao), broken into pieces

½ cup plus 2 tablespoons cacao or cocoa powder

½ cup raw walnut pieces

½ teaspoon baking soda

½ teaspoon kosher salt, or less if topping with flaky sea salt

2 large organic eggs, at room temperature

¼ cup coconut sugar

½ cup melted virgin coconut oil

¼ cup honey

1 tablespoon pure vanilla extract

Flaky sea salt (optional)

1. Preheat the oven to 350°F. Line two rimmed baking sheets with parchment paper.

2. Mix the oats, oat flour, dark chocolate pieces, cocoa powder, walnuts, baking soda, and salt in a medium bowl.

3. In a large bowl with a hand mixer, or in a stand mixer fitted with the paddle attachment, beat the eggs and coconut sugar until smooth. Add the melted coconut oil, honey, and vanilla and continue to mix until well blended.

4. Fold in the dry ingredients and mix until combined. Allow the dough to stand for 10 minutes to firm up if it seems sticky.

5. Scoop golf ball-sized balls of the dough onto the prepared baking sheets, leaving about 3 inches between them, and use your fingers to push flat until they are about ½ inch thick. Top with flaky sea salt, if desired. Bake for 9 to 10 minutes, until firm.

6. Remove the cookies from the oven and allow to cool on the baking sheets until the molten chocolate solidifies. (This could take up to 2 hours if you used larger chocolate chunks. Placing the pans in the refrigerator will hasten this process.) Store at room temperature for a few days or in the freezer for up to a month…if they last that long.

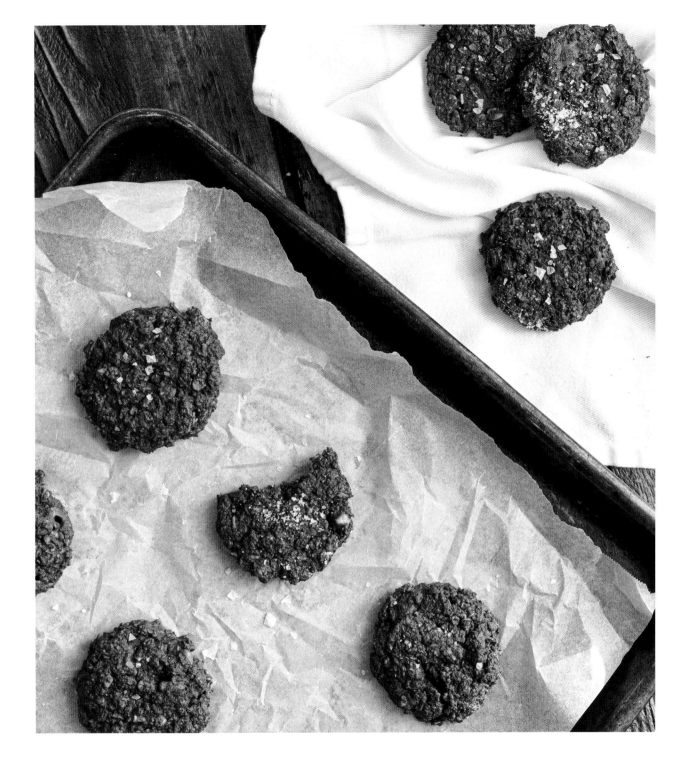

LIFE KITCHEN TIPS:

You can easily make homemade oat flour from rolled oats by pulsing them in a food processor. Use less salt in the dough if you're topping the cookies with flaky sea salt.

VARIATION:

For a twist, add 1 teaspoon of almond or peppermint extract. For a crunchy treat, add ½ cup of crispy rice cereal.

SUMMER MANGO AVOCADO SALSA

SERVES 4

PREP TIME: 20 minutes

Fruit is Nature's candy, and nowhere is this more evident than in a sweet mango. We know that mangoes are naturally higher in sugar, but they're packed with vitamin C and polyphenols, both antioxidants that protect our cells from damage due to oxidative stress. Eating too much uber-sweet tropical fruit by itself could lead to ups and downs in blood sugar, but keeping portions reasonable and pairing the fruit with the slow-burn monounsaturated-rich fats in avocados make it a nutritional win. This recipe also calls for sea vegetable granules, the naturally occurring iodine-rich ocean plants. Many of us are a little under-supplemented with iodine, an important mineral for thyroid health, due to the introduction of specialty salts into our diets. (Table salt contains iodine, but many specialty salts do not.) Adding a kick of raw red onion to the sweet mango and creamy avocado makes this salsa a must-have at your next summer gathering. It's delicious as a topping to brighten up salads or grilled seafood.

---

1 mango

2 medium Hass avocados

¼ cup minced red onions

¼ cup chopped fresh cilantro

Grated zest and juice of 1 lime

1 tablespoon extra-virgin olive oil

½ teaspoon dulse or kelp granules

½ teaspoon ground cumin

¼ teaspoon fine sea salt

¼ teaspoon freshly ground black pepper

Seed crackers, cassava flour tortilla chips, or plantain chips, for serving

Following the method described in the tip below, remove the pits from the mango and avocados, then cut the flesh into cubes. Combine all the ingredients in a medium bowl. Divide the salsa among four bowls and serve with crackers or chips.

LIFE KITCHEN TIP:

Removing the pits from stone fruits like mangoes and avocados can be challenging. For mangoes, I find the best way is to cut off a tiny bit of one end to create a flat surface and then stand it on the flat end and cut the mango "cheeks" from the long, narrow pit. Then slice around the pit to get the last bits of mango goodness. For avocados, I slice the avocado in half lengthwise and twist the halves apart while the skin is still on. Then I hold the pitted half in my hand, carefully whack the pit with the knife, and wedge it out. To make cubes of mango and avocado, simply hold the unpeeled "cheeks" in your hand and use your knife to slice it into the desired shapes while still in the peel. Then simply invert the peel or use a spoon to scoop out the segments.

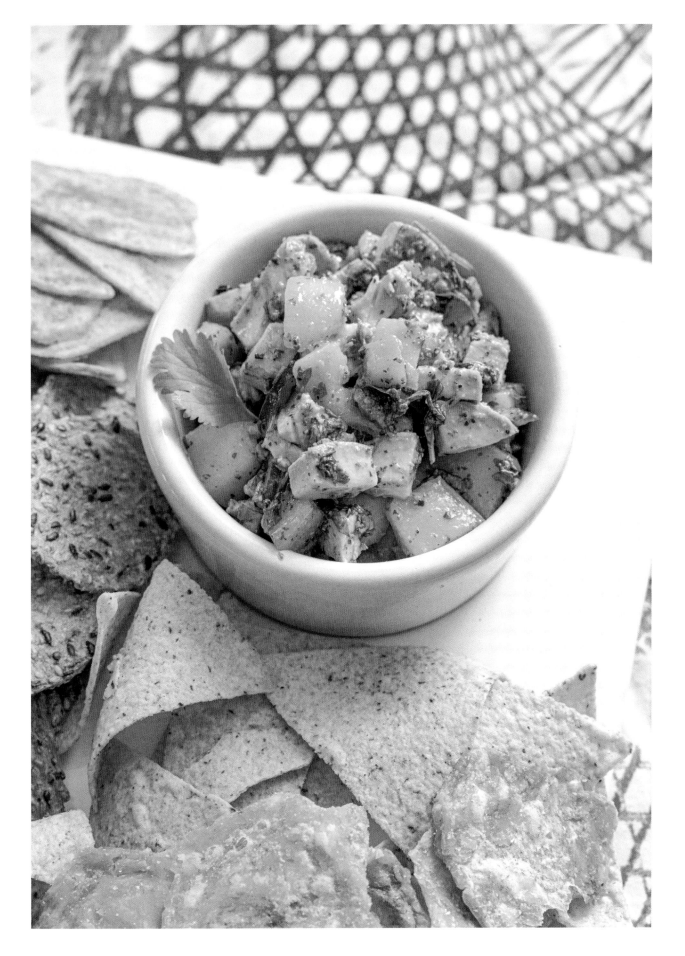

GINGER MANDARIN ALMOND TORTE

SERVES 12 to 16

PREP TIME: 20 minutes

COOK TIME: 45 minutes

This cake will knock your socks off for days…and by that I mean it tastes just as good, or maybe even better, for a few days after it's made. Thanks to the satiating fat in the almond flour and ghee, a little slice goes a long way toward satisfying your sweet tooth while keeping your blood sugar relatively stable and anchoring your appetite. Ghee gives the cake a buttery flavor without the milk solids of butter that give some people digestive woes. Ghee is also one of the few sources of the anti-inflammatory short-chain fatty acids, which are the by-products of happy probiotic bacteria that munch on fiber. My family likes Satsuma mandarins because they are easy to peel, very juicy, and seedless, but you can substitute any juicy tangerine or clementine. I like adding the bourbon to this torte because it lends a smoky oak and vanilla flavor that anchors the lightness of the citrus. Bob's Red Mill makes a great gluten-free 1:1 flour, but if you're not gluten sensitive, you can use all-purpose flour.

2½ cups unblanched natural almond flour, divided

¾ cup gluten-free 1:1 flour or all-purpose flour

2 teaspoons baking powder

1¼ teaspoons fine sea salt

½ cup organic ghee or unsalted butter

¾ cup plus 1 tablespoon coconut sugar, divided

Grated zest and juice of 5 mandarin oranges, divided

Grated zest and juice of 1 lemon, divided

1½ tablespoons grated fresh ginger

1 tablespoon pure vanilla extract

5 medium organic eggs, at room temperature

½ cup ginger-flavored kombucha, at room temperature

1½ teaspoons bourbon (optional)

1 (3-ounce) bar dark chocolate (85% cacao)

1. Preheat the oven to 325°F. Lightly grease a 9½-inch springform pan and line the base and sides with parchment paper.

2. Put the almond flour, gluten-free flour, baking powder, and salt in a bowl and mix well. Set aside.

3. Put the ghee, ¾ cup of the sugar, the zest of four of the mandarins (reserving the fifth for garnish), the lemon zest, and ginger in a large bowl or the bowl of a stand mixer. Using the paddle attachment, beat until creamed, then add the vanilla and mix until combined. Mix in half of the dry mixture. Add the eggs one at a time, scraping down the sides of the bowl as needed. Add the rest of the dry mixture alternating with the kombucha and mix until smooth.

4. Spread the batter in the prepared pan and level with a knife to promote even baking. Bake for 35 to 40 minutes, until a toothpick comes out a little moist. Do not overbake.

5. When the torte is almost done, combine the mandarin and lemon juices with the remaining tablespoon of sugar in a medium saucepan and bring to a boil. Lower the heat and allow to simmer for a few minutes. Remove from the heat and stir in the bourbon, if using. Immediately after the torte comes out of the oven, while it's still in the pan, pour the glaze over it, rotating the pan and using a rubber spatula to make sure it soaks through evenly. Let cool in the pan.

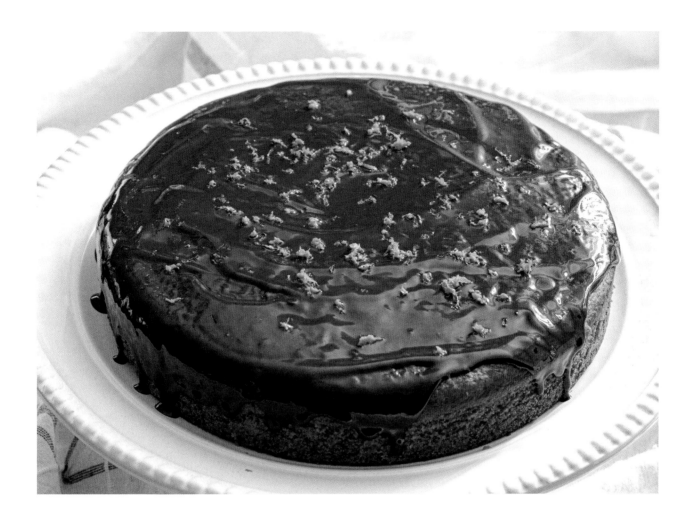

LIFE KITCHEN TIPS:

I prefer unblanched natural almond flour and coconut sugar because they are less processed than blanched almond flour and granulated sugar, but those substitutes will work just fine. Bringing eggs to room temperature takes about 2 hours, but you can speed up the process by placing the eggs in a bowl of warm water for about 10 minutes. One of my all-time favorite baking secrets is using kombucha for extra moisture when the recipe already has enough fat from oil or butter. Kombucha adds lightness due to its effervescence and works in everything from muffins and waffles to this torte. My favorite is GT's Gingerade, but any brand of ginger-flavored kombucha will work.

6. Break the chocolate bar into small pieces and place in a microwave-safe bowl. Microwave on high in 20- to 30-second intervals until melted, stirring after each interval. Alternatively, melt the chocolate in a heatproof bowl set over a pan of simmering water until smooth, stirring occasionally. If the chocolate breaks, add 1 teaspoon of water and whisk until smooth.

7. Remove the cooled torte from the pan and spread the melted chocolate over it, allowing some to drip down the sides. Garnish with the remaining mandarin zest. If you don't eat all of the torte within 3 days, I recommend freezing individual slices for those times when you want a sweet treat.

COCONUT WHIPPED CREAM

MAKES about ½ cup

PREP TIME: 10 minutes, plus 4 hours to chill milk

Coconut whipped cream is so easy to make, and it's a great dairy-free alternative to traditional whipped cream. Refrigerating a can of full-fat coconut milk upside down makes it easy to separate the cream from the liquid, or you can just use a can of pure coconut cream, which is more convenient because the separation has been done for you. Use this delicious topping on Sweet Potato Pancakes (page 242), Maca Cacao Hot Chocolate (page 310), or Extra-Dark Chocolate Avocado Mousse (page 320). Choose a brand of coconut milk that doesn't contain emulsifiers like guar gum.

---

1 (13.5-ounce) can full-fat, unsweetened coconut milk

½ teaspoon pure vanilla extract

¼ teaspoon ground cinnamon (optional)

Smidgen of fine sea salt

1. Vigorously shake the can of coconut milk for 5 to 10 seconds, then store it upside down in the refrigerator for at least 4 hours or overnight to chill and encourage the separation of the cream from the milk. Place a medium metal bowl in the freezer to chill, if desired (see Tips).

2. When ready to make the whipped cream, turn the can right side up and open with a can opener. Drain the thinner liquid and save for thinning, if needed, or for another use (see Tips). Spoon the thick cream into a metal bowl. Add the vanilla, cinnamon (if using), and salt. Whip with a hand mixer for 30 to 60 seconds, or until smooth, using 1 to 2 tablespoons of the reserved coconut liquid as needed to achieve the desired consistency. Use immediately.

LIFE KITCHEN TIPS:

After chilling and separating the cream from the liquid-y milk in a can of coconut milk, don't discard the liquid. It adds a delicate coconut flavor to a soup or smoothie. If the coconut cream is thicker than usual, you can use a small amount of the reserved liquid to thin the whipped cream to just the right consistency. Whipping the cream in a chilled bowl is best but not necessary. And if you're really pressed for time, don't whip the cream—just spoon it out!

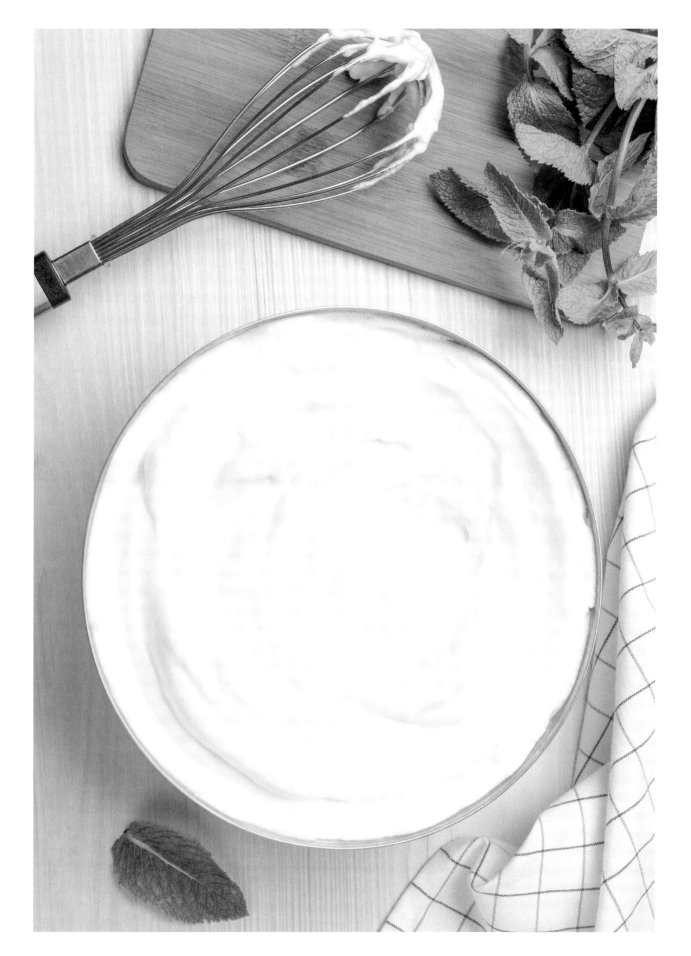

CHAPTER 12

THE DR. KATIE DETOX

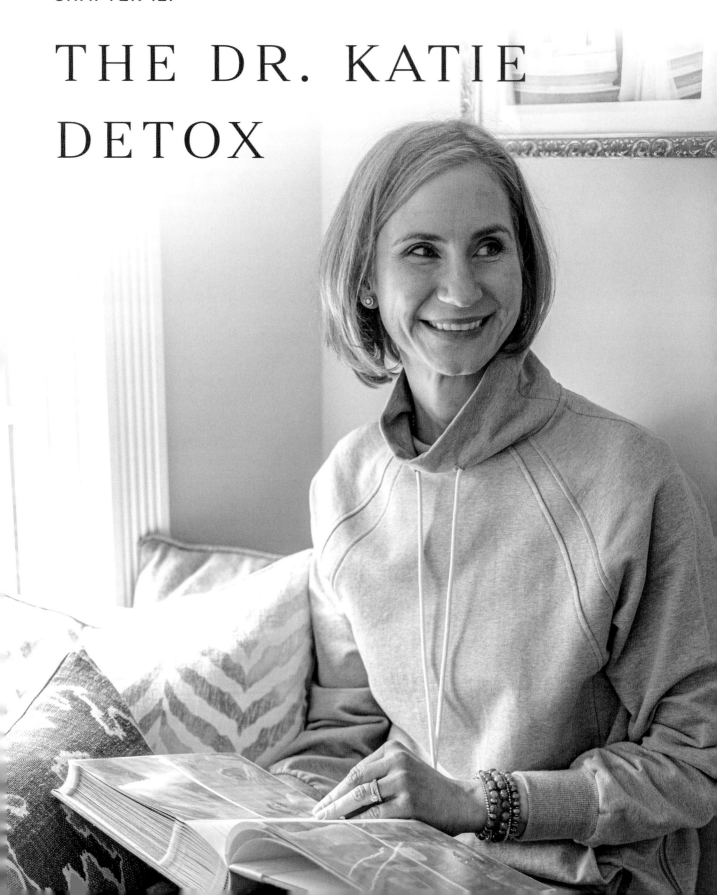

Our bodies deal with so many insults on a daily basis. Unhelpful compounds from the air, water, food, and home-care products barrage our bodies with toxins that can build up over time. While we have a beautiful, innate wisdom that allows for detoxification, sometimes following an 80/20 rule of plant-rich, nutrient-dense food is not enough to feel your best. That's when you know your body needs a reset.

Our bodies are like cars in a way. We are obviously more complex and idiosyncratic, but our bodies need the equivalent of regular brake fluid flushes, tire rotations, oil changes, and tune-ups. We need time to allow our bodies to do the good work of natural detoxification.

The good news is that our bodies inherently know how to detoxify. It's part of the way we were designed and evolved over time. Our intestines, liver, kidneys, skin, lymphatic system, and lungs are the key organs that aid natural detoxification. The problem is that we don't create space for this essential maintenance in regular life because our bodies are so busy keeping up with the day-to-day.

It takes considerable energy to digest not-so-healthy foods, sustain intense exercise that breaks down your muscle fibers, function on shortchanged sleep patterns, or feel like your real Self when you're not paying attention to the voice inside your head saying, "I can't keep feeling this way."

It's hard to pay attention to your *Wellness Intuition.* Our bodies talk to us, but often we don't listen because it's inconvenient. But if you don't pay attention to the smaller signals, your body will wake you up with a heart attack, or a cancer diagnosis, or the development of an autoimmune disease—or you will not wake up at all. If you don't make space for wellness, you'll have to make time for illness sometime in the future. We need to listen to the signals our bodies send us telling us it's time for maintenance and repair.

Speaking of cars, let me tell you a story. In the last few months, I started hearing a noise from my car while I was driving. I figured out that I heard the noise only if I was driving about 20 miles per hour with my foot off the accelerator in a quiet car without music playing, while paying attention and not being distracted by random thoughts. Insert life metaphor here, my friend. When do we ever live a little more slowly without pedal-to-the-metal speed, spending time in quiet, and actually listening to what our bodies need? Um, never. Could you be missing the signals your body is sending you?

Over the years, I have figured out what it is that allows the body to come back to its naturally rhythmic, grounded state in tune with its *Wellness Intuition.* I call my approach the *Dr. Katie Detox.* It is my invitation to take your foot off the accelerator and give your body, mind, and heart what they really want: the opportunity to do the good work of maintenance and repair.

My detox is grounded in the four pillars that I hold to be true in health: supportive nutrition, restorative sleep, joyful movement, and connection to the Spiritual Self and surrounding community.

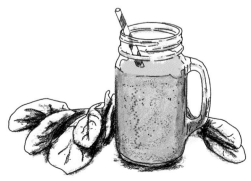

My approach is gentle and flips the switch in our diet culture from restriction and doing *more* to holistically repairing and rebuilding the structure for whole-body support by doing *less*. I flex into the space of detoxing when I feel like I need *more space* to recalibrate my body rhythms. It's not the recipes or the routines that do that work; it's the break you give your body from extra stressors that allows it to resume its premium function.

To detox Dr. Katie–style, all you need to do is take what you've already been doing in this book and elevate it. You need to take your foot off the accelerator and coast, paying attention to your daily rhythms. You need to lighten the load so your body can do its good work.

This chapter outlines the *Dr. Katie Detox Intensive,* a shorter five-day approach to rebalancing the body. I also recommend my longer seasonal ten-day *Dr. Katie Detox* at least once, as it gives you more time to refine your daily rhythms and learn what your body has to teach you, ultimately giving you a way of sustaining positive change.

HOW OUR BODIES NORMALLY DETOXIFY

Over time, toxins from our environment and lifestyle choices build up and can compromise the way our bodies work. It's valuable to spend time prioritizing anti-inflammatory lifestyle choices to enhance the incredible detoxification work our bodies naturally do on a daily basis.

On its own, the body detoxifies using six major organs: the intestines, liver, kidneys, skin, lymphatic system, and lungs. This shows up in our lives as stools, urine, sweat, and exhalations.

The waste products that come out of your body are like a daily report card for how your body is functioning. Ever notice after a night of eating rich food or drinking too much alcohol that your stools, urine, and sweat are...*different*? That difference is your body attempting to get rid of the extra toxins it took on in the form of creamy clam chowder, marbled steak, and a few glasses of red wine.

So let's talk about natural detoxification. To do that, we need to get down and dirty with our bathroom habits and other excretions.

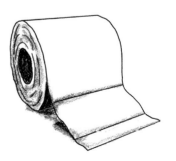

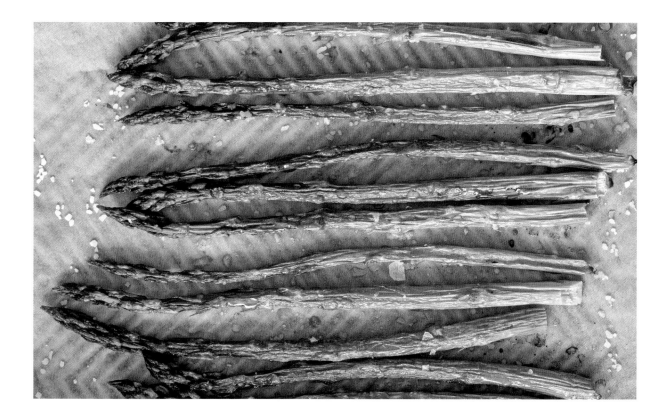

- **Stool:** Our stools tell us exactly how the good work of digestion is going and involve the intestines and liver. Bowel movements should be happening about once daily, and evacuations should be easy, non-urgent, comfortable without straining. Stools should be a medium brown color and come out in one long, smooth piece with a few cracks on the surface and only a faint odor. You should be able to stool within a minute or two of sitting down on the toilet. And you should feel good after you poop. While it's most normal to stool about once daily, some stool every other day or more than once daily. If you notice urgency, abdominal cramping or rectal discomfort, undigested food, straining, little hard pellets, or anything that loses its shape in the bowl, things are not optimal.

- **Urine:** Our urine tells us how our kidneys are filtering our blood. Urine should be generally odorless (unless you've just eaten asparagus) and near colorless (unless you've recently eaten beets), like the color of fancy champagne. Most people urinate six to seven times in twenty-four hours, or about every two and a half to three hours while awake with one or no nighttime awakenings. Urination should be painless and without urgency, taking less than about thirty seconds to completely empty the bladder.

- **Sweat:** Our ability to sweat helps our bodies cool off when we are in danger of overheating and is only minimally involved in detoxification. Sweat is 99 percent water with small amounts of electrolytes, metabolites, and unmetabolized substances.[1] It's

---

[1] Y. L. Chen, W. H. Kuan, and C. L. Liu, "Comparative study of the composition of sweat from eccrine and apocrine sweat glands during exercise and in heat," *International Journal of Environmental Research and Public Health* 17, no. 10 (2020): 3377.

normal to sweat anytime your body feels warmer than is comfortable for optimal function, especially during cardiovascular exercise or fevers. Sweating is also hormonally driven, like during pregnancy, breastfeeding, or perimenopause, or related to endocrine disorders.

- **Lymphatic drainage:** The lymphatic system is part of the immune system and has several functions. It protects the body from infection, maintains fluid balance, absorbs digestive fat, and removes cellular waste and abnormal cells. This network collects the extra fluid that seeps out of the circulation into our tissues, cleans it up, and then sends it back to the heart through the veins. You are probably most familiar with lymph nodes, which are the little bean-shaped glands that monitor the lymphatic fluid and swell up intermittently. But other organs like the spleen, thymus, tonsils, and appendix also play important roles in the lymphatic system.

- **Lungs:** Simply breathing in and out accomplishes a lot of detoxification. With each inhale, our lungs sort out valuable oxygen from the air and do the good work of purifying the blood by exchanging it for the metabolic waste product carbon dioxide that's then exhaled. The contraction and relaxation of the diaphragm muscle to move air into and out of the lungs also massages our lymphatic system, increasing our ability to move toxins out of the body.

You know you're adequately detoxifying when your stools, urine, sweat, and breath are normal while you also have sustained energy and concentration, an appetite that appropriately supports your metabolism, restorative sleep, and a feeling of authentic connection to your life.

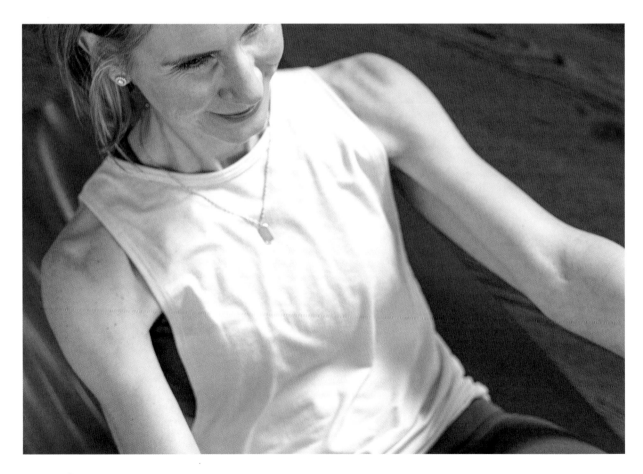

DO YOU NEED A DETOX?

How do you know you're not detoxing well on your own? It's simple: you don't feel well.

Not feeling well is different for everyone. Some of us are more finely tuned in to specific feelings, while others just globally know that they don't feel as great as they used to. Here are some common feelings that may clue you into needing a reset:

- **Waning energy,** especially after meals
- **Trouble concentrating** and an inability to focus
- **Unsatisfiable sugar and salt cravings** and overreliance on comfort foods
- **Poor digestion** with symptoms like reflux, diarrhea, constipation, bloating, gas, and/or abdominal pain
- **Questioning** if you have food sensitivities or if certain foods aren't serving your body

- **Unrefreshing sleep,** with difficulty falling asleep or maintaining sleep
- **Lack of connection** to your authentic Self
- **Not feeling as connected** to friends and family as you want to feel
- **Congestion,** rashes, joint pain, headaches, swelling, or other signs of inflammation that don't seem to make sense

I'm not going to pretend that doing a five- or ten-day reset will make all of these symptoms go away. What generally happens during a reset is that you start to notice improvements in some of these symptoms, and then you're better able to make connections between some of the lifestyle changes you've made and improvements in symptoms, which leads you on a path to your own Authentic Healing.

WHO SHOULD NOT DETOX

Generally, the *Dr. Katie Detox* is gentle enough that most people should be able to give it a go. That said, I always recommend that you talk with your healthcare team about whether a reset is a good idea for you. I do not recommend detoxing for anyone who is pregnant or breastfeeding, who is undergoing active treatment for a condition like cancer, or who struggles with disordered eating patterns or has a history of an eating disorder.

HOW TO DETOX
WITH DR. KATIE

Remember that our bodies are designed to detox naturally. Most of this detoxification happens while we're sleeping at night, but it also happens during the day. You don't have to do anything fancy to get into a space of enhanced detoxification, which is why almost anyone can do it.

You can boost your health by making a conscious choice to crowd out toxic foods, shift away from unhelpful habits, and prioritize yourself for a period of time.

At the very least, you'll want to have periods in your life without major toxins like tobacco, recreational drugs, and alcohol. If you do nothing else laid out in this chapter, start with these.

CHOOSE THE RIGHT TIME

I like the experience of spending ten days gently attending to our natural rhythms and coming back to center, but so much can be accomplished in just a few days. My business partner, Integrative Health Coach Courtney Evans, and I have developed a way to take the most important components of my real-time guided ten-day detox and make it more approachable in a self-paced five-day *Dr. Katie Detox Intensive*.

I generally recommend at least five days of finely tuned habits, but ten days is better because it allows for a more gentle transition on the front end and gives you more time to settle into these habits to make them stick, which establishes accountability. If you really want to soar, I recommend continuing your detoxification for twenty-one or even thirty days to ensure that what you've learned about your body continues to be a part of your self-care.

Doing the *Dr. Katie Detox Intensive* is not hard, but it does require some effort. It's my hope that during a period of detox you will

- **Eliminate processed and inflammatory foods** in favor of nourishing plant-rich meals that deliver energy and inspiration

- **Develop an understanding of intermittent fasting** and connect with what works best in your body

- **Emphasize sleep** by compressing your eating window, limiting device usage, giving up night-owl habits, and creating a supportive bedtime routine

- **Add more movement** to your daily routine and discover exercise that brings you joy

- **Spend five minutes in connection with your Spiritual Self** through meditating, writing In a Gratitude Journal, or grounding yourself in the breath

- **Examine your existing daily rhythms and relationships,** developing a sense of belonging to yourself and your broader community in the spirit of refining your *Wellness Intuition*

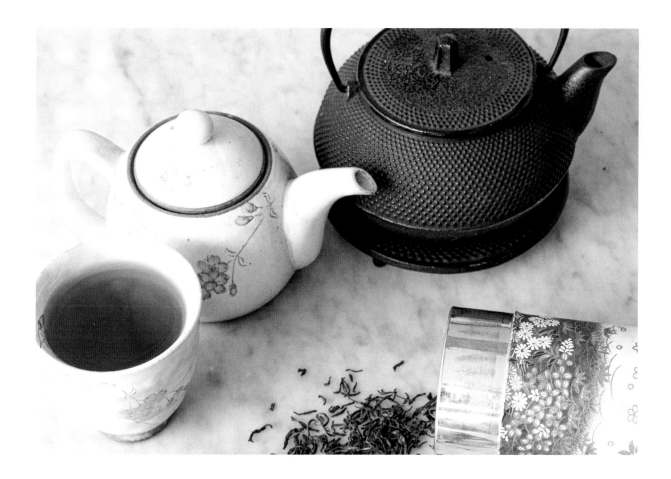

ELIMINATE THESE FOODS

One of the biggest hurdles to overcome is wrapping your mind around the food eliminations that I recommend to allow your body to fully detoxify. It's a little intense, I'll admit. And that's why I don't advocate that you follow this protocol all the time–it's just too limiting.

I see a lot of women in my practice who are trying to be perfect with their food all the time, and this effort leads to patterns of orthorexia and unsustainable, unhealthy relationships with food. Recognize that all of the following foods have a place in your diet at the right time and in the right amount. Even sugar can be a part of your life now and then if done with care.

I want you to use your detox time to lean into your *Wellness Intuition* and remind yourself how to eat to feel well. Use the strategies of mindful eating that I talked about earlier in this book (see page 87) to guide your listening.

During detox time, I'd like you to completely eliminate the following:

- Alcohol
- Beef, lamb, and pork
- Citrus
- Corn
- Dairy
- Eggs
- Gluten and wheat
- Nightshades like white potatoes, tomatoes, peppers, and eggplant
- Nonnutritive, noncaloric sweeteners (this is a category to eliminate forever, in my opinion)
- Peanuts
- Processed foods, which usually come in packages
- Refined sugar and natural sugar alternatives
- Shellfish
- Unhealthy fats, like canola oil and other inflammatory vegetable oils

Caffeine is allowed at a maximum of 1 cup of coffee (about 95 milligrams) per day, though I advocate limiting yourself to gentler sources like tea if you can.

Why does the detox cut out so many foods? The short answer is that these are the foods that people are most commonly allergic to or intolerant of.

Some of these foods, like eggs, peanuts, and shellfish, are common allergens. Some are almost universally hard to digest, like corn, dairy, gluten, and meat. Others, like processed foods, unhealthy fats, refined sugar, and alcohol, are inherently not good for anyone. Nightshades are problematic for some who have digestive, inflammatory, allergy, and arthritic-type conditions. And citrus can be bothersome to digestion, leading to symptoms like chronic cough and acid reflux.

By eliminating all of these foods, you're giving yourself your own version of a hypoallergenic diet, which eases the work of digestion for your body so that it can reroute its efforts to doing the good work of natural detoxification. If you suspect that there are other foods that don't serve you, I recommend eliminating those at the same time, even if they are not listed here.

You may be wondering what you are left with after eliminating all of these foods. Don't worry, my friend. You can eat all other vegetables, fruits, and animal proteins as well as all plant proteins, gluten-free whole grains (which is most of them), and a variety of healthy fats. Constructing detox-friendly meals is easier than you'd think.

Thankfully, all of the recipes in this book are designed to be used during a detox. All of the recipes are demarcated as being *Dr. Katie Detox Friendly* at the top, so you can figure out if you need to make any easy substitutions. You'll use the knowledge you gained in prior chapters to stock your kitchen and propel yourself forward.

Note: You may want to prioritize organic foods in your budget during the detox to give yourself the best nutrition possible.

"You may want to **prioritize organic foods** in your budget during the detox to give yourself the best nutrition possible."

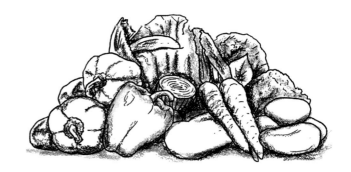

SET YOURSELF UP FOR SUCCESS

I recommend you set yourself up for success by planning ahead with the following:

- **Meals:** I believe strongly in connecting joyfully to time spent in the kitchen. Dedicating time to preparing all or most of your meals during your detox ensures ingredient control and building healthy habits that will extend beyond the end of the program. Figure out when you want to start your detox and make yourself a meal plan using my recipes. My family loves leftovers, so consider that over the course of five days, you really need to make only *two* morning meals and *two or three* midday or supper meals, most of which could be fashioned with batch cooking done on a Sunday. Spend time laying out a meal plan for yourself based on which recipes sound good to you and going to the grocery store. I've included two examples at the end of this chapter to help you along. Plan to eat your last meal of the day earlier than usual so that your body has adequate time to recharge overnight.

- **Exercise:** If you don't already include daily physical movement in your life, you'll need to create space for twenty minutes of gentle exercise each day. Most people feel better doing this movement earlier in the day and outdoors. Walking is one of the best exercises, doesn't require any fancy equipment, and is free. Spend time figuring out when you're going to build in exercise.

- **Sleep:** Leaning into how much rest your body needs to feel rejuvenated might be the most important part of allowing for natural detoxification. Attending to your sleep drive requires planning ahead, understanding that it takes forty-five to ninety minutes to wind down after a busy day. Relinquishing to rest takes effort because we are culturally wired to perform. Developing a bedtime routine might be the best planning you can do and could include restorative activities like a cup of chamomile tea, a warm bath with magnesium salts, passive yoga poses, or some mindful breathing.

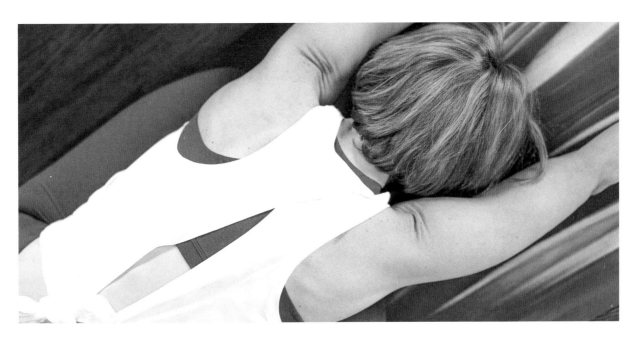

- **Connection to your Spiritual Self:**
  It's tough to listen to what the heart wants because the heart and the head sometimes disagree. Planning ahead in this realm means scheduling time in your day for tuning in to your Spiritual Self. For some, finding a space of stillness at the start of the day, before they're off to the races, works best. Others find that time between other activities. And for others, including meditative time as part of their bedtime ritual makes the most sense. If you're new to listening to your Spiritual Self, I advocate starting with a Gratitude Journal. Simply write down three people or circumstances you are most grateful for on each of the five days of your detox. You'll be amazed. Feel free to use the Gratitude Journal model that I've laid out for you on page 352.

Do you see the theme here? It's *planning ahead.* Planning is the key to changing unhelpful patterns in your life that aren't serving you and creating space for the rhythms that propel you into the life you want and deserve.

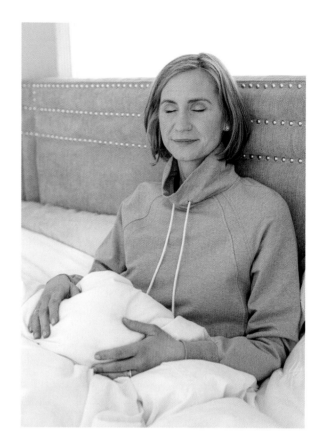

RECOGNIZE DETOX SYMPTOMS

Everyone responds differently to detoxing from inflammatory foods and bad habits, and most of your personal response depends on how you lived prior to starting the detox. If you're generally a plant-forward eater who enjoys home-cooked, nutrient-dense food along with positive lifestyle habits like moderation with caffeine and alcohol, regular exercise and meditation, and prioritization of sleep, then you might not feel too different. That said, I do all of those things and almost always feel a shift in my body at the start of a detox.

Almost universally, I hear from Detoxers that they can have mild fatigue, headaches, changes in bowel habits, bloating, achiness, and/or nausea. The clue here is that the symptoms are mild and tolerable and seem to pass with time and proper hydration. If you ever feel frankly ill, then something is not right, and you should call your doctor. And remember that the goal of the detox is not starvation or weight loss, so acknowledge your hunger and satisfy it with a well-balanced meal or snack.

TRY INTERMITTENT FASTING

A powerful tool that we use during the *Dr. Katie Detox* is intermittent fasting: the purposeful use of periods without food to aid detoxification, support cellular regeneration, balance hunger hormones, and reset the metabolism. I encourage you to maintain a minimum twelve-hour overnight fast during your detox.

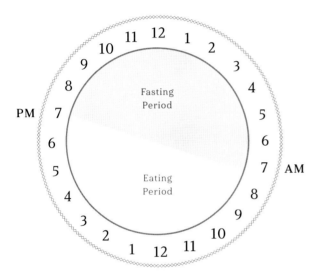

You are welcome to experiment with extending your nightly fast to fourteen or sixteen hours for a more significant metabolism boost, but I recommend doing so by pushing up your last meal to earlier in the day rather than skipping breakfast. It makes much more energetic sense to eat food when you need the fuel, especially in the early hours of the day.

Some Detoxers find it helpful to do one twenty-four-hour fast on the fifth day. This period without food allows for a more intense experience and a deeper reset of the body. I've seen Detoxers do well with going dinner-to-dinner (meaning not eating breakfast or lunch on day five) or breakfast-to-breakfast (meaning not eating lunch or dinner on day five).

If you're new to intermittent fasting, a more successful strategy could be fasting for sixteen hours after your midday meal on day five and resuming breakfast on day six. I leave this to your discretion based on how you're feeling.

Recognize that intermittent fasting takes a bit of metabolic flexibility, so if you're stressed, then you should not attempt to fast for more than twelve hours overnight because it will only further tax your adrenal glands and make you feel worse.

> "Remember that the *goal of the detox* is **not starvation or weight loss,** so acknowledge your hunger and satisfy it with a well-balanced meal or snack."

CONSIDER ELIMINATING OTHER TOXINS

I recognize that we're exposed to a lot of other environmental and social toxins on a daily basis that are not covered in this detox. If you want to step it up, consider evaluating environmental factors such as your water supply and air quality, cosmetics and personal care products, kitchen tools like the microwave, factory-farmed meat and fish consumption, plastic use, and proximity to power sources and electromagnetic fields. Social toxins can include interactions with people who don't bring you joy and overreliance on electronic devices. The world is your oyster. Do what feels right in your *Wellness Intuition*.

AFTER THE DETOX

After you finish your five days, you'll want to add back eliminated foods like sugar, eggs, dairy, gluten, and meat very thoughtfully. Don't pound a Snickers on day six and expect to feel well. Ease back into the eliminated foods category by category. Pay attention to the way you feel. If you don't feel well, then maybe it's an opportunity to explore with your healthcare team, as it could be a sign of something bigger going on or a more profound food sensitivity or allergy. If you suspect an allergy or intolerance, you may want to avoid that food for a longer period to eliminate more of the proteins in your immune system that are reacting to it. Generally, it takes at least three weeks of consistent elimination to really appreciate a difference, but if you're tapped into your *Wellness Intuition*, you may notice a change after just five days.

"**Pay attention** to the way you feel. *If you don't feel well,* then maybe it's an opportunity to explore with your healthcare team."

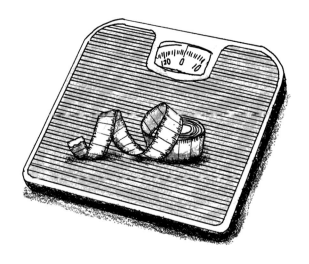

TWO DETOX MEAL PLANS

You could create so many different permutations of a meal plan using the recipes in this book. These are just two ideas to get you going. Use your imagination and your tolerance of leftovers to work in your favor. My personal best strategy for success is meal planning and preparation on Sunday afternoons so that I have a structure set for the entire week. Check out more strategies for preparation in Chapter 10.

   Note that I give you the option of fasting after lunch on the fifth day until lunch on the sixth day, but you could also fast through breakfast and lunch on the fifth day if that schedule suits your rhythm better.

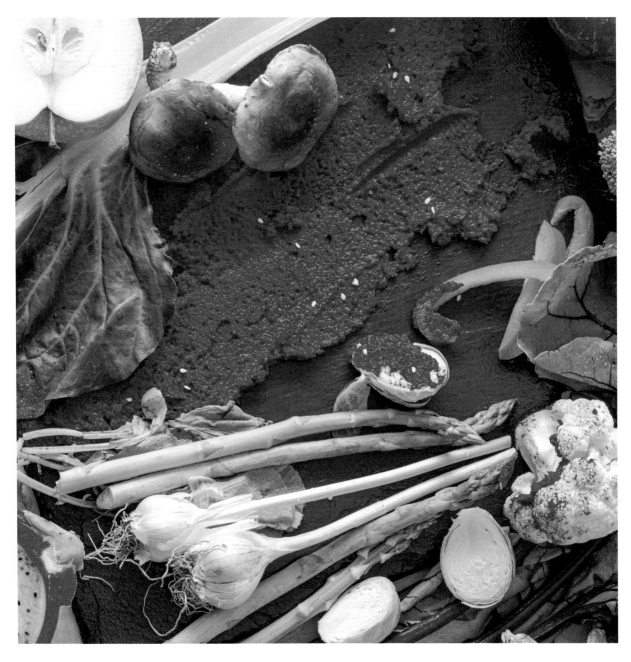

MEAL PLAN 1

	MORNING	MIDDAY	SUPPER	SNACK/DELIGHT
DAY 1	Morning Glory Muffins	Intensive Salad Shaker + Carrot Ginger Dressing	Sheet Pan Roasted Chicken with Pears, Figs & Swiss Chard	Sweet Beet Hummus with Crunchy Vegetables
DAY 2	Sweet & Savory Butternut Squash & Spinach Porridge	Creamy Roasted Broccoli Soup	Sheet Pan Roasted Chicken with Pears, Figs & Swiss Chard	Celebration Granola Bark
DAY 3	Celebration Granola with coconut yogurt	Intensive Salad Shaker with Carrot Ginger Dressing	Thai Coconut Curry Noodle Soup	Sweet Beet Hummus with Crunchy Vegetables
DAY 4	Sweet & Savory Butternut Squash & Spinach Porridge	Creamy Roasted Broccoli Soup	Almond Furikake Crusted Halibut with Roasted Vegetables, Black Rice & Coconut Lime Cream	Chamomile Lavender Antioxidant Dream Milk
DAY 5	Morning Glory Muffins	Roots & Greens Salad	*Fast* or Thai Coconut Curry Noodle Soup	Celebration Granola Bark

MEAL PLAN 2

	MORNING	MIDDAY	SUPPER	SNACK/DELIGHT
DAY 1	242 Sweet Potato Pancakes with Warm Berry Compote	252 Kale & Quinoa Greek Salad	276 Mushroom Burger with Parsnip Fries	326 Spiced Nut Mix
DAY 2	LEFTOVER Sweet Potato Pancakes with Warm Berry Compote	260 298 Intensive Salad Shaker with Carrot Ginger Dressing	LEFTOVER Mushroom Burger with Parsnip Fries	295 330 Whole-Grain Nut & Seed Crackers with Summer Mango Avocado Salsa
DAY 3	246 Omega Avocado Toast	LEFTOVER Kale & Quinoa Greek Salad	272 300 Tempeh "BLT" Collard Wrap with Lemony Basil Cashew Cream	LEFTOVER LEFTOVER Whole-Grain Nut & Seed Crackers with Summer Mango Avocado Salsa
DAY 4	248 Recovery Smoothie	LEFTOVER LEFTOVER Intensive Salad Shaker with Carrot Ginger Dressing	LEFTOVER LEFTOVER Tempeh "BLT" Collard Wrap with Lemony Basil Cashew Cream	LEFTOVER Spiced Nut Mix
DAY 5	246 Omega Avocado Toast	284 LEFTOVER Salad with leftover vegetables, Harvest Wild Rice, and Lemony Basil Cashew Cream	274 282 LEFTOVER *Fast* or Roasted Salmon with Miso Shallot Jam, Crispy Parsley, and Harvest Wild Rice	310 Maca Cacao Hot Chocolate

YOUR GRATITUDE JOURNAL

You're invited to use this space to start your daily habit of recognizing the three people or circumstances that you are grateful for in the service of connection to your Spiritual Self.

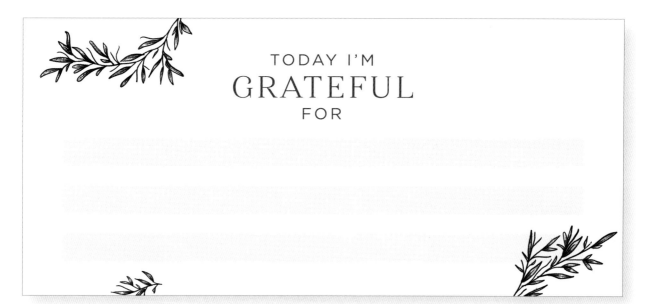

TODAY I'M
GRATEFUL
FOR

TODAY I'M GRATEFUL FOR

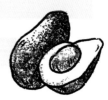

TODAY I'M GRATEFUL FOR

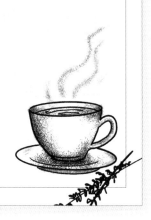

TODAY I'M GRATEFUL FOR

TODAY I'M GRATEFUL FOR

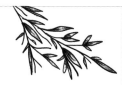

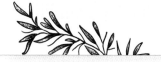

CONCLUSION

"Get **busy living,** *or* get busy dying."

—*The Shawshank Redemption*

This is your time.

You've taken the time to read my thoughts on living a plant-forward life, and now it's time to put your knowledge into action.

You can do it. Little by little. Choice by choice.

Maybe this week you think about adding an extra serving of vegetables to your evening meal. And maybe next week you think about taking one processed grain in your diet and replacing it with an anti-inflammatory whole grain. And maybe the next week you incorporate a serving of omega-3-rich fish like salmon, black cod, or halibut into your protein rotation. It doesn't matter where you start; it just matters that you get the ball rolling. Because once you get the ball rolling, you'll notice that all these tiny tweaks are not that difficult, and when taken together as a whole, they amount to more than the parts.

Health comes from finding balance between surrender and agency. We all have to accept those components of our lives that we cannot shift, no matter how hard we try. Each of us has an individual constitution that is predetermined by our genetics and the time and space we live in. You can't choose your parents. There are so many reasons to get frustrated. It's okay to surrender to what you cannot change.

But we all have agency over our health. Almost all of what happens in our lives is influenceable in some capacity. It starts with taking better care of ourselves on a daily basis and attending to the rhythms that allow us to succeed.

We know that we'll all die someday. It's a virtual certainty.

It's true that we'll still die even if we eat more plants, exercise every day, go to bed on time, and try to find space for meditation.

But what we'll get in exchange for our efforts is a higher quality of life and the satisfaction that we did the best we could with the knowledge we had. And knowing that about ourselves imparts an integrity that is so critical to our self-worth and identity that it seeps into our hearts.

Our daily decision to fuel our authentic selves with plant-rich foods and holistic lifestyle choices makes an imprint on our physical, emotional, mental, and spiritual bodies that shifts us into a higher awareness.

Let's get there together.

"*Health* comes from **finding balance** between surrender and agency."

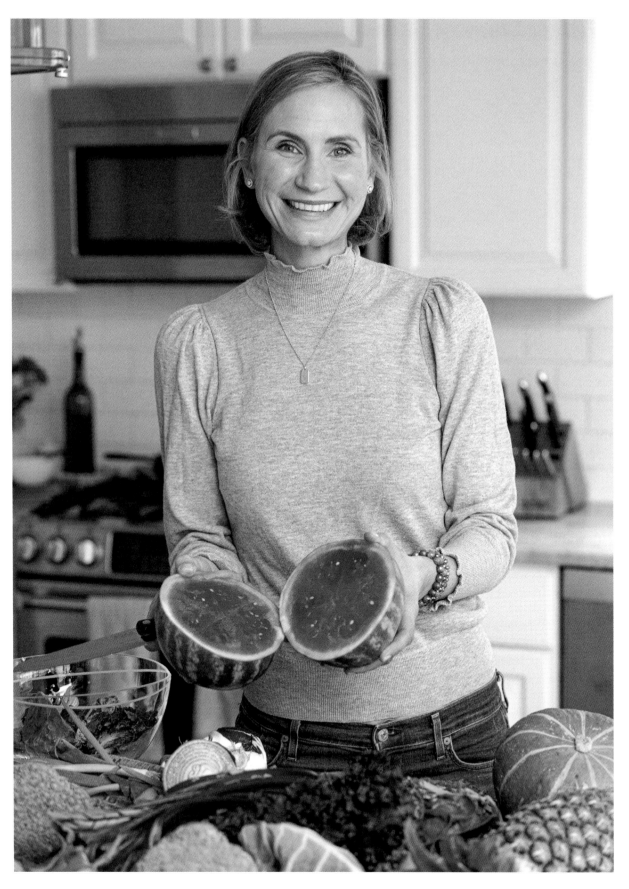

ACKNOWLEDGMENTS

I couldn't have written this book without a community of support. It's only fitting that I relied upon my community to fuel me with ideas and positive encouragement.

I'm grateful for all of my patients who asked about my book, for my extended family members across the country who trialed recipes and sent me positive thoughts. I'm grateful for the social quiet of the COVID pandemic to give me space to collect my thoughts and execute this huge project. I'm grateful for all of the people along the way who said how excited they were to read the book.

There are some special people who rose above and beyond, and those people I'd like to acknowledge by name.

To my community cooks and recipe makers for the photographs in this book, Jennifer Buchholz, Aparna Sahgal, Courtney Evans, Lisa Clarke, Alison Dickinson, Sara Terry, Marisa Chadda, Melissa Kirby, Cathrin Bowtell, Paola Ayora, Mel Hook Shahbazian, Alex Hall, Sara Swanberg, Courtney Metzler, Marissa Herbers, Katy Kinsella, Meaghan Hetherington, Pat Keenan, Suzanna Papajohn, Ashling Keenan, Alison Dickinson, Linda Felcyn, Dorothy Lammers, Nadia Saldanha, Aya Takayasu, Ulli Neugebauer, and Adam Shabana: Thank you for your enthusiasm about buying nutritional yeast, kombu, and mangoes in the middle of winter. Thank you for dropping food off at my doorstep so that it could be photographed, or experimenting in your own kitchens to find the tastiest, most delicious Creamy Roasted Broccoli Soup, or telling me how you made tastier versions of ideas I had. You're all amazing humans, and I'm grateful for you.

To Aya: It was your encouragement that got the DK ball rolling in the first place. It all started with the question of how to share my medical knowledge and experience in the kitchen with others who might be interested in going deeper. Thank you for perfecting the Carrot Ginger Dressing recipe and trialing so many others.

To Dad: You taught me what it means to have dedication to something worthwhile. I couldn't have persevered through the writing of this book without that model of excellence through my formative years.

To Julia D'Agostino and Sydney Sheehan: Your energy is warm and fun, but at the same time calm and reassuring. Thank you for your gorgeous work on the photography for this book.

To the Victory Belt Team: Wow, what a team you are. From that first conversation in the summer of 2020 to the birth of this book a year later, I am in utter amazement of how well you all work together and included me in every part of the process. Thank you for letting my vision shine. To Lance, thank you for your can-do attitude and for agreeing that every recipe needed a photograph. To Justin and Kat, thank you for indulging me in the design process and being respectful of my tiny tweaks. To Susan and Kristen, thank you for your enthusiasm and helping the book to come to life after it was a Word document. To Holly, thank you for sharing your gift of understanding recipes and the Life Kitchen. And to Pam, thank you for your sage advice, for your reassuring voice and emails, and for formatting all of my citations. Working with all of you has been a pleasure.

To Gina, Melissa, Stephanie, and Emily: Thank you for being my local marketing team. I am forever touched by you coming on board to support not only the book and the DK brand but me as a person. Surrounding myself with high-performing women is certainly part of the special sauce.

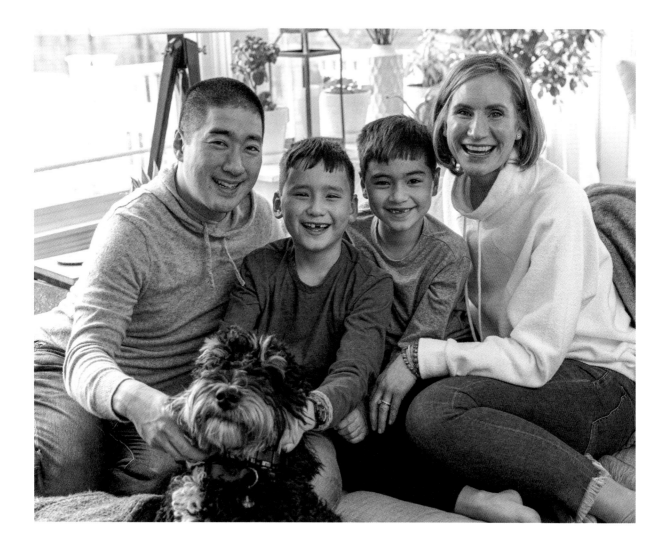

To Cathrin: Everyone needs a director, and you swooped in during the most crucial hours of the photo shoot to streamline our creative efforts. You're always there for me when I need a big cup of tea, a distraction for my kids, or whole cloves and nutmeg. Thank you for trialing recipes and perfecting the Crispy Parsley recipe. I'm glad you live so close.

To Courtney: Thank you for keeping the back burner going with the *Dr. Katie Detox* so that I could focus on what's bubbling over in my real Life Kitchen. Your partnerships, collaboration, and gentle but directive spirit are what's elevating the Detox to the vision we both had back on a rainy day in September 2019.

To Ashling: Your cheerleading of DK has been evident from the start. Thank you for encouraging me to write the Detox back in winter 2019 so that we could all trial it before our first family trip to Mexico. Do you remember how good that first margarita tasted after ten days of detoxing?! Thank you for the family dinners when I was tired, for watching my kids while I worked on weekends, and for helping me to figure out Instagram back when I had no idea what a story was.

To Alison, our "Tomato Fairy": The recipe part of this book wouldn't have been possible without you. Your knowledge of flavors and enthusiasm for trialing new ideas made sharing them with you so fun. Thank you for trialing every single recipe, many of them more than once. You are a rare gem.

To Melissa: I will forever simultaneously think of you as both my favorite Central Park running buddy and also the best person to give me feedback on this book. Thank you for using your charming wit and eagle eye to help me edit.

To Mindy: Our early morning "Tuesdays with Mindy" conversations helped me build the philosophy and overarching themes of this book. Thank you for sharing your incredible knowledge of the healing science of Ayurveda and yoga with me over the course of the last ten years. Being on my mat with your voice and inspirational words reminding me to come back to my Center is what makes my light shine so bright.

To Lisa: Could there be any more positive person than you? Your glass-half-full approach to life is good luck to anyone who has the joy of calling you a friend. Thank you for supporting me personally and professionally with your top-notch chef skills. You always show up with a smile on your face and genuine joy in your heart. We are certainly sisters in another life.

To Angie: You may be the boys' nanny in name, but you're my nanny too. Thank you for keeping our household running smoothly, for roasting vegetables until the cows come home, for making sure the boys eat balanced meals, and for trialing so many of the recipes over and over and over again. I bet you could make Morning Glory Muffins and Celebration Granola in your sleep! Most of all, thank you for taking care of our boys so that I can do my job. Having the security of your care allows me to do the good work of doctoring.

To Stephanie: Oh my, where to begin? You were the most helpful friend to me while writing this book. Thank you for answering my crazy middle-of-the-night emails with thoughtful, well-researched responses or letting me pontificate about vegetables and complain about the writing process on our prized walk-talks. Thank you for sending me packages overflowing with dark chocolate. You are a true-blue friend. You're so humble that I'm sure I'm making you blush, so I'll stop gushing about you. But know that I could go on forever. You are my greatest friend.

To Maggie: Working with you is the experience of a lifetime. I think the Universe sent you to me back in 1993 to show me how to be a good caretaker, a role model, and how to accept help from the next generation of thinkers. Your creative genius made the photography of this book possible and is taking DK to the next level. I never knew that I would have this rich of a relationship with my baby sister.

To Mom: You quietly taught me how to nurture others with delicious food. You also taught me that making family meals for seven people doesn't have to be complicated. Your use of a slow cooker is really bar none! You lead by example, and I'm grateful to have a strong woman in my life who showed me how to get things done.

To William and Oliver: Thank you for making me giggle, for the back rubs on your beds with the massage scraper and lotion, for reminding me what's most important at the end of a long day: a hug, a kiss, and a high-five. I will be your greatest supporter. Please know that I always have your back because you always had mine. Thanks for giving me space to write and starstruck eyes when I told you I was done, even though you know I'll never really be done. The night you were born the stars twinkled with delight, and it's my greatest mission in life to parent you into the amazing spirits I know that you are.

To Jun: You're the one who cleans up, who puts life back together when it falls off the pantry shelf and shatters on the basement floor. You're my glue, my grounding, my sense of stability. Your gentle smile and warm hugs are enough to fill me up for decades. I can't believe we found ourselves at a blackjack table back in 2001 and are lucky enough to be continuing on this journey together. I will never stop loving you.

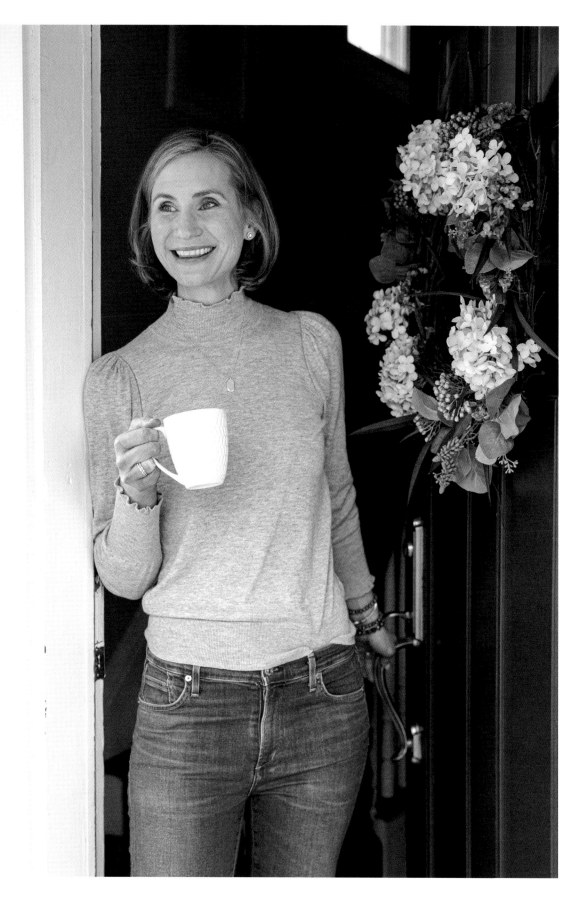

INDEX